PRAISE FOR

CHOOSE RADIANT HEALTH & HAPPINESS

"You will thank your lucky stars that you have this book as your guide."
—**LENDON H. SMITH, MD, AUTHOR OF** FEED YOUR BODY RIGHT

"This is one of the most complete books I have read on how to be healthy, happy, and fully alive. In clear and beautiful prose, Susan tells us that health and peace are a conscious choice. Reading this book is a vital step in making that choice."
—**JOHN WOODEN, FORMER UCLA BASKETBALL COACH AND AUTHOR OF** WOODEN

"Susan Smith Jones understands we are threefold—body, mind, and spirit—and to be healthy, we must balance and strengthen all three. In Choose Radiant Health & Happiness, Susan gives very practical advice to achieve a healthy and happy life."
—**DENNIS WEAVER, ACTOR**

"Susan's latest book is fantastic—it's practical, motivating, and inspiring. I know it can help you to be your healthiest and I am recommending it to all my friends."
—**TOMMY LASORDA, FORMER MANAGER, LOS ANGELES DODGERS**

"Choose Radiant Health & Happiness is filled with useful information that is presented in ways that are both easy to understand and fun to read."
—**DEAN ORNISH, MD, AUTHOR OF** EAT MORE, WEIGH LESS **AND** LOVE AND INTIMACY: THE SCIENTIFIC BASIS FOR THE HEALING POWER OF INTIMACY

"Susan's book contains information on how to achieve health and happiness. I find, however, that most people aren't inspired enough to seek information. So I invite you all to wake up to life and all its potential, read her book, become informed and live a healed life."
—**BERNIE S. SIEGEL, MD, AUTHOR OF** LOVE, MEDICINE AND MIRACLES

"*Choose Radiant Health & Happiness* offers the tools you'll need to enrich every aspect of your life."
—JOHN GRAY, PH.D., AUTHOR OF *MEN ARE FROM MARS, WOMEN ARE FROM VENUS*

"*If you're ready to improve your diet, reduce stress in your life, exercise your way to radiant health, or bring sacredness into your everyday living, this book is loaded with secrets to improve your quality of life.*"
—GERALD JAMPOLSKY, MD, AUTHOR OF *LOVE IS LETTING GO OF FEAR*

"*Body, mind, and spirit—Susan harmonizes the trio in this delightful journey into being radiantly healthy on every level of our being and bringing sacredness into our daily lives.*"
—VICTORIA MORAN, AUTHOR OF *SHELTER FOR THE SPIRIT*

"*Clearly and joyfully, Dr. Susan Smith Jones guides us to wiser choices—helping us to grow beyond our fears and harmful habits and to fully embrace life. The keys to the balance you seek are in* Choose Radiant Health & Happiness."
—MICHAEL KLAPER, MD, AUTHOR OF *VEGAN NUTRITION: PURE AND SIMPLE*

"*Susan Smith Jones has created an uplifting book dedicated to everyone's health and happiness. It should be on your bookshelf. It is on mine.*"
—EARL L. MINDELL, PH.D., AUTHOR OF *EARL MINDELL'S VITAMIN BIBLE*

"*This is a beautiful, clear, uplifting book. A guide to living joyfully, passionately, heartfully, and peacefully, it is also a fine example of the heart-connectedness that brings grace to life. Outstanding!*"
—JOHN ROBBINS, AUTHOR OF *DIET FOR A NEW AMERICA*

"*Choose Radiant Health & Happiness is a wellspring of wise and heart-centered information by an author who has devoted her life to well-being. I have the deepest respect for Susan as a model of Spirit-guided, well-balanced living. This book is sure to be a welcome companion to anyone seeking to live their highest potential.*"
—ALAN COHEN, AUTHOR OF *HANDLE WITH PRAYER*

"Susan Smith Jones writes clearly and cogently about the enormous power of changing our diets and learning how to live in balance. I grew up on a diet of roast beef and pork chops, but learning to eat a healthier diet was one of the major changes in my life. Dr. Jones will help many other people enjoy the same benefits."
—**NEAL D. BARNARD, MD, AUTHOR OF** *EAT RIGHT, LIVE LONGER*

"Too frequently we forget that we are mind, body and spirit. *Choose Radiant Health & Happiness* helps us put those three facets together into a synergistic force."
—**TOMMY HAWKINS, VICE PRESIDENT, LOS ANGELES DODGERS**

"*Choose Radiant Health & Happiness is a light that can lead us out of the morass of ill health. This book inspires and empowers the reader to "seize the day" while providing a well conceived blueprint for creating a life filled with health, happiness and peace...an excellent book.*"
—**GABRIEL COUSENS, MD, AUTHOR OF** *CONSCIOUS EATING*

"I would recommend Susan Smith Jones' workshops to anyone. However, if one cannot meet in person this fabulous example of balanced spiritual and practical living, the next best thing is this book. All Susan's books are great, but this one may well be her best ever!"
—**JOHN STRICKLAND, SENIOR MINISTER, UNITY CHURCH OF HAWAII**

"Regardless of your current state of physical or emotional disrepair, you can take this dynamic book, read carefully, and begin now to Choose Radiant Health & Happiness."
—**DR. WAYNE W. DYER, AUTHOR OF** *YOUR SACRED SELF*

OTHER BOOKS BY SUSAN SMITH JONES

*Choose to Live Peacefully**
*Choose to Live Each Day Fully**
How to Meditate

And for Children
co-authored with Dianne Warren

Vegetable Soup/The Fruit Bowl

Audio Cassette Albums
Celebrate Life!
Choose to Live a Balanced Life
A Fresh Start: Rejuvenate Your Body
Making Your Life a Great Adventure
Wired to Meditate

For more information on Susan's audio cassette programs, or to purchase her books and tapes, call (800) 843-5743 PST

*also available from Celestial Arts

Choose Radiant Health & Happiness

SUSAN SMITH JONES, PH.D.

CELESTIAL ARTS

BERKELEY, CALIFORNIA

The health suggestions and recommendations in this book are based on the training, research, and personal experiences of the author. Because each person and each situation is unique, the author and publisher encourage the reader to check with his or her holistic physician or other health professional before using any procedure outlined in this book. It is a sign of wisdom to seek a second or third opinion. Neither the author or publisher is responsible for any adverse consequences resulting from a change in diet or from the use of any of the other suggestions in this book. The publisher does not advocate the use of any particular diet or health program, but believes that the information in this book should be available to the public.

Copyright © 1998 by Susan Smith Jones. All rights reserved. No part of this book may be reproduced in any form, except for brief review, without the written permission of the publisher. For information write: Celestial Arts, Post Office Box 7123, Berkeley, California 94707. Printed in the United States of America.

Library of Congress Cataloging-in-Publication Data

Jones, Susan Smith
    Choose radiant health & happiness / Susan Smith Jones. – 1st Celestial Arts ed.
       p. cm.
    Includes index.
    ISBN 0-89087-843-9 (pbk.)
    1. Health–Popular works.   I. Title.
RA776.J626   1998
613–dc21   98-23424
                                                                                CIP

COVER DESIGN BY GREENE DESIGN

TEXT DESIGN BY COLORED HORSE STUDIOS

FIRST CELESTIAL ARTS EDITION, 1998

5 4 3 2 1 — 02 01 00 99 98

Contents

Acknowledgments
Foreword by Dr. Wayne W. Dyer
Introduction

Chapter 1	A Balanced Life: The Key Ingredient of Health	1
Chapter 2	Wholesome Nutrition: The Upcoming Dietary Revolution	15
Chapter 3	Healthy Weight: Creating a Fit, Lean Body	45
Chapter 4	Fats, Oils and Flax: Telling the Killers from the Healers	68
Chapter 5	Chlorophyll and Greens: The Great Cleansers	96
Chapter 6	Juices: Radiant Health in a Glass	107
Chapter 7	Exercise for Your Life!	120
Chapter 8	Sweating Your Way to Radiant Health	136
Chapter 9	Massage: The Healing Touch	140
Chapter 10	Be More Childlike	152
Chapter 11	Living Your Highest Vision: Turning Dreams Into Reality	168
Chapter 12	Serenity and Solitude: Essential Ingredients for Quality of Life	186
Chapter 13	Acts of Kindness: The Joy Factor	194
Chapter 14	Meditation and Prayer: The Key to Transforming Your Life	207
Chapter 15	Self-Mastery: The Power to Be Your Best	223
Afterword		240
Appendix	Workbook: Self-Discovery Questions and Action Choices	243
	Questions and Answers	261
	Resource Directory	290
About the Author		302
Index		303

This book is lovingly dedicated to my Mom, June B. Smith, the most loving, forgiving, and tenderhearted person I know. You are my very best friend and greatest inspiration.

To Paramahansa Yogananda, for teaching me through your shining example and work how beautiful life can be when we choose to put God first.

To you, the reader—because you make a difference in the world. This book will renew your hope, inspire your soul, lift your spirit, make you think, and strengthen your resolve to live the life you've always wanted to live. You can be healthy, happy, and peaceful, and you can bring about a peaceful world. You are important to the well-being of planet Earth.

"The greatest romance is with the Infinite. You have no idea how beautiful life can be. When you suddenly find God everywhere, when He comes and talks to you and guides you, the romance of divine love has begun."
—**PARAMAHANSA YOGANANDA**, *MAN'S ETERNAL QUEST*

ACKNOWLEDGMENTS

Andrew Carnegie said his success was due to picking the right helpers. This is certainly true for me regarding this book.

When I think about all the people who have enriched my life, I feel such a desire to bless and honor them as I can in these Acknowledgments.

To my special friends and family who have been a steady source of support, inspiration, and love: June B. Smith, Lynn Carroll, Helen Guppy, Ralph J. Rudser, Reverend John Strickland, Junia and John Chambers, Letitia Wims, Brad and Mary A. Tomlinson, Pamela Davis, Jimmy Langkop, Jackie Day, Bill Carnahan, Gary Peattie, Dianne Warren, Rose Marie Stack, Brian Sievers, Diane Olive, Lynn Walker, Karen Olsen, Ralph Nelson, Donica Beath, Karen McGuire, Paulette Suzanne, Gary Brink, Diana Feinberg, Jim Lennon, Tahayra Manjra, Kathy Martelli, George Marks, Lisa Ray, Sandy Shirley, Wally and Gloria Hill, Doug and Bev Beath, Dee and Arch Wilkie, Bob and Jean Macy, Sol Seifer, Dean Ornish, MD, Reid Smith, Sparkie and Ad Brugger, Jackie Benoit, and Tony, Jamie, Bryce, and Tyler Carr. You all know what you mean to me and how much I love and appreciate everyone of you. I feel so very blessed to have your presence in my life, and I give thanks for the wonderful, positive influence you have been for me.

To David Hinds and Mary Ann Anderson at Celestial Arts, for recognizing the value of this book, for your commitment to excellence, and for your continual support. To Sal Glynn, my valued editor, for your sense of humor, for your loving encouragement, for always having my best interests at heart, and for being someone I can always count on.

To Paramahansa Yogananda, my spiritual teacher, who, for the last twenty-five years, has taught me that what is most essential is invisible to the eye. Only love is real and it can only be seen and felt with the heart. It is through Yogananda's teachings that I have learned the importance of beholding the Divine in everyone and everything.

To my guardian angels, my loving celestial companions, for watching over me and guiding me every step of the way with your humor, gentle touch and loving support.

To God, my love, my life, my everything. Immersed in Your Divine presence, I receive the answers I seek, the peace I long for, and the hope that springs eternal. I revel in my oneness with your Light and Love and am eternally grateful for and trust Your enduring Love and guidance.

FOREWORD

By Dr. Wayne W. Dyer
AUTHOR OF *Your Sacred Self* and *You'll See It When You Believe It*

I have long subscribed to the idea that all of life is a choice. When we let ourselves ultimately come to believe in the power of BEING a 'choice-making' human being, we begin to take total responsibility for ourselves and our unique destinies. Susan Smith Jones provides us with a beautifully useful elaboration on this theme of choosing our own greatness in virtually all life areas. She has taken great pains to provide extremely valuable information on how to take total control of ourselves, by first and foremost taking responsibility for the quality of the journey that we call life.

In simple, easy-to-read, and, most importantly, easy-to-apply language, this book outlines an approach to living that is possible for every single reader to achieve if they are willing to make it happen for themselves. Regardless of your current state of physical or emotional disrepair, you can take this book, read carefully, and begin now to *choose radiant health and happiness.*

A very strong thread of spirituality and higher consciousness thinking is woven throughout the pages of this book. Susan cannot help but write from this perspective, because I know her to be respectful of the divine forces operating ubiquitously in each and every one of us. Susan believes strongly in the importance of love in each of our lives. Not the kind of love that requires a partner in order to be fulfilled, but the divine love that is itself the harmony that holds every living cell together. Without internal harmony, a cell will attack and attempt to devour the cell adjacent to itself, and ultimately destroy the entire organism. So it is with divine love. Each of us is a cell in the body called humanity. When we have harmony within, we cooperate with the cells next to us, and when this harmony or love is missing, we fight our adjacent cells, leading to destruction of the totality of all humanity. When we fight anything, we become weaker, for in so doing we are violating the very principle of harmony and cooperation that holds the universe together. You will see Susan's enormous regard for this spiritual (not necessarily religious, but spiritual) force that guides the universe, and each life form that occupies its own unique place in this perfect universe.

Recent efforts by chemists and other scientists have produced a synthetic form of wheat that looks, tastes, smells, feels and acts like wheat. To the naked eye it appears that this product is definitely wheat. However, when placed in the ground, something quite strange happens that sets it apart from authentic wheat. It will not grow! Despite its appearance and nutritional make-up, synthetic wheat will not grow and reproduce naturally. What is missing? The absent ingredient is the life force that can never be reproduced synthetically.

So it is with each of us. We need the higher elements in order to grow, and a life plan that incorporates authentic ingredients for choosing to be healthy, happy, and fully alive. Susan Smith Jones sprinkles her writing with marvelous quotations from the masters, both historic and contemporary, all of whom have made their own unique contributions to the betterment of humankind. Her writing is concise and useful, and the subject matter is universal: improving the quality of life for all of us. *Choose Radiant Health & Happiness* can help you forget about synthetic happiness, artificial health, and phony fulfillment, and replace them with a genuine, life-enhancing formula that will not only help you feel better, but to grow and flourish just like *real wheat* does when placed in a natural setting.

Everything we experience is a choice. Our personalities are the result of the choices we make. Our level of fitness is the result of those same opportunities to choose to be healthy. Our emotional condition likewise is a consequence of our choices. When you really consider this concept of choice, it boils down to the way that we choose to *think*. We become what we think about all day long. Thus, our personality, state of health, and our emotional stability all revolve around thinking. Learn to think healthy and visualize yourself as a success, and eventually your actions will follow those internal self-pictures. It can be no other way. Our thinking is our mental practice. With enough practice you will achieve what you desire.

Susan's approach is to help you to see that you are important enough to seek your own full measure of happiness and success, and that you are divine enough, just by the nature of your existence, to be heard. As you read through the pages of this powerful book, remind yourself that you are indeed divine enough to be answered. Think of a puzzle with one piece missing and realize that the entire picture is incomplete without that one piece. Then see yourself as one piece in this entire picture called humanity and that the whole thing is incomplete without you. That is how important you are. Your completeness makes us all whole, and Susan's outstanding book will help you not only to grasp this notion, but to take action, beginning now, to correct any limits you may have placed on yourself.

INTRODUCTION

Cherish Your Visions

Cherish the music that stirs in your heart, the beauty that forms in your mind, the loveliness that drapes in your purest thoughts, for out of them will grow all delightful conditions, all heavenly environments; of these, if you but remain true to them, your world will at last be built.
—JAMES ALLEN

There is a single magic, a single power, a single salvation, and a single happiness, and that is called loving.
—HERMANN HESSE

What a joy it is to have this opportunity to share my thoughts, experiences, and research on being healthy, happy, and fully alive in *Choose Radiant Health & Happiness*. Thank you for spending time with me through my writing. I want you to feel like we are sitting across from each other and I'm talking to you personally through this book. I already know that we have lots in common since you've chosen to read a book on health and being the best you can be.

More than two decades ago I fractured my back in an automobile accident. The doctor told me that I should get used to a life of pain, inactivity, and difficulty, as I would never be able to carry anything heavier than a light purse. I was quite upset when I heard the doctor's prognosis. For me it was what I refer to as a 'wake-up call' where the universe got my attention in a big way. All I could see was a closed door. I was filled with depression, self-pity, confusion, and feelings of being victimized. After a couple of weeks, I went to a favorite spot overlooking Santa Monica Bay where I often would go when in need of inspiration. I had a heart-to-heart talk with myself.

On the one hand, I was convinced that life was meant to be a magnificent adventure. To me a full adventurous life meant living joyfully, passionately, healthfully, and peacefully. Yet the life the doctor had described didn't align with my beliefs and desires. I just couldn't accept it. I knew I had a choice to make and I made it. Helen Keller once wrote: "When one door closes, another opens; but often we look so long at the closed door that we do not see the one which has opened for us." Although I didn't know how I could change my physical condition, I recognized that there was a Higher Power within me that had the answers. So I simply made a *deep commitment to let go, live from inner guidance, and accept only vibrant, radiant health.*

The tool that makes life a truly wonderful adventure is our power of choice. It's up to us to create a meaningful life. We are all made in God's image and have the potential to make our lives extraordinary. We are all magnificent spiritual beings having a human experience here on spaceship Earth. If you don't like your current circumstances and want to live a more peaceful, healthy, and happy life, you can change it. You can choose to be radiantly healthy and filled with joy and thanksgiving. You can choose to be at peace with life. You have the power and ability to make your dreams a reality, to manifest your heart's best desires.

This is true because life constantly flows in the direction of one's choices. Knowing that helps keep me on course. No longer do I look to people, things, or circumstances as my source of happiness and fulfillment. The value in my life is what I bring to it. Henry David Thoreau knew this when he said, "There is no value in life except what you choose to place upon it, and no happiness in any place except what you bring to it yourself."

Of course, it hasn't always been an easy road. I have made many mistakes, or what I prefer to think of as simply learning what doesn't work for me. Nonetheless, in retrospect, I can see that the car accident was a valuable experience, for it was out of hitting that real low spot that my life turned around. As a result, I chose to embark on a great adventure of learning and growing and discovering how to live my highest vision.

After my experience by Santa Monica Bay, a stream of events began that assisted me in healing my condition: finding the perfect books and tapes, hearing certain lectures, meeting people who told me about healing and salutary foods, visualization, and meditation—much of which sounded kind of weird to me at the time.

During the months following the accident, and to this day, I have made several changes in my lifestyle, behavior, thoughts, and attitude. I've learned to bring more consciousness to my living, to pay attention to life and observe patterns, to use the ones that support me in new ways, and to change the ones that don't. I now choose to live more deeply, to find the intention beneath my intention, and to always talk things over with God before making any decisions.

I've also discovered the tremendous power of commitment, belief, and faith. Faith means belief in an inner knowing, appearances notwithstanding. Commitments link me, both mind and heart, to people, aspirations, and goals. When I give myself wholeheartedly to a relationship, my work,

Introduction   xv

or some plan, I do well. However, when my first commitment is to be God-centered, I bring a greater measure of love, understanding, and imagination to all my other commitments. When I am God-centered, I do my best in a new or long-standing relationship. When I am God-centered, I bring love and compassion to every interaction with others, and inspiration to every activity I undertake.

I have the following poem by Johann Wolfgang von Goethe taped on my refrigerator door so I can read it often. It inspires and beautifully expresses the impact commitment can have on your life.

> *Until one is committed there is hesitancy,*
> *the chance to draw back, always ineffectiveness.*
> *Concerning all acts of initiative and creation there is one elementary truth*
> *the ignorance of which kills countless ideas and splendid plans:*
> *that the moment one definitely commits oneself*
> *then Providence moves too.*
> *All sorts of things occur to help one*
> *that would never otherwise have occurred.*
> *A whole stream of events issues from the decision,*
> *raising in one's favor all manner of unforeseen incidents and meetings and material assistance,*
> *which no man could have dreamed would come his way.*
> *Whatever you can do or dream, begin it!*
> *Boldness has genius, power, and magic in it.*

After examining me at my six-month checkup following the accident, the doctor just shook his head in bewilderment and said, "This just can't be. There is no sign of a fracture and you seem to be in perfect health, free of pain. There must be some mistake. It's just miraculous."

Perhaps it was. Yet I've since discovered that miracles are a natural part of committing to being healthy, happy and peaceful. This magnificent universe is alive and mysterious, ultimately benevolent and orderly. Intention and consciousness, discovery and synchronicity are magical. Yet since we cannot see synchronicity or experience it directly with our senses, we become skeptical of it. Western culture teaches that events which intuition tells us are special are really only random happenstance, coincidences. We've been taught not to believe something until we see it with our own eyes, even though the most important things in life are intangible.

I believe in the magic of life, the ultimate source of creativity and love which I call God. I know I can never be separated from God. This divine presence is for me like returning home to a parent who loves me unconditionally. It is my connection to synchronicity and to miracles. The point of connection is through love and through the conscious, unconscious, and superconscious mind. It responds to our power to choose. Believe in your connection with the Divine and its power to create synchronicity.

When you choose to live an inspiring life, you make a difference in everyone's life with whom you come in contact. Every day the world presents you with miracles waiting for your awareness. Hidden beneath the wrapping of every experience is a new opportunity to know the joy and wonder of growth and love. *Carpe diem*: Seize the day. What makes certain people seize life? Why are some people open to growth, to unfolding, to deepening, and living more fully? Some people have an enormous capacity for maintaining a steady equilibrium, for accepting what they cannot change, for facing what they can, and moving on. You can choose to live that way by loving life and aligning your thoughts with God's.

One of the most important lessons I've learned is that if I'm facing a challenge—whether it's pertaining to health, relationships, finances, or whatever—all I need to do is to turn my focus from the challenge to God and let the Divinity reveal the hidden gift within it. We're given the circumstances we require for our awakening. Every situation, seen rightly, contains the seeds of freedom. You can be sure that it's there, just waiting for you to look at it from the right perspective. *A Course in Miracles* says, "When any situation arises which tempts you to become disturbed, say: 'There is another way of looking at this.'"

My auto accident taught me that dark nights of the soul can reveal the true purpose of suffering—namely that out of our pain we can rise, expand, grow, conquer, and achieve new and even better things. Like the butterfly that is strengthened by its desperate struggle to break out of a constricting cocoon, we too can emerge stronger, wiser, and more resilient because of the dark, difficult times in our lives. In those times we learn to simplify life, clarify values, sort out priorities, and discover which friends are true and which are not.

By rising out of my distress I've also come to realize that the purpose of my existence is to become truly loving. That's how we find the way back to the divine source. *Nothing will change your life more quickly for the better than the consistent feeling of love.* Everything in your life—making decisions, raising children, your lifestyle, your career, your friends, your contribution to society—will become more coherent and whole when you love life fully. Loving all aspects of your life, regardless of challenges you may be facing, opens doors and lets in

Introduction xvii

light, energy and joy. Love yourself out of sheer gratitude for existence. Love the mystery of life and the process of creating what you want. When you love, you become transformed spiritually. *A Course in Miracles* says, "Every loving thought is true. Everything else is an appeal for healing and help, regardless of the form it takes."

The more you love, the more you come to realize you don't need to force things. The *Tao-Te-Ching*, the classic manual on the art of living, is referred to simply as *The Book of the Way*. The author, Lao-Tsu, was a sage whose large-heartedness, humor, and wisdom grace every page. He teaches that the true way is "to do by not doing," a paradigm for nonaction, the purest and most effective form of action. He wrote, "The way to do is to be." For a long time, this has been one of my favorite maxims. You don't need to force things. Let go and let God. Or as the Buddha put it at the end of a long life dedicated to teaching mindfulness and peaceful living, "Be a light unto yourself."

Ultimately, your choices are what separate you from everyone else. They are the only road to becoming truly independent. Choose what you want and how you want to live. Accept and expect the best. Learn to trust your ability to make decisions. The greatest lessons often come from the ones that prove to be wrong. Taking risks is our chance to find out what works for us, what we can do well. We must learn to choose what we want and to not worry about the rest, knowing it's all in God's hands. If we are the best we can be, we learn to respect what we can become in the future. Choosing—it's the only way.

In my time of crisis, I didn't just choose health. There's more to health than a strong body, toned muscles, clear mind, and disease-free and pain-free existence. I chose to be the best I could be—physically, mentally, emotionally, and spiritually. That's what this book is about: tapping into your inner truth and power and choosing to be the best you can be. It's about living your truth and reclaiming your spirituality. And it's also about taking loving care of yourself, honoring the Divine within you, and bringing spirituality into your everyday life.

Why not become the best that we can be? *Choose Radiant Health & Happiness* will help show you the way. We owe it to ourselves to choose health and happiness—no one is going to do it for us. You may find that I suggest things that are entirely new to you such as meditation, visualization, solitude, certain foods and supplements, or a way of living that's different from your present lifestyle. When applicable, refer to the Resource Directory for more information. Don't simply take my word for it. You have all the answers within you. Always consult your inner guidance on every decision and choice in your life. Deep within our hearts, each of us knows the truth.

I hope that by reading and *participating* in this book, your life will become a magnificent adventure. Active participation is important in reading this book. It's not what we read that makes a difference in our lives; it's how we apply and experience the material that is of real value. At the end of the book you'll find Self-Discovery Questions and Action Choices for you to complete. Don't pass over these. Take time with each item. No one has to see what you've written. This should be your personal transformation workbook. This special section will assist you in getting to know yourself better. And after all, isn't that the key ingredient to living to your fullest potential?

Like you, I have a lot of things I want to accomplish in this life and I have no interest in being slowed down in any way by health problems. Because I want to be the best I can be, I want to embrace the best life has to offer. So can you. I believe in you and your ability to be the best you can be, and I salute your great adventure.

Namaste.*

SUSAN SMITH JONES

* 'I celebrate the place in you where we are all one.'

> *If one advances confidently in the direction of his dreams, and endeavors to live the life which he has imagined, he will meet with a success unexpected in common hours…If you have built castles in the air, your work need not be lost; that is where they should be. Now put foundations under them.*
> —HENRY DAVID THOREAU

> *To laugh often and much; to win the respect of intelligent people and the affection of children; to earn the appreciation of honest critics and endure the betrayal of false friends; to appreciate beauty; to find the best in others; to leave the world a bit better, whether by a healthy child, a garden patch or a redeemed social condition; to know even one life has breathed easier because you have lived. This is to have succeeded.*
> —RALPH WALDO EMERSON

CHAPTER ONE

A Balanced Life: The Key Ingredient of Health

You are not being called upon to change yourself. You are being asked to be more of what you already are. The invitation is bold, the stakes are high, and the outcome is certain. Dare to live your destiny now.
—ALAN COHEN

Man is made or unmade by himself. By the right choice he ascends. As a being of power, intelligence, and love, and lord of his own thoughts, he holds the key to every situation.
—JAMES ALLEN

Last year a man came to see me. He was and still is the president of a major corporation in America. He was impatient, aggressive, sometimes hostile, and unaware of how to make choices to support his well-being. He routinely put in six or seven fourteen-hour pressure-packed days a week at the office or traveling. He always had to be first, always had to be right, and always had to be busy with work to feel worthwhile. As a fancier of rich foods, he put away vast quantities of cheese, ice cream, steak, butter, processed foods, and cream sauces. A typical breakfast would be his favorite sausage—which was composed of pork liver, white rice, port, and hot spices—along with eggs, ham, and two cups of coffee. He knew his food was loaded with cholesterol and fat, but he loved it all the same. His exercise was shifting gears in one of his expensive sports cars.

He was usually tired and thought his hot tub and a drink were all he needed to relax. It wasn't until he began to sink into a depression that his wife encouraged him to have a medical checkup, his first in more than five years. Then came the shocker. This forty-year-old man discovered he had high blood pressure and hardening of the arteries, and was told that if he didn't make some changes in his way of life immediately, he was headed for a heart attack within six months. It was also suggested that he have quadruple heart bypass surgery.

As providence would have it, the following day a friend of his who had heard about the doctor's prognosis recommended that he follow the program outlined in my tape albums and books. That's how we met. We worked together on his wellness program. His experiences and adventures over these past twelve months have been a great inspiration to me, for I had never worked with anyone who was so stressed, so unhealthy, and who led such an unhealthy way of life. During our first visit he made a choice—and he chose to make a commitment to changing his life and to being healthy. Today both he and his family are the picture of health. Recently, the family participated together in a 10K run and left on the following day for a two-week health and fitness vacation.

Health and happiness are much more than just feeling fine. It's a quality of life, a joy and radiance for living so that every day, each and every moment, is a celebration. For most people, being radiantly healthy is simply a matter of choice. But it is not merely a matter of choosing to exercise regularly and eat wholesome, nutritious foods. The latest research discloses that what we think, believe, and expect in life powerfully influences our well-being, our immune system and our lives, and that it affects not only our own lives but the condition of the entire planet.

The idea that we have control over our wellness and that we can choose to be healthy and functioning fully is a new science that's rapidly gaining popularity. Immunologists, psychiatrists, endocrinologists, neuroscientists, microbiologists, and psychologists from around the world—who rarely step out of their own fields—are coming together to unite their expertise in this new field called psychoneuroimmunology. This new science deals with the mind's effect on the immune system's incredibly complex network of organs, vessels, and white blood cells.

Research indicates that the immune system, brain, and other vital body systems communicate, connect, and influence one another. That means that your body will be in a better position to cope with factors that can cause disease and heal itself if you are not under stress. If your brain allows your stress level to get out of control, it suppresses the immune system. Well-managed stress, however, may help keep your immune system healthy. We can't totally avoid pressure in this world but we can choose a healthy balance.

Psychoneuroimmunology researchers have looked extensively into the body/mind connection and how each of us can become masters of our lives. The fruits of this approach are already being harvested in comprehensive programs of mind/body medicine at Harvard University, the University of Massachusetts, Stanford University, the University of Miami, and the University of California at San Francisco and Los Angeles. People with such life-threatening and debilitating illnesses as cancer, AIDS, coronary heart disease, and chronic pain are learning to change their habits and attitudes—what they eat, when they exercise, and how they think. A number of landmark studies have shown that these men and women are functioning far more effectively, feeling better and, in some particularly striking instances, living longer.

Particularly impressive is the work of Dr. O. Carl Simonton in Pacific Palisades, California, and the incredible advances he has made with cancer patients using visualization. He reports that only about ten percent of the people who come to him are willing to do the work he recommends. The remainder would rather get the operation or the medication—anything to keep the reality 'out there' rather than looking within and taking charge.

There are those who receive a lot of value out of being victims. They get to blame everybody else for their problems. They hold on to resentment and are unforgiving. As research discloses, people have a difficult time processing emotions. Some scientific evidence suggests that much of the sickness we experience comes at least in part from the inability to express anger, guilt, and fear. Researchers have even gone so far as to say that our level of stress and how we deal with it is a main contributing factor to our level of health.

THE BIOLOGY OF EMOTIONS

A whole-person approach is the foundation to recovery from all ailments and diseases. Dr. Simonton's method calls on the patient to alter emotions, attitudes, and expectations. Very important to the process are daily exercises in relaxation and imaging techniques, and physical activity intended to reduce the stresses that Simonton says play a role in disease.

At its most basic, mental therapy—known in some circles as the mind-body connection—uses emotions to prod certain brain chemicals into stimulating the body's defense systems. By the same token, the repression of certain emotions can depress the body's ability to maintain a healthy immune function.

"If you get angry and that emotion doesn't get discharged, the resulting hormonal products and smaller particles such as neurotransmitters and endorphins don't get used," says Dr. Caroline Sperling, a clinical psychologist and director of the Cancer Counseling Institute in Bethesda, Maryland. "The residue remains and can become toxic in our bodies." The opposite is also true. "When you release those emotions effectively, you get real well-being and adrenal charging so that the immune system stays strong and the body stays healthy," adds Sperling.

According to Dr. Joan Borysenko, author of *Minding the Body, Mending the Mind*, and co-founder and former director of the Mind/Body Clinic at New England Deaconess Hospital in Boston, these messages are transported instantaneously between the brain and a newly discovered site called a neuroreceptor on the white blood cells. So when someone is happy or thinks a happy thought, the white blood cells—which are the body's primary defense system—receive that message immediately. Conversely, when someone is depressed, that same message is transmitted directly to the white blood cells through the nervous system. All this happens very quickly. Everything which is registered in our minds is registered in our bodies. The discovery of the neuroreceptor site on the white blood cell is an exciting breakthrough.

Following the footsteps of Dr. Simonton, Dr. Paul Rosch, president of the American Institute of Stress in New York, agrees that there is some very exciting work going on in the field, particularly in the area of visual imagery and cancer. "It has been determined that negative emotions have a high link to certain types of malignancies, and support for that comes from the observation that there are receptor sites on T-cell lymphocytes (white blood cells) for certain brain chemicals, which suggests that there is a conversation going back and forth between the immune system and the brain," says Rosch.

Sperling concurs. "Imagery works like a computer to program into the hypothalamus the directions you want. It helps open up the parasympathetic nervous system so your body gets healthy. In other words, you're giving messages to your body, which translates them into neurotransmitters...to get the immune system to work better and the hormone system to calm down a little and stop creating abnormal cells."

Along these same lines, Dr. Deepak Chopra spoke on a national television talk show about this mind-body connection and how the mind and body are inseparable. He explained that the mind is in every cell of the body and that each thought causes a release of neuropeptides that are transmitted to all the cells in the body. Thoughts of love, he said, cause the release of interleukin and interferon which help heal the body. Anxious thoughts cause the release of cortisone and adrenaline which suppress the immune system. Peaceful, calming thoughts release chemicals in the body similar to Valium which help the body to relax.

Similarly, Norman Cousins throughout his insightful book, *Head First: The Biology of Hope*, presents evidence that hope, faith, love, will to live, purpose, laughter, and festivity help combat disease. Cousins writes, "The greatest force in the human body is the natural drive of the body to heal itself—but that force is not independent of the belief system, which can translate expectations into physiological change. Nothing is more wondrous about the fifteen million neurons in the human brain than their ability to convert thoughts, hopes, ideas, and attitudes into chemical substances. Everything begins, therefore, with belief. What we believe is the most powerful option of all."

A clue to the magnitude of impact that knowledge of this inner healing/belief system may have is evident in the phenomenon of the placebo effect. Medical researchers are well aware that a certain percentage of participants in medical studies who are treated with placebo drugs or procedures (treatments of no known medical value) will improve because they believe they have received a potent treatment. In the past, researchers tended to dismiss the placebo effect as a distraction, a confounding psychological variable that interfered with the real aims of the research. Yet the fact that belief can override the non-physiological actions of placebo medicines demonstrates the remarkable capability of this inner healing force.

While the messages from the brain through the nervous system are instantaneous, there is also another transport system that's slower and more steady. Through our endocrine system, our thoughts trigger what's known as the hypothalamic-pituitary-adrenal axis, which gradually influences our body to respond to our emotional responses. Borysenko writes about the studies on neuropeptides, a group of hormonal messengers (neurotransmitters) secreted by the brain, immune system, and digestive system. Endorphins, for example, which are commonly associated with the 'runners' high' experienced by joggers, are one among several dozen neuropeptides researchers have identified. These substances represent a rich pharmacy of natural drugs that the body produces in response to various internal and external stresses.

Borysenko explains: "When you react to your boss as if he is a saber-toothed tiger, your body secretes chemicals that prepare you to die rather than helping you to live. These drugs are then pumped out into the blood stream and eventually bind to the surface of all the cells in the body the way that a key fits into a lock. They then affect the function of the cells. So, if you are fearful, for example, it is not just an emotion. It is that every cell in your body has now received a biochemical signal about fear broadcast by the neuropeptide system, and has changed its metabolism in some way."

As exciting as these insights are, Borysenko adds an important caveat when she cautions not to exaggerate the connection between personality and disease. "It is not as if everyone who is hostile and cynical will have heart disease or that everyone who acts like a doormat will develop cancer," she explains. "Personality is only one of many variables that can affect health."

British cardiologist Dr. Peter Nixon explains that increased stress and arousal cause numerous changes in body functioning that eventually interfere with immune function, protein synthesis, and cardiac functioning. Repetitive stress also uses up the body's reserves, leading to increased stress on other physiological functions. This, in turn, can result in heart disease, cancer, or depression.

These ideas about the body-mind connection are not new. Plato said that the physician who treats just the body and does not address the mind is not treating the whole patient. In 140 AD, the Roman physician Galen said that it is depressed women who get breast cancer. Our reaction to stressful situations plays an integral part in our health and illnesses.

Clearly, health represents a complex and dynamic interplay of attitudes, emotions, and physiology that affect our state of mind and sense of well-being. The amount of exercise in our lives, the foods we eat, a hug from a loved one, can all have a decided influence on our moods. In turn, anxious or worried thoughts can cause such physiological effects as tense muscles or elevated blood pressure. Emotional depression can translate into fatigue. And having fun with people we enjoy can create energy.

It is within our power to take charge of our lives, thoughts, and emotions, and our beliefs and attitudes. It is within our power to become the best we can be—physically, mentally, emotionally, and spiritually.

TWENTY-ONE STEPS TO A BALANCED LIFE

Here are some ways to live a balanced life—to be the best you can be, healthier and happier than ever before.

1. KEEP FIT AND LIVE A WELLNESS LIFESTYLE. Develop a well-rounded fitness program that includes lifting weights or body-building, aerobics, and stretching. Make it a top priority in your life and stay committed. There is nothing that will do more good for you in terms of being vibrantly healthy, energetic, and youthful than a regular fitness program. To create the body of your dreams, participate in a regular, well-rounded fitness program (see Chapter Seven on exercise).

Make sure to get enough rest, water, and wholesome foods. Eat your foods close to the way nature produced them. Get plenty of fresh air, healthy amounts of sunshine, and take saunas, too. Avoid dependence on caffeine, nicotine, alcohol, and drugs that interfere with your immune functioning. Be a good role model for your family. The only person's health and fitness you can change is your own. If you want to be an influence on the health and fitness of those you love, take care of yourself. The compelling influence of personal example will ripple outward. I love these words from George Bernard Shaw: "If you must hold up yourself up to your children as an object lesson, hold yourself up as an example and not as a warning."

Only when you approach health and fitness from a holistic perspective can you expect to achieve optimal well-being. You must include body, mind, and spirit. Here's a great question to ask yourself from Satchel Paige. "How old would you be if you didn't know how old you are?" The more healthy and fit you are, the younger you feel (see Chapter Two on nutrition).

2. GET ENOUGH SLEEP. According to a recent study by the National Sleep Foundation, even though ninety-eight percent of people know that sleep is just as important to their health as nutrition and exercise, most adults get too little sleep. Americans average seven and one half hours of sleep a night, two and one half hours less than what is ideal. In his excellent book, *Power Sleep*, Dr. James B. Maas reveals that half of the United States is sleep-deprived. Maas maintains that many Americans don't know what it's like to be fully alert, and have become habituated to low levels of alertness. If you need an alarm clock to wake up or if it's a struggle to get out of bed in the morning or you fall asleep watching television, you are sleep-deprived.

Even minor sleep deprivation causes mood changes. People get angry more easily, irritable, upset, lose patience, and snap at one another. One of the first things to go when sleep-deprived is communication skills. Maas recommends taking ten to twenty minute power naps; any longer than twenty minutes and you go into delta or deep sleep and wake up groggy. Also, if you nap too long in the afternoon, it will create nocturnal insomnia. Power naps pay back the debt we all carry in our sleep-debt banking account. Never underestimate the importance of getting enough sleep. It's clearly an essential part of living a balanced life.

3. LEARN TO ELICIT A RELAXATION RESPONSE. This means becoming deeply relaxed in mind and body. Our nervous systems are bombarded by excessive environmental stimulation. Learn deep relaxation techniques such as meditation, yoga, and breathing exercises so that stress levels are under control. Every hour, take a deep breathing break instead of a coffee break. For two to three minutes every hour, breathe slowly and deeply. This practice will do wonders to relieve stress, foster calmness, clear

your mind, and help you to see your life from a higher, more positive perspective.

4. WATCH OUT FOR STRESS ASSOCIATED WITH PROLONGED FEELINGS OF ANGER AND DEPRESSION. Beware of unexpressed feelings—especially negative ones. People who do not express feelings get sick more often, stay sick longer, and die sooner than expressive people. Nonexpression of emotion and denial of hostility or anger are two of the factors most related to unfavorable prognosis in cancer patients. Unexpressed negative feelings feed on themselves—for instance, anger can turn against the self and emerge as depression or severe anxiety (see Appendix on self-discovery).

Negative emotions also trigger the release of substances that can suppress immune function. Solve your problems in a way that lets you clear up your negative feelings as thoroughly and quickly as possible. Remember that feelings aren't good or bad; they just are. Sharing feelings with a trusted friend or other support person is healing. Have positive expectations about everything in your life, including your wellness.

There is a classic study of people about to have surgery. The first group of patients dreaded surgery and attempted to avoid it. The second group, which had the same medical problems, regarded the surgery as an opportunity to rid themselves of their illnesses. After surgery, those who had positive expectations had better post-operative experiences. Similar outcomes have been repeatedly documented.

If a person is able to integrate a loss into a broader meaning of life, and feel some loss, grief, and depression, those feelings will be relatively temporary. But if a person responds to loss with a prolonged state of depression, the body will also be in a prolonged state of depression, making that person vulnerable and susceptible to many things. When a person sees himself as a participant in life rather than as a victim of undesirable circumstances, he or she will experience a more wholesome and less stressful life.

5. BE AWARE OF YOUR THOUGHTS. Thoughts determine your experiences. Each of us has the freedom to accept and embrace whatever thoughts we choose. We possess within the silence of our being the ability to think, create and become whatever we want to become. Don't think negatively. Instead, only think about things you want to be part of your life (see Chapter Eleven on your personal vision).

6. FEEL THE FEAR AND LET IT GO. Fear is a significant, powerful force that we feel on many levels—physically, mentally, and emotionally. Whatever our fears, they are neither good nor bad—they just are. All we risk by uncovering them is becoming healthier and more fully human and tasting another part of life and love.

7. VISUALIZE YOUR GOALS AND DREAMS EVERY DAY. James Allen wrote these words seventy-five years ago, and they are still true today: "You think in secret and it comes to pass. Environment is but your looking glass." Every day we should spend a few minutes visualizing with our mind's eye not only our goals but also how we would like our lives to be. In addition to visualizing, assume the feeling of the wish fulfilled (see Chapter Eleven on your personal vision).

8. FIND TIME EACH DAY TO BE ALONE. Find some time each day to enjoy the peace of your own company. It is by spending time alone, breathing deeply and quieting everyday thoughts, that you can do the most for your health, happiness, and peace of mind. Silence nourishes your soul and heals your heart. It restores peace and takes you back home. It is always sacred. Solitude is necessary for deep silence. The word alone is derived from the Middle English phrase "all one." When you are alone, you are with the best company possible—you and God. It's in silence that I see most clearly exactly what is out of balance in my life. And it's in silence that I feel the all-providing power that is the Source of all creation. Mother Theresa writes, "We need to find God, and He cannot be found in noise and restlessness. God is the friend of silence." (See Chapter Twelve on serenity.)

9. PRACTICE SOME KIND OF MEDITATION DAILY. This goes hand-in-hand with spending time alone each day. Research by Dr. Herbert Benson of Harvard University, author of *The Relaxation Response*, has shown that meditation not only improves immune function, but is associated with a host of other beneficial physiological effects such as altered brain states, decreased heart rate, lower blood pressure, a relaxed body, and a more youthful appearance.

By spending time each day in meditation, listening to your inner guidance or intuition, you realize you are never alone. Too often we look outside ourselves for our worth and forget that nothing will ever be enough until we are enough. Meditation nourishes faith and connects us to our Source, which I call God. My spiritual teacher, Paramahansa Yogananda, taught that the most important thing in human life is to seek and do the will of God. A person who does this is living by faith. He or she doesn't have to look around trying to find faith; it springs from within. (See Chapter Fourteen on meditation and prayer.)

10. SIMPLIFY LIFE. Contrary to popular belief, we are not mere victims of our environment. When we go faster and continually push harder without keeping life in perspective, we grow more and more insensitive to our needs and the needs of those around us. Slow down. Find joy in simple pleasures. Breathe deeply, smell the flowers, talk to the animals, sing with the birds, be with friends, greet the sun, scratch behind your kitty's ear, make someone smile, marvel at the miracle you are, tell someone you love them, and laugh out loud and often.

11. DEVELOP A SENSE OF HUMOR. A healthy degree of emotional detachment and hearty laughter every day can stimulate the immune system. Don't take life so seriously. Strive to move gracefully among all the activities of daily life without being ensnared by either outer things or inner desires.

Research shows that humor aids most—and probably all—major systems of the body, says Dr. William F. Fry, a psychiatrist at the Stanford University School of Medicine in California. A good laugh, he says, gives the heart muscles a good workout; improves circulation; fills the lungs with oxygen-rich air; clears the respiratory passages; stimulates alertness hormones that stimulate various tissues; alters the brain by diminishing tension in the central nervous system; counteracts fear, anger, and depression, all of which are linked to physical illness; and helps relieve pain.

12. NURTURE AND DEVELOP YOUR INTUITION. Intuition is sometimes called a sixth sense, a hunch, a gut feeling, going on instinct or just knowing deep inside. Psychologists call it intuition—an obscure mental function that provides us with information so that we know without knowing how we know. I believe it's the voice of God within each one of us. The word 'intuition' means to guide and protect. Intuition can be nurtured in a variety of ways—through contemplation, gazing out a window, relaxing or by taking walks in nature. The best way is to be still and listen. The more we act on our intuitive hunches, the stronger and more readily available they become.

13. EMBRACE AN ATTITUDE OF GRATITUDE. An attitude of gratitude creates blessings. Be grateful for everything that's going on in your life, no matter the circumstances, for it's this kind of attitude that will help foster happiness and peace of mind and assist you to live more fully. There is power in difficulty and challenge—it forces you to tap reserves of courage, hope, faith, surrender, and love you weren't aware you possessed. In my life, I clearly see that pain and heartache accelerate the learning and growing process and foster personal power and peace. We don't have to have problems to grow. We can grow in spiritual maturity as we turn to God. But it seems to me that only a faith and belief in God and His goodness can give us the understanding and strength to be grateful in the midst of challenge. In *A Course in Miracles*, it says: "Love cannot be far behind a grateful heart and thankful mind...These are the true conditions for your homecoming."

14. BECOME MORE CHILDLIKE. Young children seem to know how to celebrate life, live fully, and create magical moments. They see the everyday world as full of wonder and mystery, and with this perception, they infuse the most ordinary things with magic. Children know how to open the door to the kingdom of wonder. Take their example. Be more flexible, practice forgiveness, leave time for spontaneity in daily activities, don't plan your calendar minute-to-minute, and let go of being critical and judgmental. Let your inner child come out and play (see Chapter Ten on being more childlike).

15. LIVE IN THE PRESENT. Living in the moment is different from living for the moment. Don't compare the present with the past. Children live in the timelessness of the present. To be fully present each moment, we must free ourselves from the past. To achieve this freedom, we must heal our past. If we don't, the past will repeat itself and keep us trapped in it. When we're trapped in the past, we're not here now; we're not fully present and we can't pay attention to what's happening all around us. We must stop living our lives mechanically and unconsciously and start paying attention to the present moment. Every step you take is upon holy ground. Every moment is imbued with wonder and miracles.

16. SHARE YOUR LOVE AND KINDNESS. Being loving and kind improves health. We all need love—and I'm not just talking about romantic attraction. That warm, loving feeling you get from

hugging a child, counseling a friend, being a good listener, or even treating yourself to a luxurious bubble bath boosts the immune system. Petting a dog or watching fish in a tank lowers your blood pressure. In one study, people watching a film of Mother Theresa tenderly caring for sick children experienced the same heightened immune response as people who had recently fallen in love.

Whether we are at work or at play, with friends or with strangers, a friendly smile and a kind word can go a long way toward brightening someone's day. Every day, we also have opportunities to express our responsibility to our environment. Take care of your home, planet Earth. Act in caring, loving ways for your own sake and for the future sake of your children and of all children.

Led by divine guidance, welcome every opportunity to express love and kindness (see Chapter Thirteen on acts of kindness).

17. LIVE WITH INTEGRITY. To live with integrity means that who you appear to be is who you really are. Your inner realities—your beliefs, your commitments, your values—are all reflected in how you live your life on the outside. The more you live with synchronicity in what you believe, think, feel, say and do, the more peace and happiness you will invite into your life. It takes a lot of energy to live without integrity. It is emotionally and intellectually exhausting when who you are on the inside and how you behave on the outside are not aligned or congruent with one another. It's enervating to be dishonest.

Honesty and integrity go hand-in-hand. It was Thomas Jefferson who said, "Honesty is the first chapter in the book of wisdom."

To be honest is to be genuine, authentic and real. To be dishonest is to be partly forged, fake, or fictitious. Honesty is best cultivated by being honest. The more you choose to be real and honest, the more it becomes a habit.

18. REVERENCE FOR LIFE AND JOY FOR LIVING. Live your life with joy and reverence. Greet each day with joy and enthusiasm regardless of circumstances. Be thankful for everything that touches your path—the warm sun on your face, the food that you eat, your family and friends, for nature all around you, and for the air that you breathe. Living with reverence brings happiness and fulfillment and makes every moment sacred. Take notice and enjoy the everyday miracles that make up your life. Behold the divine in everyone and everything.

19. DEVELOP HIGH SELF-ESTEEM AND SELF-LOVE. High self-esteem is important for your well-being, as well as for the well-being of your children. You are the most powerful influence on your children. Your children learn from watching you live. When you are the best, you are a positive model for them to emulate. "Nothing has a stronger influence psychologically on their environment, and especially on their children, than the unlived life of the parents," says Carl Gustav Jung. Heal your emotional wounds of the past. Release your emotional baggage and treat yourself with respect and kindness. Your life is a reflection of how you feel about and treat yourself.

Be true to yourself. This means following your heart. We just need to have enough confidence in ourselves to follow our inner guidance. Being true to yourself is to be in a state of grace. To find out if you are being true to yourself, ask yourself these questions: If I weren't getting paid for what I'm doing, would I continue to do it? If I only had one year to live, would I continue to do what I'm doing? If the answer is "no," carefully consider what you can do to make different choices that will change your answer to "yes."

20. LIVE IN GOD'S LOVING PRESENCE. The whirlwind of life may suggest that you are at the mercy of other people or random circumstances, but you're not. With practice, you can withstand any turbulence by keeping your thoughts centered on God.

God's loving presence is with us at all times. No matter where we go or what activities are before us, God's presence is right there in the midst of each person and event. The light of God shines where the darkness of doubt once existed. This guidance illumines the paths we walk and shows us the best way to go.

What is the single most important relationship we can have? Our relationship with God. We are always in God and God's life nourishes us and provides for us. Our peace is founded on God's eternal presence and love. No problem is too big or too small, no question too unimportant to place in His hands. Turn to Him for everything. Give everything to God. Ask that only God's purposes be served in every situation. Ask Him to show you the love and innocence within all people. Be honest and humble. Honor your holiness. Participate in a divine love affair with God. His loving presence is who you are. I love this Sufi saying: "I searched for God and all I found was myself. I searched for myself and all I found was God."

21. LIVE PEACEFULLY. What would be a greater goal in life than peace of mind? What asset could be of more value to us than unshakable calmness and tranquillity? What better evidence of spiritual strength could we have than a peaceful mind and heart?

Peace of mind comes from accepting what you can't control and taking responsibility for what you can. It grows out of faith in your higher power and your spiritual nature. It comes when you let go of guilt, fear and doubt. It is the result of forgiving yourself and others for all human imperfections. When you let go of the delusion that something will someday make you happy, you can concentrate on the peace and contentment of the present moment. Inner peace is always found in the here and now. It waits quietly for you to discover it.

A healthy lifestyle is more than eating right and exercising regularly. Make a commitment to yourself to enrich each day physically, mentally, emotionally, and spiritually. By choosing to put this balance into your life, you'll reap the rewards of living—healthfully and happily.

CHAPTER TWO

Wholesome Nutrition:
The Upcoming Dietary Revolution

Let food be your medicine and medicine be your food.
—HIPPOCRATES

Your body is composed of over sixty trillion cells. Think of each cell as a little engine. Some of these engines work in unison, some work independently, and they all work twenty-four hours a day. In order for engines to work right, they require specific fuels. If the engine is given the wrong fuel blend, it won't perform to maximum capacity. If the fuel is of a poor grade, the engine may sputter and hesitate, creating a loss of power. If the engine is given no fuel, it will stop.

Much of the fuel for our cells comes directly from the things we eat. The food we eat contains nutrients in the form of vitamins, minerals, water, carbohydrates, fats, proteins and enzymes. Just as a car requires different forms of energy for the brakes, transmission, and battery to run smoothly, the cells of the body require different amounts and types of nutrients depending on their location and function in the body. These nutrients allow us to sustain life by providing our body's cells with the basic materials needed to carry on.

Each nutrient differs in form, function, and amount needed; however, each one is vital. Nutrients are involved in every body process, whether it be combating infection or repairing tissue or thinking. Nutrients have different functions such as to provide energy or promote tissue repair, but their common goal is to keep us going. To eat is one of the most basic and powerful of human drives. Although eating has been woven into many cultural and religious practices, essentially we eat to survive.

A fundamental problem with most of us is that our bodies simply do not get what we need from our modern diet. Consistent absence of the proper nutrients eventually causes great harm to the body by impairing its normal functions. Even if you are not sick, you may not necessarily be healthy. It simply may be that you are not yet exhibiting any overt symptoms of illness. Unlike a car engine which immediately malfunctions if you put water into the gasoline tank, the human body has tremendous resilience and often camouflages the repercussions of unhealthy fuel choices. By understanding the principles of holistic nutrition and knowing what nutrients and foods you need, you can improve the state of your health, stave off disease, and maintain a harmonious balance in the way nature intended.

There is a huge industry in the Western world working to convince us that it doesn't matter what we eat. Fast food chains try to convince us that what we eat has no effect on our health. We are told that any combination of heated, treated, processed, chemicalized 'foods' will meet our nutritional needs so long as we take plenty of vitamin pills, heartburn medicine, headache pills, and other remedies.

"Call it science. Call it the state of the art of medicine. I now believe," writes Dr. Lendon H. Smith in his excellent book, *Feed Your Body Right*, "what I learned in medical school in the early 1940s was a calculated effort by the pharmaceutical industry to get fledgling medical doctors to use drugs, their drugs. We were taught to make a diagnosis, clear and simple. Once a label was attached to the patient, a drug was attached to the disease label. It was neat and clean. If we could not remember the name of the drug, the pharmaceutical representative who came to our offices one or twice a month reminded us. Ads in the medical journals kept the name alive in our memory storage banks."

Last year over a million people left the same suicide note:

Shopping List
Sausage, whole milk, cake, hot dogs, margarine, eggs, mayonnaise, potato chips, sour cream, hamburger, pastries, ice cream, ham, cookies, bacon, cheese, chicken, donuts, luncheon meats.

HEART-HEALTHY LIFESTYLES PAY OFF

It's tough to pick up a newspaper these days without reading yet another article about some strange factor, like baldness or short stature, that might cause a heart attack—factors that we often can't do anything about. That's why a major study published in the *British Medical Journal* is so redeeming. Investigators from Finland have found that all those headline-catching items aren't worth a moment of worry. In tracking the lives of 14,257 men and 14,786 women for twenty years, the researchers concluded that the reductions in mortality rates from heart disease that Finland has experienced over the past two decades were brought about primarily by changes in three main coronary risk factors: cholesterol levels, blood pressure, and smoking.

Finland had a vested interest in finding the keys to coronary prevention. In the early 1970s middle-aged Finnish men had the highest mortality rates from cardiovascular disease in the world. They also consumed some of the highest amounts per capita of full-fat dairy products.

Early on, government officials took action, instituting health education programs and tracking the results of various preventive measures. The researchers recruited a random sample of close to 30,000 Finnish men and women ages thirty to fifty-nine. In surveys conducted every five years from 1972 to 1992, they kept close track of their medical history, current health, socioeconomic factors, and lifestyle habits. Specially trained nurses measured height, weight and blood pressure, and took blood specimens to determine cholesterol concentrations. Nonsmokers were defined as those who had never smoked regularly as well as those who had smoked regularly but had quit at least six months before the start of the survey.

During this same two-decade period, the rate of heart disease in Finland began to drop dramatically. The investigators knew it was the perfect opportunity to see just how much the country's reductions in risk factors had influenced that decline. They predicted that, among their 30,000 subjects, a nonsmoking lifestyle and decreases in cholesterol and blood pressure levels would be associated with decreases in mortality from heart disease of forty-four percent in men and forty percent in women. It turns out, to their delight, that their estimates were conservative. The observed decline was fifty-five percent in men and sixty percent in women.

"Most of the decline in mortality from heart disease," the authors concluded, "can be explained by changes in the three main coronary risk factors."

Atherosclerotic vascular disease is a buildup of fat in the blood vessels. The associated heart attacks and strokes caused by this fat buildup prematurely cause half of all deaths each year. Cancer of the breast, colon, prostate, lung, and other organs cause another twenty-five percent of deaths each year. Diabetes, cirrhosis of the liver, and emphysema also kill many people prematurely.

All these conditions have one thing in common: they are caused or greatly influenced by what we put or don't put into our mouths. Of all the things human beings put in their mouths, says Dr. Alan Goldhamer, co-director of the Center for Conservative Therapy in Penngrove, California, tobacco, alcohol, caffeine, and recreational and prescription drugs are perhaps the most harmful. Attempts by people to modify their internal chemistry through powerful chemical agents and quick fixes is an ever-widening tragedy. More and more people are suffering and dying from the consequences of using and abusing chemicals.

Headaches are not caused by an aspirin deficiency. There are better ways of modifying moods than with pills, potions, and elixirs.

THE IMPACT OF ANIMAL PROTEIN

'Nothing will benefit human health and increase the chances for survival of life on earth as much as the evolution to a vegetarian diet.'
—ALBERT EINSTEIN

Perhaps the second most destructive habit Dr. Goldhamer sees is the use of animal products. Meat, fish, fowl, eggs, and dairy products all have much in common. In addition to economic, environmental, humanitarian, and, for many, spiritual reasons, there are well-documented health reasons that support the adoption of a vegetarian diet.

In their search for evidence on how food affects health, researchers have often considered Asian countries because, statistically, their longevity surpasses other more developed countries. While they do not have a perfect diet, they do a much better job of holding cancer, heart disease, and many other serious conditions at bay than do Western countries.

One of the most ambitious nutrition research projects ever undertaken is the China Oxford Cornell Project (called the Grand Prix of epidemiology). Conducted by Dr. Colin Campbell of Cornell University and his colleagues, Drs. Chen Junshi and Li Junyao of Beijing, China, and Dr. Richard Peto of Oxford University, the Project looked in detail at China as a natural laboratory. Diets vary significantly from one part of the country to another, yet people in China tend to stay in the same place all their lives, allowing observable relationships between diet and health to emerge. Beginning in 1983, the team collected information about the typical foods of sixty-five Chinese provinces. They studied records of health and illness, took blood samples, and made other tests. In 1991, they published an 896-page monograph filled with data from this and subsequent and even larger studies which they continue to analyze.

The Project's hypothesis was that a diet substantially enriched with good quality plant foods prevents a variety of chronic degenerative diseases, and that the more the diet contains plant-source foods, the lower the disease risk. "In a sense," explains Dr. Campbell, "one might say that we are testing whether a diet which contains no animal products and is low in fat, is better than, say, an average vegetarian diet which usually contains dairy and egg products and nutrient compositions which are not too different from non-vegetarian diets. Our study suggests that the closer one approaches a total plant food diet, the greater the health benefit."

Their first finding was that, overall, Chinese diets are extraordinarily healthy by Western standards. Rice and other grains, vegetables, and legumes are consumed in much greater quantity than in the United States. While Americans get around forty percent of their calories from fat, the Chinese get much less—ranging from six to twenty-four percent—and their health is much better.

The study placed much emphasis on protein (how much and what kinds) and its influence on heart disease, cancer, and other diseases. There is a tremendous difference between the two countries in source of protein. The average protein intake from animal sources in the United States is seventy percent. In China, only seven percent comes from animal sources. But in spite of the generally low levels of protein intake from animal sources in China, those Chinese who add just a little bit of animal protein to their diet register increases in cholesterol levels, heart disease, and cancer. This suggests that it doesn't take much animal protein to start changing cholesterol levels and consequently increase the risk of heart disease and cancer, explains Campbell.

"There is strong evidence in the scientific literature that when a reduction in fat is compared to a reduction in protein intake, the protein effect on blood cholesterol is more significant than the effect of saturated fat," says Campbell. Animal protein is a hypercholesterolemic (cholesterol-increasing) agent. He adds, "We can reduce cholesterol levels either by reducing animal protein intake or exchanging it for plant protein. Some of the plant proteins, particularly soy (see *White Wave Tofu* in the Resource Directory), have an impressive ability to reduce cholesterol. I really think that protein—both the kind and the amount—is more significant as far as cholesterol levels are concerned than is saturated fat, and certainly more significant than dietary cholesterol itself."

Animal protein is about as well correlated with overall cancer rates across different countries as is total fat. Of course, animal protein is tightly coupled with the intake of saturated fat, so a lot of these associations between saturated fat and various cancers could just as easily be accounted for by animal protein. "The consumption of animal protein has a profound effect on enzymes that are involved in the metabolism of cholesterol and related chemicals and this occurs very quickly—within hours after the consumption of the meal," explains Campbell.

Protein is so highly regarded by everyone, including investigators themselves, that there is a tremendous bias against considering its implication in disease. "It is easy to see that fat is greasy and nasty," says Campbell, "so most people more readily accept the idea that fat might have something to do with the emergence of disease. They do not want to imagine that animal protein does the same things as excess fat intake. But it turns out that animal protein, when consumed, exhibits a variety of undesirable health effects. Whether it is the immune system, various enzyme systems, the uptake of carcinogens into the cells, or hormonal activities, animal protein generally only causes mischief. High fat intake still can be a problem, and we should not be consuming such high fat diets. But I suggest that animal protein is more problematic in this whole diet/disease relationship than is total fat."

Many Americans are switching from beef to skinless chicken breasts and other animal-based foods, simply to reduce their intake of fat. However, the evidence suggests that this makes little or no sense. It may reduce fat intake a bit, but even lean cuts of meat or poultry still contain around twenty to forty percent of total calories as fat, or even more. This is not going to get us very far. We might get our fat intake down a bit, but our protein intake is not going to change; if anything, the already high level may go even higher. As Campbell says, "One really has to change the total diet."

If you want to see big changes in your health, you must make big changes in your life. Only dramatic reduction or elimination of all animal products merits your consideration. If you are accustomed to a high salt, high fat, high animal protein diet, you might not like healthier foods at first. But with a little patience, you will find that after two or three months, perhaps longer, you adapt to new tastes. And then you discover new tastes that you never realized were there before.

Since heart disease is the leading cause of death in this country, it is appropriate to also describe a landmark study in heart disease, the Lifestyle Heart Trial, conceived by Dr. Dean Ornish of the University of California, San Francisco. This interventional study, conducted on patients with documented coronary artery disease, split participants into two groups, a control group and an intervention group. All of the patients in the study had cardiac tests before beginning the study. These tests were repeated a year later to document the effect of the intervention.

The control group was placed on the American Heart Association recommended diet, which is similar to the diet recommended by the American Diabetic Association for diabetics. This diet includes limited red meat, chicken, fish, and substitutes margarine for butter, resulting in a reduction from the American norm of about forty percent of calories from fat down to thirty percent, and reducing cholesterol to less than 300 mg daily (the norm is higher). These patients also were advised to exercise and to stop smoking. To the surprise of many, the majority of participants in this control group that was following the American Heart Association recommendations showed worsening of their cardiac status on the one-year follow up.

The intervention group did dramatically better. These patients were placed on a low-fat vegetarian diet, with less than ten percent of calories from fat. To achieve this, they ate—without restriction in quantity—plant foods, such as fresh fruits, vegetables, legumes, and grains, with a limited amount of egg whites and non-fat milk or yogurt. They also engaged in light exercise and stress management. After one year, researchers found reversal in atherosclerotic plaque in eighty-two percent of this intervention group, all of whom were coronary disease patients.

The Lifestyle Heart Trial is just one of several impressive studies that show that standard dietary recommendations, utilizing thirty percent of calories from fat, allow the progression of heart disease and that heart disease is reversible with vegetarian diets. Studies such as this one were initiated after numerous population-based studies showed that cardiovascular deaths were virtually non-existent in rural populations consuming vegetarian diets, and that deaths from heart disease increased gradually as populations gradually increased their consumption of animal-based foods.

In addition to bacterial infestation, carcinogenic agents, toxic poisons, free radicals, and parasites, animal products all suffer from the problem of biological concentration. Animals consume large quantities of grain, grass, and other foods that are, to a greater or lesser extent, contaminated with herbicides, pesticides, and other agents. In addition, animals often are fed antibiotics and treated with other drugs and toxic agents. These poisons concentrate in the fat of the animal and are present in the animal's milk and flesh. This biological concentration of poisons poses significant threats to the health of humans who consume animal products. If you still desire eating burgers, check out *Boca Burgers*. They've won numerous taste tests and they're vegetarian. My favorite is the vegan Boca Burger. These are available in your health food stores as well as your local supermarket.

In spite of the millions of dollars the meat and dairy industry spend on advertising to try to make you believe otherwise, it is excess protein, not inadequate protein, that is the threat to health. Animal products are extremely high in protein. Excess protein, especially the high sulfur-containing amino acids found in animal products, has been strongly implicated as a causal agent in many disease processes, including kidney disease, various forms of cancer, a host of autoimmune and hypersensitivity disease processes and osteoporosis.

Osteoporosis is a condition common to postmenopausal women. Bones become weak and fracture easily. Campbell found in his study that osteoporosis is not caused by a calcium deficiency, and calcium supplementation does not prevent it. In osteoporosis there is a loss of the bone matrix that holds calcium. A diet high in animal protein can cause osteoporosis by creating toxic nitrogenous wastes that must be neutralized by calcium drawn from the body's reserves, creating a negative calcium balance where more calcium is lost in the urine than is taken in. Thus, no matter how much calcium is taken, if the individual is on a high animal protein diet, the calcium balance remains negative. To prevent osteoporosis, a low animal protein diet and regular weight-bearing exercises are essential. It's a misconception that you have to eat dairy products to prevent osteoporosis. Dairy products are implicated in many diseases, including autoimmune disorders, heart disease, arthritis, and cancer.

THE NON-DAIRY ALTERNATIVES

I choose not to eat dairy. When I announce this at my workshops, hands inevitably go up to ask, "What do I use in place of milk?" I either use White Wave Silk (soy or rice beverage) or I make fresh nut milk.

Nut milks are also an excellent replacement for dairy products. You can use a variety of nuts and seeds to make milks, ice cream, dips, and dressings. Here's a simple recipe:

ALMOND MILK
3 1/4 cups pure water
1/3 cup organic raw almonds
1 tablespoon Omega-Life fortified flax seed meal (see Resource Directory)
1 teaspoon lecithin granules
2 tablespoons sweetener (optional—I use pure maple syrup)

In a two-quart saucepan, heat the water to almost boiling. Turn stove off and allow to sit. Place the almonds in a blender and grind to a fine powder. Add flax seed meal, lecithin granules, and sweetener. Then add 3/4 cup of the warm water and blend on medium speed to a smooth, pudding-like puree. Add the remaining water and blend on high speed until creamy. Use three cups water per recipe for extra creamy nut milks.

Pour the contents of the blender through a fine mesh strainer into a bowl or pitcher. Serve immediately or refrigerate for up to seventy-two hours. It's delicious when you blend in fresh fruit or a frozen banana. This is a basic recipe that's simple to use. Here's an excellent book I recommend, containing more than forty delicious nut and seed milks recipes: *Not Milk...Nut Milks!* by Candia Lea Cole.

Why do I choose to avoid dairy products? For many reasons, the least of which is the case linking dairy products with a greater risk of breast cancer is gaining momentum. One of the latest studies to confirm this connection was published June 20, 1997 in the journal *Medical Hypotheses*. Researcher Jessica Outwater of the Physicians Committee for Responsible Medicine (see Resource Directory) found that estrogens, IGF-1 (insulin-like growth factor), and organochlorines, which are routinely found in dairy products, are all cause for concern.

In-vitro studies have revealed that breast cancer cells multiply by as much as four to five times in the presences of IGF-1. IGF-1 has growth-promoting effects in concentrations as low as 1ng/ml. Milk has approximately thirty times that concentration. IGF-1 is believed to be absorbed through the digestive tract into the blood.

Bovine growth hormone (bGH) doubles the concentration of IGF-1 in milk. Although the Food and Drug Administration has reported bGH to be safe for use in milk production and that pasteurization reduces its levels, research suggests the contrary. Additionally, dairy products contain both fat and estrogens, naturally produced hormones that have been implicated in increased breast cancer risk.

Don't take chances with your health! The health risks associated with milk and dairy products, from clogging arteries to allergies, are well documented. If these products still play a role in your diet, start cutting back. Check at your local health food store for more healthful substitutes, such as soy cheese, and White Wave Silk non-dairy beverages. The cookbooks I recommend offer ideas for making the transition to a vegetarian or vegan diet. Check at your health food store or bookstore for these and other books geared toward helping you change your diet.

It's ironic that the chief argument used to promote the use of animal and dairy products—the purported need for large quantities of protein—is one of the greatest reasons for avoiding them. If animal and dairy products are included in the diet in significant quantities, it is virtually impossible to design a healthful diet that is consistent with the overwhelming evidence in the scientific literature on nutrition.

CHANGING TO A HEALTHY DIET

I'm often asked, "If I have to avoid drugs (including alcohol, coffee, cola, and chocolate) and animal products (including meat, fish, fowl, eggs, and dairy products) and refined carbohydrates, what's left?" The answer is: a diet derived from whole natural foods—fresh fruits, vegetables, whole grains, legumes, and the variable addition of nuts and seeds.

Sometimes, however, when changing from an animal-based diet to a plant-based diet, you'll experience headaches, indigestion, and other uncomfortable symptoms. Have no fear—what you are experiencing is actually encouraging! People who initially experience severe symptoms when changing over to a healthy diet usually find that these symptoms resolve within the first two weeks. From that point on, they generally feel better and are more energetic than they have been in years. The fact that changing your diet exacerbated your headaches illustrates how necessary it was for you to improve your diet.

Keep these points in mind:

1. When you remove something harmful from your system, withdrawal symptoms can occur, especially headaches. People who discontinue the use of alcohol, cigarettes, caffeine, and other drugs also temporarily experience unpleasant symptoms, especially headaches. Having these diet-related headaches appear, then resolve, is a very common experience. The exacerbated headache brought on temporarily by dietary change is a withdrawal symptom and is a necessary step toward recovery.

2. The average American consumes a low-fiber diet, and the digestive tract of the typical person is unaccustomed to the higher fiber and water content of stools that result from an improved diet. These stools contain more weight, allowing them to pass through the digestive tract at a faster rate. The peristaltic waves that propel the food have to adjust for the new type of stool. It can take two weeks or longer for this adjustment to take place. During the transition time, you might experience diarrhea, bloating, gas, or other digestive discomforts.

3. When you switch to a lowered protein, low-fat diet, the body starts to eliminate retained proteinaceous wastes. Fat cells also are broken down, and the toxins stored in the fat cells are released into the bloodstream. In this manner, the body is able to 'clean house' more effectively. It's not uncommon to feel enervated and lethargic. The above symptoms are the temporary result of this detoxification. Do not let any temporary discomfort lead you to abandoning your new eating habits. You cannot accomplish healing overnight. It will be helpful to eat slowly and chew the vegetables very well, or temporarily eat a few leaves of lettuce with each meal rather than one big raw salad at dinner. If you are experiencing indigestion and cramping, do not eat asparagus or the cruciferous vegetables (cabbage, cauliflower, broccoli or Brussels

sprouts) for the first two weeks as they may produce bloating and gas. Fruit juices and other sweet drinks also can increase gas, so these also should be avoided temporarily if you are experiencing this problem.

4. Be informed. Educate yourself as much as you can on nutrition and an optimum diet. There are numerous excellent books and magazines available to give you support, inspiration, motivation, and delicious, nutritious recipes. Some of my favorites include:

Foods That Fight Pain and *Food for Life* by Neal Barnard, MD
Love Yourself Thin and *Get the Fat Out* by Victoria Moran
Diet for a New America by John Robbins
The McDougall Plan by John McDougall, MD
Quick and Easy Cookbook* by John McDougall, MD
Think Before You Eat by Diane Olive
Conscious Eating by Dr. Gabriel Cousens
Everyday Cooking with Dr. Dean Ornish* and *Eat More, Weigh Less* by Dr. Dean Ornish
A Diet for All Seasons by Dr. Elson Haas
The American Vegetarian Cookbook* by Marilyn Diamond
Fasting and Eating for Health by Joel Fuhrman, MD
Vegetarian Magic* by John Nowakowski
Spontaneous Healing and *8 Weeks to Optimum Health* by Andrew Weil, MD
Intuitive Eating and *Food Enzymes* by Humbart Santillo, ND
3 Days to Vitality by Pamela Serure
The Health Promoting Cookbook* by Dr. Alan Goldhamer
Anti-Aging Plan by Roy Walford, MD
Health Science Magazine (see American Natural Hygiene Society in the Resource Directory)

*cookbooks

Some excellent books on raising healthy children include the book I co-authored with Dianne Warren titled *Vegetable Soup/The Fruit Bowl*, *Hyper Kids Workbook* by Dr. Lendon H. Smith, *Good Food Today Great Kids Tomorrow* by Dr. Jay Gordon, *Pregnancy, Children, and the Vegan Diet* by Dr. Michael Klaper and *Dr. Attwood's Low Fat Prescription for Kids* by Charles Attwood, MD.

The long-term rewards of improvement to your diet—increased vitality, improved sleep, more energy, regular and soft bowel movements, lower cholesterol and a healthy heart, lower cancer risk, and stronger bones—are well worth any temporary discomfort. A longer and healthier life, free from compulsive, addictive behavior and the occurrence of degenerative diseases, can only be realized by avoiding the dietary causes of illness and adopting a plant-based diet.

Why do we find it so difficult to eat what we should eat and avoid what we shouldn't? To eat well, we have to understand the factors that drive us to eat unhealthfully. Very often we eat for the wrong reason. One reason is genetics—we are programmed to eat concentrated foods when they are available. That is an important survival trait. In a natural setting, there are no ice cream cone trees, hot dog vines, or candy bushes. But today, surrounded by unlimited access to concentrated foods, we must overcome instincts with intellect.

We might eat because we are emotionally distraught. Instead, take a walk, listen to relaxing music, or do some deep breathing. We might feel fatigued and eat for stimulation. But when we are tired, we should sleep. Fear of being different is another factor that drives us to make poor food choices. Friends can create a lot of pressure with comments like, "You're no fun anymore," "You're so thin," "Don't you think you're carrying this a little too far," "I made it just for you," or "A little won't hurt." Thank them for their concern and stay committed to your health program. Often a short explanation is all that is necessary. You don't need to justify yourself or your health habits.

Your body is a wonderful feedback machine. It is continually giving you messages about what's working and what's not. Pay attention to the signs and symptoms, the emotions and stressors. I really like what Dr. Lendon H. Smith has to say about this in his book *Feed Your Body Right*. "The more we investigate the origin of symptoms, signs, and diseases, the more we find that nutrition—and specifically, the chemical imbalances in the blood and tissues—is at the bottom of what ails us. The triggering event that precipitates an actual disease may be an emotional upset or a physical injury. Something has stressed our body chemistry beyond its ability to compensate; our ability to buffer the changes accompanying stressors has been compromised by our lifestyle, which includes our diet. We are all at risk—some more, some less."

THE UPCOMING DIETARY REVOLUTION

Health is the result of healthful living. This is the philosophy known as Natural Hygiene (see American Natural Hygiene Society in the Resource Directory). Natural Hygiene is about health promotion and I've practiced this way of living for over twenty years, although I do take a few nutritional supplements as described in this book which strict hygienists do not advocate. Hygienists believe that the body heals itself if you give it a chance. The method is to remove the factors that interfere with healing and provide the requirements for health. That is what you do whether you are trying to get healthy or stay healthy. The emphasis may be slightly different for different conditions, and it might need to be fine-tuned for different individuals.

One of the phenomenal things about the hygienic approach is that it teaches people about the power of their own vitality. Acute symptoms are the direct expression of this vitality and the most expedient means to recovery. Hygienists fully realize the integration of the body and how to really allow the body to function at its highest potential.

Science keeps supporting Natural Hygiene. A growing body of scientific studies on the disease-preventing and healing properties of food confirms the value of a vegetarian diet and even validates the nutritional teachings of the spiritual leader Paramahansa Yogananda, as well.

In 1929 Yogananda gave a talk in Washington, DC about renewing and transforming your body, mind, and spirit. He said: "We must also understand about food values. Meat is detrimental to your system; but so is an improperly cooked vegetable dinner of killed vitamins. Resurrect your mind from the bad habits of wrong eating. Start with carrots. Don't forget them. They are hard and nice—you have not to chew bones to get strength. When you chew carrots they give power to the teeth. Carrots contain valuable vitamins. Wash them, but do not do anything else to them. I ordered some raw carrots at a place I was visiting, and when they were brought in they didn't have any heads or feet. The tops and bottoms are rich in vitamins."

He went on to say, "A lemon a day; an apple a day; an orange a day; half a glass of orange juice with two tablespoonful of ground nuts (preferably almonds); and eight leaves of raw spinach...Grapefruit, too, is very good. Then a little piece of banana—about one-fourth. Then unsulphured figs and raisins...Eat these things every day. I do not mean that you shall live only on this regimen; you may eat more or less. But if you remember these basic rules—an abundance of fresh fruits and vegetables, not denatured by improper cooking or storage, and nuts, and some whole grains—you will not be making any transgression on nature...Nature will not listen to your excuses of your years of transgression against her health rules. If you eat sensibly, then if you are in the habit of breaking some laws occasionally, it will not hurt you so much." He added, "Since you have to eat, why not eat rightly?" Good question!

Scientists are actually proving that some of the old folklore medicine is absolutely true. According to a program called "Everyday Healing Food," broadcast on the American Public Radio (APR), "Medical science is now discovering an entire hidden world of disease-fighting substances that nature quietly deposited in everyday produce. Foods like garlic, onion, carrots, broccoli, beans, and citrus fruits contain an amazing network of natural ingredients that may help you prevent heart attack, cancer, and other serious illnesses."

Because a broad consensus of medical authorities recognizes the disease-preventing properties in fruits and vegetables, this knowledge is revolutionizing the way we think about food and health.

In 1992 the National Cancer Institute (NCI) published a review of 156 specific studies on how foods safeguard us from disease. They were done in a variety of countries, used a variety of methods, and looked at a variety of fruits and vegetables. Of these studies, eighty-two percent showed that fruits and vegetables have a protective effect against cancer. "Overall, the evidence of an association between fruit and vegetable consumption and cancer prevention is exceptionally strong and consistent," the NCI report said.

To gain this protection, "you should eat at least five servings of different fruits and vegetables every day," said Dr. Jerianne Heimendinger at the NCI. "A medium apple would be one serving, whereas a large apple or a large salad would be two servings," she explained.

Dr. Paul Talalay of Johns Hopkins University School of Medicine said on the APR broadcast that scientists have become interested in the potential of food to fight cancer and other illnesses at a time when the success of medical efforts at treatment generally has not been encouraging. Despite extraordinary advances in our understanding of the cancer process and breakthroughs in the treatment of some specific forms of the disease, Dr. Talalay said that the overall incidence of cancer and the mortality rate of victims have not changed significantly in the last twenty years.

Dr. Talalay heads a team that studied a compound called sulforaphane in the much-maligned broccoli. This compound significantly reduces the development of mammary cancer in lab animals. Sulforaphane activates a process that, in effect, kicks carcinogens out of cells. The results, which Dr. Talalay described as "dramatic," were reported in the Proceedings of the National Academy of Sciences.

The food substances that have scientists excited are called phytochemicals ('phyto' comes from the Greek word for plant). Plants produce these chemicals to protect themselves against such hostile elements as fungi, insects, and too much sunshine. By a benevolent act of nature, phytochemicals also seem to protect us. "We just borrow the compound that they use for their diseases and use it to treat our own diseases," said a US Department of Agriculture researcher, Dr. James Duke, on APR.

"At almost every one of the steps along the pathway leading to cancer there are one or more compounds in vegetables or fruit that will slow up or reverse the process," said Dr. John Potter of the University of Minnesota.

Here's some good news for tomato lovers. Dr. Joseph Hotchkiss and other scientists at Cornell University reported last year that two of the tomato's estimated 10,000 phytochemicals stop the formation of cancer-causing substances. You don't like tomatoes? These same phytochemicals also exist in green pepper, pineapples, strawberries, and carrots, which should give almost everyone something to chew on.

There's more help from our food friends. Besides the sulforaphane in turnips, they also have a phytochemical that inhibits or 'disarms' cancer, as does cabbage. Another phytochemical called ellagic acid, found in strawberries, grapes, and raspberries, performs a similar service. When harmful substances enter the body through food, drink, smoke, or air, certain cell enzymes feed on them. These enzymes are messy eaters and leave small fragments. The fragments can cause mutations in critical genes and sometimes initiate an explosive growth of cancer cells. Before this occurs, ellagic acid feeds itself to these enzymes and neutralizes them, a self-sacrifice that works to our benefit.

Dr. Duke confided on the APR broadcast that he smoked three packs of cigarettes a day for thirty years. Although he has stopped smoking, Dr. Dukes' long indulgence left him more at risk to develop cancer. As a result of his food research, he now eats two carrots daily. These contain enough beta-carotene to halve his chances of getting lung cancer, he asserted.

All this adds up to very hopeful news for those concerned about life-threatening chronic diseases. As Jean Carper, author of *Food, Your Miracle Medicine*, put it: "We see that our modern drugs are not going to solve those chronic diseases, because they have to be prevented rather than cured. Food seems to me one of the absolute best preventive medicines we could have."

ENZYMES AND FIBER FOR HEALTH

The old saying "You are what you eat" is only half true. We are actually no more than we can digest. The key is effective assimilation of what we eat through good digestion. Optimal digestion depends on more than just eating the right foods. The key to good digestion is the class of complex chemical substances known as enzymes.

Three types of enzymes have been identified: digestive enzymes (which digest our food), food enzymes (available only in fresh, live food) and metabolic enzymes (which science has discovered no means of replenishing). When we eat cooked food over a period of many years, we eventually deplete our digestive enzymes and have to rob our pool of metabolic enzymes to assist the digestion process. As the metabolic enzymes are depleted, deterioration of the body sets in. The aging process begins.

Food enzymes are necessary in order to break large food components into smaller ones which the body can absorb. Each enzyme has a specific job and can only break down certain components. The three main components that we consume are fats, proteins, and carbohydrates.

Most nutritionally aware people take care to get a daily ration of fruits and vegetables, grains and legumes. But unless they are eaten raw, the fresh-food nutrients may not be effectively absorbed by the body. Once a piece of food is steamed, baked, fried, boiled, broiled, barbecued, toasted, roasted, sautéed, poached, grilled, or microwaved, it is in many ways as good as dead. Fresh, raw food's 'life force,' its vital energy, is lost. If you take a handful of raw sunflower seeds, bury them in the earth, and water them, chances are good they will sprout. If boiled first, they will rot in the ground. The difference between raw and cooked is the difference between life and death.

The reason a cooked seed won't sprout is because the enzymes have been destroyed by the heat of cooking. "Enzymes are substances that make life possible," explains one of the world's leading experts in enzyme research, Dr. Edward Howell in *Enzyme Nutrition, The Food Enzyme Concept*. "They are needed for every chemical reaction that takes place in the human body. No mineral, vitamin, or hormone can do any work without enzymes.

"Our bodies, all of our organs, tissues, and cells, are run by metabolic enzymes. They are the manual workers that build the body from proteins, carbohydrates, and fats, just as construction workers build our homes. You have all the raw materials with which to build, but without the workers (enzymes) you cannot even begin," he says.

Among many important enzymes so far identified, three start out as major league players in the assimilation of food. The body needs protease for the digestion of proteins, amylase for breaking down carbohydrates and starch, and lipase for digesting fats. These and other enzymes can be gotten from raw foods, in which naturally present enzymes tend to correlate with the nutritional factors of the food itself. Raw fatty foods such as oils and nuts, for example, contain lipase. But if these same fatty foods are cooked, the lipase and other enzymes are destroyed, placing extra demands on the body (especially the pancreas) to produce more enzymes in order to facilitate digestion.

The human body will produce its own enzymes, but only in a limited quantity over the course of a lifetime. When the enzyme potential is depleted beyond a certain point, according to research documented in Howell's book, a given life is effectively over. Researchers in Chicago have found that enzyme levels in the saliva of young adults are thirty times higher than in persons over sixty-nine years of age. Research in Germany has found that the urine of young people contains nearly twice the amount of the starch-digesting enzyme amylase than the urine of old people. An individual's enzyme potential, maintains Howell, not only determines the length of that person's life but is directly related to good health and resistance to disease.

According to Humbart Santillo, ND, author of the excellent book I highly recommend, *Food Enzymes: The Missing Link to Radiant Health*, a diet of mostly cooked foods is a disservice to the body. The pancreas must borrow enzymes from other parts of the body to properly digest cooked food. Inadequately digested food can putrefy in the intestines, creating gas and toxins and further impede nutrient assimilation.

Unfortunately, we don't always have time to eat right. We are too busy to buy and prepare several servings of fresh fruits and vegetables a day. Those we do eat tend to be overprocessed, overcooked, or too far removed from the field, and thus lack much of the nutrition and enzymes provided by fresh, raw fruits and vegetables. And, let's face it, many people complain about the taste of some fruits and vegetables. Enter *Juice Plus+*. Juice Plus+ is a "live" whole food supplement, made from a wide variety of nutritious fruits and vegetables. Each natural ingredient has been specially selected for its unique nutritional make-up, then combined with all the others to provide many of the nutritional benefits of eating a wide variety of fresh fruits and vegetables. Most of the active plant food enzymes and other vital nutrients found in the fresh, raw fruits and vegetables they use remain intact, making Juice Plus+ a healthy choice and sound nutritional insurance (see Resource Directory).

It's also important to get enough fiber in the diet. While not a source of fuel, fiber is an essential component of an effective health program, especially if you want to lose weight. You should try to get about thirty to fifty grams of fiber per day. That's not really difficult if your diet contains plenty of fruit, vegetables, grains, and legumes.

The typical American diet derives forty to sixty percent of its calories from fats, thirty percent from carbohydrates (mainly refined sugars), and twenty percent from protein. Its fiber content is a mere ten grams. Obviously, this is a diet tailor-made to produce obesity and ill health since a health-promoting diet is exactly the reverse.

Dietary fiber helps digestion and elimination. It adds bulk to your diet and provides a feeling of fullness that may help you be more moderate in your food intake. Fiber also increases the amount of necessary chewing, thus slowing the eating process. When you eat too quickly, without chewing well, it places extra stress on the digestive system. Fiber stimulates the release of intestinal hormones that, along with its bulk, satisfies your appetite by giving a feeling of fullness. Fiber is also helpful in disease prevention. Diets rich in fiber appear to decrease risks of constipation, coronary heart disease, hemorrhoids, diverticulitis, and colon cancer. (See Chapter Three for more on fiber.)

Dietary fiber consists of insoluble types, which are not digested in the gut, and soluble types, which are. Soluble forms of fiber include pectins, gums, and certain hemicelluloses, and are found especially in oats and oat bran, barley, dried beans, and other legume foods. Soluble fibers help lower blood cholesterol by trapping it in the gut and preventing its absorption. These fibers are often useful in the treatment of heart disease and diabetes.

Insoluble forms of fiber include complex carbohydrates such as cellulose, lignins and some hemicelluloses, and are found in wheat bran, whole grain breads and cereals, and the skins of fruits and vegetables. Insoluble fibers are useful in promoting elimination. Rates of colon cancer risk are quite low in populations that subsist on diets high in insoluble dietary fiber, perhaps because of the ways in which it speeds the passage of carcinogens through the intestine and/or changes the metabolism of bacteria residing in the gut.

The Standard American Diet (SAD) consists of a high intake of refined carbohydrates such as pastries, cakes, cookies, candy, fries, and so on; foods that are often stripped of vitamins and minerals, but are full of simple sugars, salt, fats, and chemicals; animal products that are excessively high in protein and loaded with cholesterol, saturated fats, and hormones; and an extremely low intake of fiber, complex carbohydrates, and fresh fruits and vegetables.

Not surprisingly, a natural weight loss diet turns out to be the same as the one which promotes health. Whether your goal is long life, lots of energy and/or a lean youthful body, your diet should be high in dietary fiber (thirty to fifty grams) and complex carbohydrate foods (sixty to seventy percent), sufficient in protein (ten to fifteen percent), and low in fat (ten to twenty percent). Whole grains and legumes, along with lots of fresh fruits and vegetables, will provide you with generous amounts of vitamins, minerals, soluble and insoluble fibers, fuel for sustained energy, and more than adequate amounts of protein and essential fats.

ANTIOXIDANT AIDS

We have been hearing a lot in the 90s about the importance of eating foods rich in antioxidants to reduce the risk of certain diseases. Beta-carotene, vitamin C, vitamin E, and selenium belong to a group of vitamins called dietary antioxidants. The scientific evidence is undeniable. One of their roles includes the prevention of a certain undesirable chemical event in the body called a 'free radical reaction,' which may be associated with several disease processes (see Chapter Four on flax seed for more information). Some studies have shown that daily consumption of vegetables and fruits rich in antioxidants (or high blood levels of these vitamins) is associated with a decreased risk of some forms of cancer and heart disease. Antioxidants have been shown to be effective in fighting disease, slowing the aging process, and supporting the body's natural defenses, which are often weakened by environmental pollution, poor diet, and stress. However, it's difficult to pinpoint exactly which components of these foods account the most for their beneficial effects. For example, fruits and vegetables high in beta-carotene and vitamins C and E also tend to be high in fiber and some minerals, and low in fat. These qualities may also affect risk in the same or different ways.

You may want to consider supplementing your diet with a good all-around supplement with antioxidants. I recommend these four products—*Bio-Strath, Green Magma, Juice Plus+*, and *Sun Chlorella*. (See Chapter Five on chlorophyll and greens.)

Bio-Strath is an excellent herbal food supplement in liquid and tablet form. A result of accurate, scientifically-based work and based on plasmolysed yeast and wild herbs, Bio-Strath has been available for decades in over forty countries around the world. I've included Bio-Strath in my health program for over fifteen years and highly recommend it. From numerous scientific studies, it has been found to combat fatigue, lethargy, and nervousness, increase physical and mental efficiency, improve concentration, reinforce the immune defense system, and restore vitality. I also like the fact that it is 100 percent natural, virtually manufactured by nature without chemicals, synthetic vitamins, or heat. The Bio-Strath herbal yeast contains a great variety of vital substances such as antioxidants, amino acids, nucleic acids RNA and DNA, vitamins from the B-complex, and various minerals and trace elements. Bio-Strath also comes in yeast-free drops. Available in health food stores or order from the number listed in the Resources Directory.

Green Magma is a powdered juice made from barley grass that offers nature's own perfect balance of nutrients. Grown in some of the world's most fertile soil near the Pacific Ocean, young barley grass is harvested, then transported to a state-of-the-art processing facility just minutes away. Barley grass is flowing with antioxidants, beta-carotene, live enzymes such as superoxide dismutase (or SOD), vitamins C, E, B_1, B_2, B_3, B_6, (B vitamins are catalysts essential for converting food into energy), amino acids, chlorophyll, and much more. Powdered brown rice, grown without pesticides or chemical fertilizers, is mixed with the concentrated juice. The rice increases the levels of B vitamins and helps the fine powder bind together after it is spray-dried at low temperatures. I appreciate that it is a 'live' whole food concentrate.

People who drink Green Magma frequently say they notice a boost in their energy, especially in the afternoons when they need it most. I agree. That's probably because of the supplement's active live enzymes, which are essential for proper digestion and assimilation of the valuable vitamins and trace minerals in the foods we consume. Green Magma is available in health food stores, nutrition centers or through the number listed in the Resource Directory. Look for it, along with Veggie Magma, Magma Plus, Barley Dog and Barley Cat—all excellent supplements. For more information, see the Resource Directory.

I also highly recommend Juice Plus+. This is a super food concentrate of pesticide-free fruits and vegetables that have been picked ripe and juiced and never heated—with the water and sugars extracted—and the remaining powder is encapsulated. Each capsule contains lots of antioxidants, vitamins, minerals, fiber, enzymes, and phytonutrients—all the things nature gives us in seventeen raw fruits, vegetables, and grains: apple, cherry, cranberry, date, orange, papaya, peach, pineapple, prune, beet, broccoli, cabbage, carrot, kale, parsley, spinach, barley, oats, plant enzymes, and acidophilus.

This whole food supplement has been tested in major bio-availability studies and findings are very impressive. The results show increased plasma antioxidant levels in users of Juice Plus+. In fact, independent laboratory analyses show that four capsules (the daily recommendation is two Juice Plus+ Orchard Blend capsules —fruit juice powders—and two Juice Plus+ Garden Blend capsules—vegetable juice and grain powders) contain the Vitamin C of four oranges, the beta-carotene of three raw carrots, and more Vitamin E than several servings of spinach and broccoli, as well as many of the other nutritional components found in the fruits and vegetables from which they're made. Results of another study showed marked and consistent increases in plasma alpha tocopherol (Vitamin E) and similar significant increases in plasma beta-carotene and related carotenoids such as retinol, lycopene, zeanthin, lutein, and alpha carotene. The study's conclusion: "Long-term supplementation with Juice Plus+, if resulting in a sustained high level of the above antioxidants, may offer significant potential health benefits in terms of reducing risk of major age-related disorders."

Juice Plus+ is not a processed, fragmented vitamin-mineral pill, nor is it an extraction. Juice Plus+ combines the latest advances in nutritional science and food processing technology to give you added daily nutrition from fresh, raw fruits and vegetables in an easy-to-use capsule or chewable form for adults and children. This product is not available in health food stores. For more information or to order, please refer to the Resource Directory.

I believe that one of the reasons I have not been sick in years is because I eat a very healthy diet and take these supplements (also Sun Chlorella) on a regular basis, in addition to *Ester* C and *Kyolic*.

C POWER

Vitamin C is fundamental for health and disease prevention. In fact, many researchers believe that vitamin C's role in the body goes far beyond that of a nutrient. The evidence comes from studies of animals and the health benefits people derive from taking high doses of vitamin C. Most animals produce their own vitamin C—literally hundreds of times the amount people routinely obtain from food. In addition, scientific studies on people show that a high intake of vitamin C extends life span, fights infections, lowers blood pressure and cholesterol, as well as reducing the likelihood of dying from heart disease and cancer. According to Linus Pauling, "Vitamin C is different because, at one time, all animals made their own vitamin C in their livers. All of this extra vitamin C must be important—otherwise, the majority of animals wouldn't be producing so much of it."

So, why don't people make their own vitamin C? One theory holds that a genetic accident millions of years ago left the ancestors of human beings and a handful of animals—including the guinea pig—unable to produce this vitamin in their bodies. If true, it means people have hobbled from one generation to the next totally dependent on meager dietary sources of vitamin C.

In animals—and in people—vitamin C maintains homeostasis, the term biologists use to describe staying on an 'even keel' when faced with stress, infections, heart disease, cancer, and other conditions. Vitamin C is essential for a smooth-running immune system, and is also an antioxidant.

New methods of preparing this vitamin have added to its effectiveness and tamed it for those who have been put off by its acidity. This new family of mineral ascorbates is called Ester-C, a trademark for a product made by the Inter-Cal Corporation of Prescott, Arizona (see Resource Directory). Ester-C can be found in hundreds of products sold by dozens of distributors. It is non-acidic, so the harshness that might upset your stomach is gone. The unique manufacturing process creates a patented vitamin C complex consisting of ascorbate and C metabolites. These metabolites, naturally present in Ester-C, are the same ones that your body makes at much smaller concentrations. They enhance cellular absorption and utilization of the ascorbate in Ester-C supplements. Inter-Cal is actively investigating new therapeutic uses for this new form of vitamin C, and they are getting exciting results.

Dr. Anthony Verlangieri of the Department of Pharmacology at the University of Mississippi, and Dr. Seth Rose of the Department of Chemistry at Arizona State University, have been the trailblazers in identifying the C metabolites and investigating their role as cellular 'door-openers' that allow ascorbate to build intracellular levels not possible with ordinary supplements.

By now, it's well accepted that stressful situations and illness can tax our immune systems to the limit. One of the reasons for this is the rapid depletion of ascorbate from our cells in response to stress and infection. So it makes sense to combat this threat by taking ascorbate supplements like Ester-C that have a good chance of getting into the critical cells, such as the white blood cells that are the first-line defense against bacterial and viral attack.

Research conducted by the Life Management Group of San Diego has provided new evidence that Ester-C is a more effective way of building intracellular levels of ascorbate. Their study used male subjects receiving a one-gram dose of vitamin C in the form of Ester-C calcium ascorbate or ordinary ascorbic acid. They found that after twenty-four hours, Ester-C had delivered and maintained significantly higher amounts of ascorbate to the white blood cells. These are the cells that really count and they need ascorbate to maintain their essential functions in stress and infection.

Scientists often use animal models to answer questions about vitamin C when it's not possible to conduct clinical trials. Dr. Verlangieri showed that Ester-C ascorbate was better than ordinary ascorbic acid at preventing scurvy in a type of laboratory rat that has a requirement for this vitamin. We have known for a long time that humans cannot manufacture their own ascorbate and require it in their diets. Many investigators are now discovering that even some animals may benefit from additional ascorbate, even though they can survive without it in their diets and don't get scurvy the way people do. Studies with dogs and horses with various musculoskeletal disorders—from lameness to hip dysplasia to joint inflammation—are showing that large doses of Ester-C ascorbate can relieve pain and restore mobility in these animals after several weeks.

Dr. L. Phillips Brown, a Massachusetts veterinarian, has compared Ester-C calcium ascorbate to ordinary ascorbic acid in a large population of old, lame dogs in the Best Friends Animal Sanctuary in Kanaab, Utah. He fed different doses of ascorbate supplements to the dogs several times a day and then scored the degree of improvement in pain relief, lameness, and mobility. The results were remarkable. Not only did nearly eighty percent of the dogs improve clinically, but Ester-C ascorbate was significantly more effective than ordinary ascorbic acid. Similar results had been obtained several years earlier by Dr. Geir Berge in Norway. Dr. N. Lee Newman, a Virginia large-animal veterinarian, is beginning to show very similar results with Ester-C supplementation for horses with degenerative joint diseases such as ringbone and hock spavin.

It's tempting to dismiss these results by saying that animals don't require vitamin C because they make ascorbate in their own tissues. But do they make enough? Can their internal supply keep up with the increased demands of aging and with a degenerating circulatory system? At the very least, these intriguing results suggest—for both humans and animals—that the vitamin C requirement may increase with age. It is beginning to look as though certain joints and connective tissue may not get enough vitamin C unless it is supplied as Ester-C ascorbate.

Ester-C can also give you a reason to smile! Researchers have learned that Ester-C ascorbate in the zinc form is just as effective an antiplaque agent as some of the ingredients in your favorite mouthwash. Dr. Steven Silverstein of the School of Dentistry at the University of California in San Francisco has shown that Ester-C zinc ascorbate is very effective at inhibiting the growth of the types of bacteria known to produce dental decay and plaque formation on tooth enamel. In another study, Dr. Silverstein used a high-resolution microscope to produce shockingly explicit photographs of the process of tooth erosion by acid—ascorbic acid! Can you imagine the countless numbers of children who have been biting into chewable Vitamin C tablets and losing their tooth enamel in the process? The good news is that Ester-C ascorbate, which is neither acid or alkaline, doesn't affect enamel in the least. With results like these, you can bet you'll be seeing more Ester-C in oral health products in the near future.

Ester-C mineral ascorbates put the technology of C metabolites at your service to achieve and maintain higher intracellular levels of ascorbate than ordinary vitamin C supplements. Ester-C products are backed up by strong research support and pioneering scientific discovery. If you believe as I do that extra vitamin C can enhance your health and well-being, Ester-C mineral ascorbates are the way to get it. I take Ester-C by itself and in a formula that includes an aged garlic extract called Kyolic Formula 103 available in health food stores. For more information, see Resource Directory.

GREAT GARLIC

Garlic can do more than make food taste good—it can save your life, say the experts. Numerous studies show that garlic—and especially an aged garlic extract called Kyolic—may help prevent several types of cancer, reduce the risk of heart disease, lower cholesterol, help prevent Alzheimer's disease, improve memory, boost the immune system, and much more.

These studies, explains Dr. Herbert Pierson, a top nutrition expert formerly with the National Cancer Institute, "clearly showed garlic's effectiveness in lowering the incidence of cardiovascular disease and drastically reducing stomach and colon cancer. I was amazed at the number of studies showing how garlic actually can reverse the effects of aging, including memory loss."

Most researchers used Kyolic in their studies because of its potency and purity. Since the development of Kyolic almost four decades ago, aged garlic extract has attracted the attention of some the world's most promising researchers. A wide range of research and clinical studies confirming the superiority of Kyolic have been conducted by various research institutes worldwide. Over 100 studies on aged garlic extract have been presented at various symposiums, including the First World Congress on Garlic in 1990, and published in various scientific journals. Kyolic is also covered by more than a dozen patents and patents pending worldwide.

Here are some of the exciting findings.

CANCER: "Garlic significantly lowered the risk of getting breast and prostate cancer and slowed its progress in subjects who already had the disease," according to Dr. John Pinto, director of the Nutrition Research

Laboratory at Memorial Sloan-Kettering Cancer Center. A Michigan State University study confirmed that garlic can lower the risk of breast cancer. Several Chinese studies have found garlic also helps prevent stomach cancer. And Dr. Vivenne Reeve, a researcher at the University of Sydney in Australia, revealed that she was able to greatly reduce skin cancer in mice by applying aged garlic extract on affected rodents.

HEART AND CIRCULATORY DISEASE: Garlic reduces the risk of heart disease and stroke, according to research by Dr. Robert I-San Lin, who has worked with the US government to help establish nutrition standards. "My research shows that garlic unclogs blocked arteries and prevents cholesterol and other deposits from sticking to the arteries, reducing plaque formation," he said. "Since plaque is the major cause of heart attacks, I think garlic should be mandatory medicine for anyone at risk for heart disease."

ALZHEIMER'S DISEASE AND AGING: "Garlic enhances blood circulation to the brain, which helps prevent senility, Alzheimer's, and even Parkinson's disease," said Dr. Lin. A Japanese study showed that garlic can combat age-related memory loss and brain cell deterioration. A French study found that garlic improves memory and relieves symptoms of depression and fatigue.

IMMUNE SYSTEM: Garlic contains compounds that boost the activity of white blood cells—the cells that help ward off disease—reveals research by Dr. John Milner, head of the department of nutrition at Pennsylvania State University.

I have been taking Kyolic aged garlic extract for the past twenty years. While I use some garlic in my cooking, too much raw garlic is irritating to the digestive system, not to mention its effect on the breath. That's why I take Kyolic. It's the most scientifically researched garlic supplement, rather than a commercial food additive or flavoring. Kyolic is organically grown and aged naturally. During aging, the concentrated active compounds are mellowed and the harsh, irritating, odorous compounds found in raw garlic are converted to dozens of valuable, stable, safe, and odorless compounds, including S-allyl cysteine, that make Kyolic so beneficial. It is the only truly odorless garlic product available.

Kyolic comes in a variety of excellent formulas (see Resource Directory). One of my favorites is Kyolic Formula 103, which is a combination of Kyolic aged garlic extract, Calcium, Ester C, and Astragalus.

(The herb astragalus is an excellent energizer. It has been used by athletes for building energy reserves, especially in the arms and legs. It is also useful in cold climates for keeping the body warm. And it's a natural interferon support, immune stimulant, and overall tonic.)

FABULOUS FLAVONOIDS

You should choose a diet containing at least seven servings of fruits and vegetables each day. Dark green leafy or yellow, orange, and red vegetables (such as spinach, squash, carrots, and peppers) and some fruits (such as apricots, cantaloupe, mangos, and papayas) are good sources of beta-carotene. Fresh citrus fruits and some vegetables (such as peppers, tomatoes, collard greens, and broccoli) are rich in vitamin C. Green leafy vegetables, nuts, and wheat germ contain vitamin E.

What we're seeing here is the importance of eating foods with a variety of colors, which will help prevent diseases like cancer, heart disease, and other illnesses. Blackberries, blueberries, strawberries, plums, squash, pumpkin, apples, oranges, grapefruit, tomatoes, and other fruits and vegetables colored purple, blue, black, red, orange, or yellow are nearly all rich sources of carotenoids and flavonoids.

You may have heard of citrus flavonoids including rutin and hesperidin. Biochemical dictionaries say there are 3,000 or more naturally occurring flavonoids, of which only several hundred are colored. However, even colorless flavonoids often contribute to plant coloration by interaction with other flavonoids. As some of the specific effects of individual bioflavonoids are researched and documented, a few of the better known—including quercetin and pycnogenol—have joined rutin on the health food store shelves.

A 1994 report in the prestigious medical journal *Lancet* states that "flavonoids in regularly consumed foods may reduce the risk of death from coronary heart disease in older men." In this study, 805 men, ages sixty-five to eighty-four years, were studied over a five-year period for flavonoid intake and incidence of heart attacks. The highest risk of heart attacks was found in those with the lowest flavonoid intake. Conversely, those men who consumed the most flavonoids had the lowest risk of heart attacks. It was also reported that flavonoids also interfere with cancer growth and development.

EAT AT THE BOTTOM OF THE FOOD CHAIN

Fruits and vegetables are clearly main ingredients of health, but try to get them free of pesticides and herbicides. These are among the most toxic chemicals known to science, designed to kill living creatures.

Along with other industrial metals and chemicals, pesticides run off into our lakes, rivers, and oceans, polluting both water supplies and marine animals. All of these toxins become more concentrated as they move up the food chain. From phytoplankton to zooplankton to small fish to larger fish, the metals and chemicals concentrate as they move up. That's why a large fish like tuna has more mercury than a smaller fish like cod: tuna is further up the food chain.

Livestock animals also concentrate toxic chemicals in their fat and livers. This toxic concentration as we move up the food chain is confirmed in tests. Compared to the average pesticide residues found in plant foods, dairy foods have about three times as much; meat, fish, and poultry have about six times as much.

If you want to lower your ingestion of harmful toxins, eat lower on the food chain. The closer we come to being vegans (vegetarians who eat no animal products including dairy or eggs), the fewer harmful metals and chemicals we take in. I have been a vegetarian for over twenty-five years and a vegan for a few years. A plant-based diet is also a safe, simple way to re-establish a relationship with nature and practice environmental awareness. Eating these foods is eating at the bottom of the food chain. The lower you eat on the food chain the less energy it requires to produce food and the less damage it does to the environment. And it's more economical, too.

Whenever possible, choose organic food. This is a loose term, but generally means fruits and vegetables grown without pesticides or herbicides.

LOOK AT THE LABELS

Read labels when you are grocery shopping. In its top ten list of the "Best Science of 1994," *Time Magazine* included what it termed a 'radical idea' implemented by the US Food and Drug Administration: food labels that actually are useful to consumers. Indeed they are. On packaged foods—cereals boxes, breads, crackers, potato chips, ice cream, just about everything, in fact—manufacturers must now display data on cholesterol, total fat, sugars, sodium, and saturated fat. Gone is a lot of the deception behind health claims. 'Fat-free' really does mean fat-free. Gone also are serving sizes so small they wouldn't satisfy a rabbit. Life in the supermarket aisles has definitely gotten easier.

Ironically, those foods that are best for us—the ones naturally lowest in fat, cholesterol, and sodium, and highest in fiber and other rich nutrients—are the very foods that don't have any labels on them. They're your fresh fruits and vegetables.

A good rule of thumb when reading labels is that if you find it difficult to pronounce one or more ingredients on a label, it's probably best to pass that food by. The label does provide two key pieces of information to help you judge the nutritional attributes of the product: the ingredients list and the nutrition information panel.

Ingredients are listed in descending order by dry weight, so you can get a good idea of their relative proportion. For example, if salt is listed before the vegetables in a package of dehydrated soup mix, the soup contains a lot of salt and very few vegetables. Similarly, if sugar (sucrose) is listed as the first ingredient, or sugar appears in several other forms (corn syrup, fructose, molasses), then a large portion of the product's calories comes from sugar. There's no shortage of 'fat-free' products on the shelves, but it appears, in an effort to retain flavor while removing fat, manufacturers have poured on the salt—sometimes quadruple the sodium of the original higher fat product—and have added sugars. Optimally, the total number of milligrams of sodium should not exceed the total number of calories. Simple sugars pump glucose into your bloodstream at breakneck speed, driving up insulin levels, which then trap fat in your fat cells, forcing the body to burn less fat. That's right, the very product that's supposed to help you get rid of fat tissue is actually promoting fat storage.

The nutrition information panel provides details about the nutrients in the food. The number of calories, the grams of carbohydrates, protein and fat, and the milligrams of sodium per serving size are at the top of the list. In foods where a large proportion of the calories comes from fat, the grams of unsaturated and saturated fat and the milligrams of cholesterol may also be provided. But it's easy to be misled. For example, there is a lot of confusion about two percent low-fat milk. Although people assume that 'two percent' means the milk is ninety-eight percent fat-free, this is not so. The percentages are based on weight, not total calories. An eight-ounce glass of 'low-fat' two percent milk has 120 calories and 4.7 grams of fat with thirty-five percent of the calories coming from fat. Skim milk, on the other hand, has only eighty-five calories and 0.4 gm of fat with a mere four percent of the calories coming from fat. Although I don't recommend eating dairy products, if you choose to, skip the two percent and use skim milk.

The new food labels don't always tell you the percentage of calories from fat, but it's now easier to figure out. Just go to the nutrition panel and find the calories from fat. Divide that number by the total calories—ending up with the percentage of calories from fat. If division trips you up, go by grams, using this easy rule: if a product has 1.5 fat grams or less per 100 calories, its fat content is within healthy guidelines; the fat, per serving, is fifteen percent or less of total calories.

There's a catch. Though the nutrition panel lists the amount of cholesterol and saturated fat for each serving, it does not tally up under either of those categories the amount of trans-fatty acids in the food—those fatty acids which do not contain saturated fats, per se, but can act like saturated fats in your body, driving up blood cholesterol levels. Trans-fatty acids pop up all over the place—in breads, chips, crackers, cookies, microwave popcorn, and other packaged foods. Manufacturers like them because they give margarines and other foods a creamy consistency and they prolong shelf life. On your ingredient list, they're known as hydrogenated or partially-hydrogenated fats. If you see the word 'hydrogenated' on an ingredient list, don't even bother reading further. Just put it back. It's a product that can raise cholesterol levels and clog arteries.

Under 'sugars,' the nutrition panel will give you a fairly good sense of the number of sugar grams you're eating. It gets a little tricky, though, because that number includes both added and natural sugars. Your best bet is to stick with the ingredient list. If on the list you're seeing natural sugars, like raisins, date sugar, figs and other fruits, that's good. Your insulin levels won't shoot up nearly as high as with added sugars. However, if the ingredient list sports a lot of "ose" words—like sucrose, glucose, fructose—or if there are other added sugars, like corn syrup, sorghum, honey, and mannitol, it's prudent to limit your intake to less than 1.5 grams for every 100 calories. If you're eating 2,000 calories a day, then your 'budget' is around thirty grams of added sugar.

The nutrition information panel is especially important if you are interested in controlling calories by trimming the fat content of your diet or in limiting the amount of sodium you consume. However, when making product comparisons, bear in mind that serving sizes are specified by the manufacturer and may vary substantially between similar products.

I also suggest that you do some housecleaning in your kitchen cupboards and refrigerator. This is one of the things I do in my counseling with individuals and families. I actually go to their homes and lend guidance on what to throw out or keep—with the goal of optimum health.

MY KITCHEN ESSENTIALS

There are some appliances and other essentials which make being healthy a little bit easier, such as a top quality set of knives, a juicer, salad spinner, Vita-Mix Nutrition Center, and Neova Cookware. These items are very important in my kitchen. They help me prepare the kinds of foods that I want to eat, and they compliment the look of my kitchen—cleaner and healthier, reflecting my feelings about myself. For over twenty-five years I have been teaching classes on vegetarian cooking. After taking my vegetarian lifestyle courses, everyone chooses to get the above items to make their healthy lifestyles more convenient and simple. Refer to the Resource Directory for more information on some of the above items or to order.

In Victoria Moran's wonderful book, *Love Yourself Thin*, she says, "Start with small things. Delight in your dishes or your herb plants or the needlework saying on the wall. You'll soon delight as well in how your eating has changed. It's all connected...When you're eating the purest, most healthful foods available to you, you feel good about your body, your thinking is more lucid, and your outlook more positive."

Healthful behaviors are more likely to increase if they are easy and convenient. Have healthy foods easily available. When I come home from being out all day and am tired and hungry, there is a greater possibility that I will include a raw vegetable salad with my evening meal, or as my evening meal, if I washed the vegetables and perhaps partially prepared or trimmed them earlier. Sometimes it's harder to stay on track when you have to start from scratch. Do you know what I mean?

Plan Ahead. I usually bring some fresh fruit to the movie theater and I've been known to take in vegetarian sandwiches, bottled water, and even homemade fresh juices.

Enjoy your food. But remember, food is fuel. Eat to live. Don't live to eat. There is more to life than food. Honor the divine temple that you are and support your self-esteem by selecting foods that support your body and promote optimum health.

CHAPTER THREE

Healthy Weight: Creating a Fit, Lean Body

The body is ultimately a reflection, a reflection of what is going on inside: emotionally, intellectually, and spiritually.
—VICTORIA MORAN

You've seen the headlines on supermarket tabloids: "Use your zodiac sign to pick the perfect diet," or "Lose ten pounds in one week on a dessert diet!" Americans are preoccupied with their waistlines and fat. We spend more than thirty billion dollars a year on diet foods, diet programs, diet pills, and other 'guaranteed' weight-loss regimens and products. Yet according to the National Center of Health Statistics, we're getting fatter all the time.

While millions of people starve to death in many parts of the world, the United States has the dubious honor of being the fattest country on the globe. The unhealthy numbers show no signs of lightening up. Experts call obesity an epidemic—one that encourages major health problems. Heart disease, endometrial (uterine) cancer and possibly breast cancer, high cholesterol, high blood pressure, immune dysfunction, osteoarthritis, stroke, gout, gallstones, and diabetes are all associated with overweight. Put in a more positive way, losing even a little weight may significantly improve your health and well being. Even if you're only interested in losing ten or twenty pounds to look better, you'll also benefit in many other ways.

Your body has an unlimited capacity for storing fat. Fortunately, it also has ample capacity to use and reduce it. Losing excess fat reduces crowding of your organs and the strain on your lower back, hips, and knees. It also boosts your mood, self-esteem, and energy levels, helps you sleep better (being overweight is often associated with sleep disorders such as sleep apnea—temporary cessation of breathing), and improves your appearance and attractiveness.

Eating disorders such as anorexia and bulimia are on the rise, and women's magazines are not helping when they continue to use models who are embracing the waif look. Take Barbie, a doll that's part of most little girls' upbringing. This model of good looks and perfect body is giving the wrong message about what a healthy woman's body should look like. Barbie's body fat, were she an actual person, would be so low that she probably wouldn't even be able to menstruate. As little girls swarm to Barbie and teens try to emulate her, she has one accessory missing—food.

So how do you know what's an ideal weight for you?

Until recently, we have usually referred to height and weight tables provided by Metropolitan Life Insurance Company (MetLife). Yet, according to Dr. William P. Castelli, medical director of the famed Framingham Heart Study, these MetLife tables, which were revised in 1983 to allow for more weight, have become too lenient. In fact, the American Heart Association has urged people to ignore those guidelines. According to the current MetLife tables, 155 pounds is within the desirable weight range for a 5' 5" woman. That may be fine for a female bodybuilder with lots of lean muscle tissue, but it's too high for a normal non-bodybuilder female. These MetLife tables are based on death rates and vital statistics from millions of insurance holders in the United States. They don't account for the fact that many thin people with high death rates are cigarette smokers or otherwise ill. If those people had been eliminated from the current tabulations, says Dr. Castelli, the desirable weights would be lower. Dr. Castelli and other experts are exploring better ways to evaluate optimal body weight based on the latest research on weight-related health risks.

WHAT YOUR SHAPE SAYS ABOUT HEALTH RISKS

Two approaches, when used together, are emerging as the new 'gold standard' for weight: Body Mass Index and Waist/Hip Ratio.

Body Mass Index (BMI) is a ratio of height to weight. It's determined by a mathematical formula: first divide your weight (in pounds) by your height (in inches) squared, then multiply the resulting number by 705. You should get a BMI that's somewhere between 19 and 30. For example, let's say you weigh 140 pounds and you are 5' 8" tall. You would first figure out your height (68") squared which is 4624. Then take your weight (140) and divide it by 4624 which gives you .030. Multiply this number by 705 and you get 21 (see figure 1).

Numerous studies have already been conducted to validate the efficacy of the BMI and weight-related health risks. The conclusion is that 21 to 22 is the optimal body mass index because there are no weight-related health risks at this level.

One large-scale study indicates that a BMI below 22 is ideal for preventing heart disease in women. This Nurses' Health Study, co-directed by Dr. JoAnn E. Manson and conducted at Brigham and Women's Hospital and Harvard Hospital in Boston, followed 115,886 initially healthy American women ages thirty to fifty-five for eight years.

Healthy Weight

During that time, 605 of the women experienced coronary-artery disease, of whom eighty-three died. There was no elevated risk of heart disease among women whose BMIs were under 21; the risk was thirty percent higher than that of the lean group for women whose BMI was between 21 and 25, eighty percent higher for a BMI 25 to 29, and 230 percent higher than the lean group for those with a BMI greater than 29. The researchers concluded that "obesity is a strong risk factor for coronary heart disease in middle-age women." They reported in the March 1990 issue of the *New England Journal of Medicine* that "even mild-to-moderate overweight is associated with a substantial elevation in coronary risk."

There's no consensus yet among the experts on how much is too much. Some insist that although a BMI between 23 and 25 isn't ideal, the excess risk for cancer and other weight-related diseases seems to be

---

FIGURE ONE

CALCULATING BODY MASS INDEX (BMI)

HEIGHT	BODY WEIGHT IN POUNDS										
4'10"	91	96	100	105	110	115	119	124	129	134	138	143
4'11"	94	99	104	109	114	119	124	128	133	138	143	148
5'0"	97	102	107	112	118	123	128	133	138	143	148	153
5'1"	100	106	111	116	122	127	132	137	143	148	153	158
5'2"	104	109	115	120	126	131	136	142	147	153	158	164
5'3"	107	113	118	124	130	135	141	146	152	158	163	169
5'4"	110	116	122	128	134	140	145	151	157	163	169	174
5'5"	114	120	126	132	138	144	150	156	162	168	174	180
5'6"	118	124	130	136	142	148	155	161	167	173	179	186
5'7"	121	127	134	140	146	153	159	166	172	178	185	191
5'8"	125	131	138	144	151	158	164	171	177	184	190	197
5'9"	128	135	142	149	155	162	169	176	182	189	196	203
5'10"	132	139	146	153	160	167	174	181	188	195	202	207
5'11"	136	143	150	157	165	172	179	186	193	200	208	215
6'0"	140	147	154	162	169	177	184	191	199	206	213	221
BMI	19	20	21	22	23	24	25	26	27	28	29	30

To find your BMI, locate your height in the left column. (If you've lost inches over the years, use your peak adult height.) Move across the chart (to the right) until you hit your approximate weight, then follow that column down to the corresponding BMI number at the bottom of the chart.

small. Approximately around a BMI of 26, these health risks appear to rise, although it's not quite clear to scientists where to draw the line. Jean Pierre Despres, Ph.D., associate director of the Lipid Research Center at Laval University in St. Foy, Quebec, says that between 25 and 27 is a gray zone. "A lot of people in this range are perfectly healthy, but others have a substantially higher risk of developing diabetes and premature coronary disease." Most scientists do agree that a BMI over 27 increases risk for many people. But their risk also depends on other factors, including their waist/hip measurement, notes Dr. Despres.

Although less common than overweight in the United States, excessive thinness can also be a problem. It is linked with osteoporosis and other health problems, even early death, especially if weight loss is sudden. The experts feel that someone with a BMI under 19 should be evaluated. "That doesn't mean everyone low is going to be unhealthy, but it's worth taking a closer look," says James O. Hill, Ph.D., associate director of the Center for Human Nutrition at the University of Colorado Health Sciences Center.

In addition to knowing your BMI number, it's equally important to be aware of your Waist/Hip Ratio (WHR). You get this number by measuring your waist (at the midpoint between your bottom rib and hip bone) and your hips (at their widest point). Then divide the waist measurement by the hip measurement. For example, if your waist is 29 inches and your hips measure 38 inches, then your WHR is 0.76.

Why is this ratio important? In the last few years, researchers have determined that the fat most associated with health risks is on the upper body—the abdomen and above, rather than the thighs and hips. (This pattern of upper-body fat is often called 'central obesity.') "Central obesity is turning out to be the most lethal risk factor associated with excess body weight," says Dr. Castelli. That's because upper-body fat is strongly correlated with visceral fat, which is fat that is packed around our internal organs.

The WHR, though not perfect (it isn't very reliable for women who are very thin, very overweight, or for bodybuilders) can in most cases be used to predict cardiovascular disease risk, especially in women. Researchers at the University of Miami School of Medicine and the University of Minnesota School of Public Health examined data on 32,898 healthy women ages fifty-five to sixty-nine. As reported in the January 1993 issue of *Annals of Epidemiology*, there were nearly three times as many heart-disease deaths in a four-year period among women with the greatest waist/hip ratio (0.86 and over) than those under .80. A high waist-to-hip ratio has also been associated with diabetes, hypertension, stroke, breast and endometrial (uterine) cancers, and high cholesterol.

If the ideal BMI is around 21 or 22, let's see what the experts say about the ideal WHR. Most target 0.80 as desirable. If you're a woman, a number greater than 0.85 indicates higher health risks. If you're a man, health risks are related to a ratio greater than 1.0. Dr. Castelli believes that the WHR measurement is even more important than BMI in predicting risk. "If someone has a healthy BMI but a high WHR, it is important to try to bring that WHR down," he explains. "Someone with a higher BMI but a low WHR might not be quite as bad off."

There's another point to consider. Are you overweight or overfat? Weight tables can classify you as overweight when you actually have average or below average body fat. Athletes are often overweight because of a large frame or muscle development, but they aren't overfat.

Obesity means an excess accumulation of body fat. Usually, obesity and overweight are related. If you're twenty-five pounds or more overweight by most weight charts, you're probably overfat. At this point, the health risks of obesity surface. When you are twenty-five pounds overweight, your heart must pump blood through nearly 5,000 extra miles of blood vessels.

An easy way to judge whether you're overfat is by looking in a mirror. If, despite good BMI and WHR numbers, you look flabby, you probably are. You'd do well to measure your body fat and to embark on an exercise regimen that burns fat and tones muscles.

Exact standards don't exist for how much body fat a person can carry without increasing risk. I suggest aiming for body fat of eighteen to twenty-eight percent of total weight for women as optimal, slightly higher than for men who optimally have body fat of twelve to twenty-two percent.

There are several ways to determine your body fat. You can get calipers that pinch skin folds or use a special fat monitor/scale. You can use a bioelectric impedance test (running a mild current through the body to measure resistance) or do underwater weighing. Unfortunately, the latter two methods are not widely available outside health clubs or specialists' offices and are not always reliable. All methods only give you a ballpark figure. The older and fatter you are, the less reliable the measurement may be. Whatever method you pick, stick with the same one over a year or so. I usually check my percentage of body fat four times a year with the Omron Body Logic Model HBF-301 (see Resource Directory).

Obesity in infancy and childhood can lead to a life battling the bulge. During the first few years of life, you form new fat cells rapidly. As the rate of fat storage increases, so does the number of fat cells. In obese children, the number of fat cells is often three times that in normal-weight children. As a result, overfeeding children, especially in infancy, can lead to a lifetime of obesity. After adolescence the number of fat cells remains almost constant throughout the rest of life.

Although the extra pounds and less than ideal BMI and WHR numbers could be explained by exercise-induced muscle (which, inch for inch, weighs more than fat), unless you're an avid fitness enthusiast or athlete, it's not likely. "The people in this country are still geared toward overeating," says Margaret McDowell, RD at the National Center for Health Statistics. If you don't want your eating habits to get the best of you, consider raising your basal metabolic rate.

METABOLISM AND WAYS TO INCREASE IT

Your basal metabolic rate is the rate at which your body utilizes energy. Put another way, it has to do with how efficiently your body burns calories. Calories are the measuring unit of heat energy. When your metabolism is higher, you burn more fat and have an easier time losing weight (fat) or maintaining your ideal body weight.

Statistics reveal that most people are not happy with their weight or the shape of their body. Half of the women and a quarter of the men in this country are currently trying to lose weight and reshape their bodies. The sad thing is that a majority of these people are going about it in the wrong way, like swimming upstream. Most people try to lose weight by dieting, which usually involves eating certain foods and cutting back on calories. Diets don't work!

Statistics also reveal that two out of three people who go on a diet will regain their weight in one year or less; ninety-seven percent will gain the weight back in five years. To make matters worse, a majority of dieters who lose weight will gain back even more fat than they had before they started the diet. They have all violated an important rule in creating and maintaining a healthy, fast metabolism: they lost lean body mass, or muscle.

Lack of exercise is a major reason for the rise of obesity in the United States. Between our desk jobs and our automobiles, we don't move our bodies enough to ward off the gain in fat that naturally tends to come with aging. The problem is, many people do not realize that they need to include deliberate exercise in their daily routine.

In my workshops around the country, people tell me they get plenty of exercise doing household chores or walking around at work. I emphatically tell them that it's not enough! You need intentional exercise, like fitness walking and lifting weights or cycling, to call yourself anything but sedentary.

Most adults lose about one percent of their muscle every year after about age forty. At the same time, many people gain about a pound of fat a year. But the slide to fat really doesn't have to happen if you participate in appropriate physical activity programs that include both some aerobic and some strength-training exercise, and if you select the proper foods.

So let's go over fifteen ways for increasing your metabolism, selecting the right exercises and foods, and making healthy choices for creating a fit, lean body. I call this my *Aliveness Program*.

FIFTEEN STEPS TO A FIT, LEAN BODY

1. MUSCLE BURNS FAT. Decreased activity leads to muscle loss. Why is lean muscle tissue so important? More muscle means a faster metabolism because muscle uses more energy than fat. That is because muscle is a highly metabolic tissue: it burns five times as many calories as most other body tissues, pound for pound. In other words, muscle requires more oxygen and more calories to sustain itself than does body fat. When you have more muscle on your body, you burn more calories than someone who doesn't, even when you're both sitting still. So it's easy to understand how people who build muscle have an easier time maintaining a healthy weight. They're simply more efficient calorie burners.

Why does it seem that men can eat more of everything than women without gaining weight? One explanation is that men have more muscle and less fat than women. Because men have more muscle, they burn ten to twenty percent more calories than women at rest.

The addition of ten pounds of muscle to your body will burn 600 calories per day. You would have to run six miles a day, seven days a week to burn the same number of calories. Ten extra pounds of muscle can burn a pound of fat in one week—that's fifty-two pounds of fat a year. If you increase muscle mass, you increase the number of calories your body is using every moment of the day, not just during exercise, but also at work, play, and even when sleeping.

The best way to increase lean muscle mass is through resistance training, which means weight lifting or resistance machines—barbells, dumbbells or machines, cables, or even 'free-hand' movements such as push-ups and sit-ups. All it takes to add ten pounds of muscle is a regular weight training program involving only thirty minutes, three times a week for about six months. Isn't that fantastic? The wonderful thing about increasing your metabolism through increasing your muscle mass is that you don't have to restrict your calorie intake.

2. AEROBIC EXERCISE CAN INCREASE METABOLISM. While the best exercise for permanent fat loss is resistance training (lifting weights) because it increases muscle which burns more calories, low intensity aerobic exercise such as walking is also an excellent way to burn fat efficiently. Cutting 250 calories from your daily diet can help you lose half a pound a week (3,500 calories equals one pound of fat). But add a thirty-minute brisk walk four days a week, and you can double your rate of weight loss. Aerobic exercise increases your metabolic rate for hours after exercising.

In a study conducted at the Cooper Aerobic Center, Dr. John Duncan took 102 sedentary women and divided them into three groups. Each group walked three miles, five days a week for six months. The first group walked five mph, the second group four mph, and the third group three mph. He found that the slowest walking group lost the most weight. Any aerobic exercise that raises heart rate above eighty percent of maximum (220 minus your age times 0.8) will cause you to burn more muscle and less fat. An exercise heart rate kept closer to sixty percent of maximum (220 minus your age times 0.6), or 108 beats per minute for a forty-year-old person, will burn mostly fat. This is why walking is superior to overzealous running as a fat-burning exercise. Walking is one of the most underrated of exercises. The risk of injury is lower than for many other exercises, it's inexpensive, and you can do it just about anywhere. All you need is a good pair of walking shoes.

Other good aerobic/endurance activities include hiking, jogging, skating (ice, roller, or in-line), cross country skiing, swimming, aquarobics (aerobic exercise in water), bicycling, rowing, and stair climbing.

For healthy adults, the American College of Sports Medicine recommends fifteen to sixty minutes of aerobic exercise three to five times a week. The intensity or level of effort will depend on the goals and condition of the person exercising. Simply walking at a moderate pace (two and a half to three miles per hour) for thirty minutes or more on a regular basis can do wonders to improve body composition and appearance, cardiovascular risk factors, mood, self-esteem, sleep quality and perceived energy level. And that's just for starters.

3. BREAK UP YOUR EXERCISE. The news from the American College of Sports Medicine and the US Centers for Disease Control and Prevention is that exercise need not necessarily occur in one continuous bout (unless you have extra weight to lose, which might make exercising longer more effective). The daily training can be broken up—with equivalent health benefits—into segments. For example, in lieu of spending forty-five minutes doing aerobics at the gym in either a class or on the aerobic equipment, you can take a ten-minute walk in the morning, walk up and down stairs during the day instead of taking the elevator, take a ten-minute walk during your lunch hour and finish up with a relaxing twenty-minute walk after dinner. Even house and yard work, such as sweeping, mopping, gardening, mowing the grass and shoveling snow, count toward your daily total.

4. INTENSE EXERCISE HELPS BURN FAT. Take the hills on tomorrow's walk. They could give you greater fat-burning power than you got on the level today. A report suggests that a few bouts of high-intensity exercise mixed with low-intensity exercise (that might be a few short hills and some easy walking in-between) may be strikingly more effective in burning fat than one long lower-intensity bout, even if the long bout burns more calories.

Case in point: Seventeen exercisers on stationary bikes followed a moderate-exercise training program (thirty to forty-five minutes, four to five times per week for twenty weeks). All burned about 300 to 400 calories per session. Ten other exercisers did only about one-third as many bouts of thirty-minute bike riding over fifteen weeks. They filled the other sessions with short bursts of high-intensity cycling—they went almost as quickly as they could for thirty to ninety seconds and repeated these bursts several times per exercise session. These folks used only about 225 to 250 calories per session, but they lost more fat (according to skin-fold measurements) than did the moderate exercisers (who technically burned more calories). When expressed as calories expended during exercise, their fat loss was nine times greater than that in subjects performing lower intensity exercise. Muscle biopsies confirmed that the important step of fat oxidation had occurred in the cells of the high-intensity exercisers to a greater degree than in the low-intensity exercisers, as reported in the journal *Metabolism*, July 1994.

It seems to be a paradox that less exercise time could result in more fat burning. Standard thinking says that high-intensity exercise burns the available carbohydrates as the fuel source before it digs into fat. Researchers think that what happens here may have to do with two things believed to happen between and after exercise. First, intermittent high-intensity exercise may encourage a higher rate of fuel burning during the recovery periods and after exercise—and that fuel may come from fat. And second, high-intensity exercise may have an anorectic effect— that is, you may feel more satisfied with fewer calories (and few fat calories) in what you eat for a while after your workout.

The high-intensity exercise levels in this study were equivalent to sprinting. That level of effort isn't appropriate for everyone, says study leader Angelo Tremblay, Ph.D., professor of physiology and nutrition at Laval University, Quebec. "Something comparable might be vigorous circuit training. Or it could be reasonable—if you are healthy and accustomed to performing vigorous exercises—to briefly increase walking to a level where speaking is not possible. You can do that for sixty or ninety seconds, three to five times during a walk." Later, he says, you can increase the number of high intensity bouts. Of course, even if this is confirmed in other studies, it's not an excuse to cut your exercise time. Even trained athletes can't sustain day-in/day-out workouts at super-high intensities.

Endurance exercise may have benefits we're just beginning to tap. Another study, for instance, found that thirty-five to forty-five minutes of endurance exercise three times a week reduced insulin levels in the blood of seventy- to seventy-nine-year-old men and women.

So pump up the intensity if your doctor says you can. Just find a way to fit that extra vigor into your regular workout program. My favorite way is hiking. I often hike in my local Santa Monica Mountains where I experience frequent bouts of high intensity when hiking up the hills, interspersed with more level or declining grades.

5. GRAZING DECREASES FAT STORAGE AND UNDERNUTRITION INCREASES LONGEVITY. Liquid meals, diet

Healthy Weight

pills and special combinations of foods aren't your answer to increasing metabolism, weight control or better health. Instead, learn how to eat.

Results of four national surveys show that most people try to lose weight by eating 1,000 to 1,500 calories a day. However, cutting calories to under 1,200 (if you're a woman) or 1,400 (if you're a man) doesn't provide enough food to be satisfying in the long term. Eating fewer than 1,200 calories makes it difficult to get adequate amounts of certain nutrients, such as folic acid, magnesium and zinc. It also promotes temporary loss of fluids rather than permanent loss of fat.

To increase your metabolism, eat several small healthy meals a day (see figure 2). This keeps your metabolism stoked. The typical dieter will often skip meals and, as research points out, the

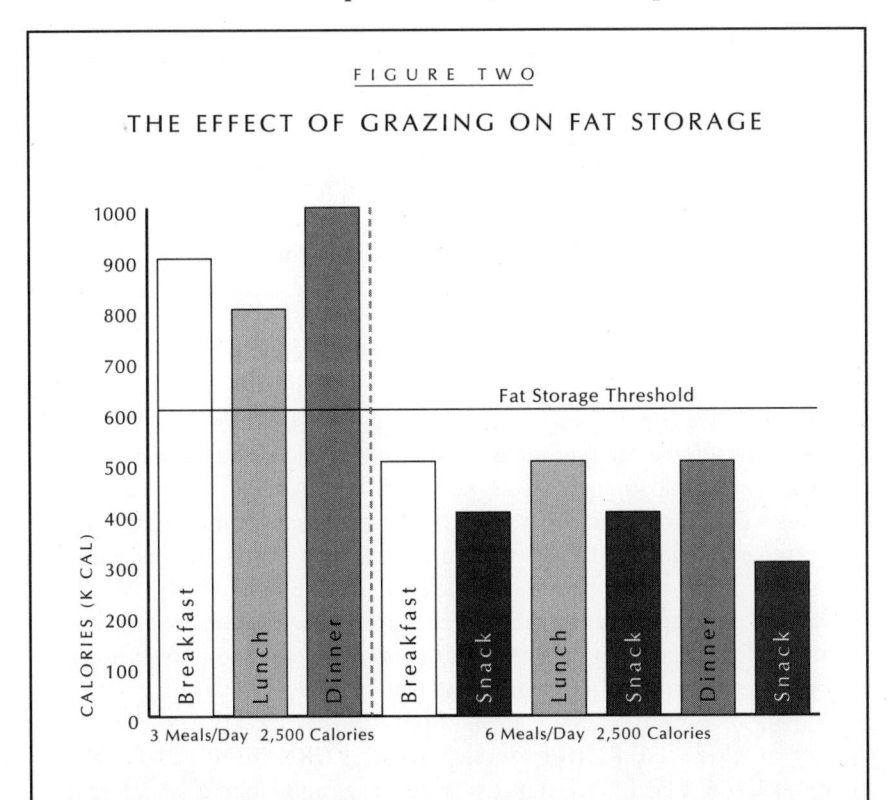

FIGURE TWO
THE EFFECT OF GRAZING ON FAT STORAGE

This graph illustrates how three meals can result in 700 calories being stored as fat. The same calorie intake spread over six meals produces no fat storage.

worst meal to skip, if you want to increase your metabolism, is breakfast. This temporary fasting state sends a signal to the body that food is scarce. As a result, the stress hormones (including cortisol) increase and the body begins 'lightening the load' and shedding its muscle tissue. Decreasing muscle tissue, which is metabolically active, decreases the body's need for food. By the next feeding, the pancreas is sensitized and will sharply increase blood insulin levels, which is the body's signal to make fat.

The secret to keeping your metabolism from slowing is to make sure that you graze throughout the day and that your diet contains at least ten calories per pound of your ideal body weight. If you are aiming for a weight of 150 pounds, your daily menu should contain at least 1,500 calories. If you have less food than this, you run the risk of slowing down your metabolism. People on restrictive diets and limited calories usually get tired of feeling deprived and hungry. Grazing throughout the day eliminates feeling deprived.

Have you ever wondered how the Sumo wrestlers get so big? They fast and then gorge themselves with food.

If this information is not enough to motivate you to eat smaller meals, maybe the following will be food for thought. One of the best things you can do to retard the aging process is simply to eat smaller amounts of the highest quality foods available, according to two professors of pathology at UCLA. In a landmark 1982 study published in *Science*, Richard Weindruch, Ph.D., and Roy L. Walford, MD (author of *Maximum Life Span* and *Anti-Aging Plan*), reported that when the food of 'middle-aged' mice was gradually restricted over a one-month period and then kept at that level, they lived an average of ten percent longer than the control group. They also had fewer spontaneous cancers than control mice. Their conclusion and recommendation is to strive for "undernutrition without malnutrition." In other words, limit caloric intake while providing adequate amounts of all the necessary nutrients. It is not absolutely clear how dietary restriction slows down the aging process, but evidence points to its retarding the age-related decline in immune function.

6. CHOOSE THE RIGHT FOODS THAT BURN MORE FAT AND INCREASE ENERGY. About twelve years ago I had a wonderful opportunity to work as the consultant for the Los Angeles City Fire Department. For thirty weeks I worked with the first group of women recruits. In the areas of motivation, holistic health, and

particularly nutrition, I saw many of the concepts and principles discussed in this book come alive.

One of the female recruits usually ate a large breakfast, high in animal protein and fat. A typical morning meal consisted of two eggs, sausage or bacon, toast with butter and jam, milk, and coffee with cream and sugar. Although she didn't have a weight problem, by midmorning she was often short on energy and had difficult in the endurance and strength aspects of her training. She also complained of an inability to think clearly for more than short periods. Within two weeks of changing her breakfast to more healthy, energy-promoting foods, however, she experienced an abundance of energy and increased mental clarity, important for participation in the rigorous training program.

What was the new breakfast I recommended? Her typical fare included fresh fruit and freshly squeezed juice, whole grain cereal and herb tea.

Another woman ate too many dairy products—lots of cheese, milk, butter, sour cream, cottage cheese, and ice cream. Other than that her diet was healthy, with an emphasis on complex carbohydrates and fresh foods. When she cut down on her dairy intake and began choosing more nondairy substitutes (soy milk instead of cow's milk), she experienced a noticeable increase in energy. Even as soon as the third day on her new nutrition program, she was able to perform the endurance events, which included running, continuous stair climbing, and the fire hose pull, more easily.

If you change what you eat, you don't have to be as concerned with how much you eat. By doing this, you can eat whenever you're hungry until you feel full. You'll lose weight without hunger or deprivation and you won't need to count calories. You need information, not willpower.

The best foods are complex carbohydrates. Low in fat, fast-burning, and rich in vitamins and minerals, they are also high in bulk, which means you can feel full on fewer calories. These foods are whole-grain cereals and grains including brown rice, whole grain breads, legumes, vegetables, fruits, and nuts (sparingly). Fruits should be eaten for breakfast or between meals. When you eat fruit with or after meals, the fructose is likely to be converted to fat by the liver.

Whole, natural foods usually have a low glycemic index. A low glycemic index means that blood sugar is not rapidly elevated after a meal. High glycemic index foods, such as sugary foods, put your blood sugar on a roller coaster. When blood sugar rises too rapidly, an overabundance of insulin is secreted. This excess insulin stimulates fat production and storage. The superfluous insulin will cause too much sugar to be stored, resulting in low blood sugar. Low blood sugar, in turn, will then cause stress hormone release, depression, fatigue, and hunger.

The high fiber in this recommended plant-based diet will actually slow digestion and absorption for a more even blood sugar level. Fiber will also bind with some fat and prevent its absorption. High fiber foods are beneficial for speeding up bowel transit time, too. This will take some stress off the liver as fewer toxins will form. The body can then more efficiently metabolize fats (see Chapter Two on fiber for more information).

There may also be a significant connection between toxicity in the body and weight problems. Toxicity in the body causes retention of fluids, called edema. The short term solution to toxicity is to drink more water. In other words, dilution is the solution to internal pollution. When toxins are eliminated, the body no longer needs to retain water, and a significant loss of fluid occurs. Water retention alters the body's energy-production systems and affects metabolism. The long term solution is to eat wholesome foods. A plant-based diet doesn't create the toxic overload in your body that unhealthy foods do.

Eating healthy foods with many nutrients (which includes a generous serving of sprouts every day—see Sprouting Guide) increases your mitochondrial bioenergetics (energy production, which helps increase metabolism). The nutritional support necessary for promoting this increase in energy production includes adequate levels of B vitamins, trace minerals (copper, iron, and chromium) and nutrients necessary for supporting proper detoxification—including molybdenum, selenium, manganese, and zinc, the antioxidant vitamins E and C, and bioflavonoids, along with pantothenic acid, biotin, and folic acid. These nutrients, together with a well-designed nutrition program, can lead to improved mitochondrial bioenergetics, which helps you reset your body weight to a lower set point by improving your body's heat-producing properties.

Investigators at the Department of Community Health at the University of Oregon recently published a paper in which they report on the use of a specific, controlled weight-loss program

SPROUTING GUIDE

VARIETY OF SEED	SOAKING TIME (HOURS)	FULL TIME RINSE & DRAIN (PER DAY)	AVERAGE TIME TO HARVEST (DAYS)	SPECIAL HANDLING	SUGGESTED USES
Alfalfa	8	3	3–4	None	Juices, Salads, Sandwiches
Beets	8	3	3–5	None	Juices, Salads
Buckwheat	8	3	2–3	Remove remaining husks	Juices, Pancakes, Salads
Chia	8	No	3–5	Mist	Casseroles, Salads, Sandwiches
Corn	8	3	2–4	None	Soups, Tortillas, Vegetable Casseroles, etc.
Cress	No	No	3–5	Mist gently with water 3 times a day or mix with other seeds	Breads, Salads, Sandwiches
Dill	8	3	3–5	None	Juices, Salads, Sandwiches
Fenugreek	8	3	3–5	Mist gently with water	Salads, Snacks
Flax	No	No	3–5	Mist gently with water 3 times a day or mix with other seeds	Juices, Salads
Garbanzo	8	3	3–4	None	Soups, Vegetable Casseroles
Lentil	8	3	2–4	None	Juices, Salads, Soups, Vegetable Casseroles, etc.
Millet	8	3	3–5	None	Juices, Salads, Soups, Vegetable Casseroles, etc.
Mung Bean	8	3	3–4	None	Omelets, Oriental Dishes, Salads, Snacks, Soups
Mustard	No	3	3–5	Mist gently with water 3 times a day or mix with other seeds	Juices, Salads
Napa Cabbage	8	3	3–4	None	Juices, Salads
Oats	8	3	2–3	Remove remaining husks	Breads, Granola, Snacks
Peas, Alaskan	8	3	3–4	None	Omelets, Salads, Snacks, Soups

SPROUTING GUIDE, continued...

VARIETY OF SEED	SOAKING TIME (HOURS)	FULL TIME RINSE & DRAIN (PER DAY)	AVERAGE TIME TO HARVEST (DAYS)	SPECIAL HANDLING	SUGGESTED USES
Peas, Special	8	3	3–4	None	Omelets, Salads, Snacks, Soups
Pichi Bean	8	3	3–4	None	Omelets, Oriental Dishes, Salads, Snacks, Soups
Porridge Pea	8	3	3–4	None	Omelets, Oriental Dishes, Salads, Snacks, Soups
Radish	8	3	3–4	None	Juices, Salads, Sandwiches
Red Clover	8	3	3–5	None	Juices, Salads, Sandwiches
Rye	8	3	2–3	None	Breads, Granola, Snacks
Sesame	8	3	2–3	None	Breads, Granola, Snacks
Soybean	24	3	3–5	Change soaking water every 8 hours	Casseroles, Oriental Dishes, Salads
Sunflower (Green	8	3	3–5 5–7)	Remove remaining husks	Salads, Snacks
Triticale	8	3	1–2	None	Breads, Granola, Pancakes, Snacks
Wheat (Wheat Grass	8	3	2 5–7)	None	Breads, Granola, Pancakes, Snacks

in moderately overweight women. In this study, reported in the 1994 *Journal of the American College of Nutrition*, eighteen sedentary, moderately overweight women followed a seven-week program consisting of a diet of whole foods containing 1,000 to 1,100 calories per day and a specific vitamin and mineral-fortified meal supplement drink, along with a progressive walking program. Mitochondrial energy production was assessed in these women before, during and after the weight-loss program. The weight loss was principally body fat, not muscle. In fact, some women actually gained muscle as they lost fat, causing their bodies to be much leaner at the conclusion of the program.

The bottom line: eat a wholesome diet with lots of nutrients, drink plenty of water between meals, and exercise regularly.

7. FAT MAKES YOU FAT. Overweight people tend to eat a higher fat diet than people of normal weight. Fatty foods slow metabolism. Your body converts dietary fat into body fat very easily. Gram for gram, fats not only have twice the calories of carbohydrates and proteins (nine compared to four), they also burn only two percent of their calories to be stored as fat. Protein and carbohydrates, on the other hand, will burn about twenty-five percent of their calories to be stored as fat. It is considerably more difficult to convert protein and carbohydrates into body fat: your body actually burns calories doing so. Even when calories are the same, a person eating a high-fat diet tends to store more excess calories as body fat than someone eating a lower-fat diet. The closer you can adhere to a low-fat diet, the less fat will remain on you. So, if you are currently maintaining your weight on 3,000 calories a day, and then decrease the percentage of fat from forty percent to twenty percent, you can lose one pound of fat in about three weeks—while at the same time eating twenty percent more food from carbohydrates and protein. The bottom line: eating fat makes you fat.

You can also fight fat with fat. Sounds paradoxical, doesn't it? Despite what I just said, not all fats make you fat. Omega-3 fatty acids can actually increase your metabolic rate (see Chapter Four on fats and oils). They also rid the body of excess fluids and can increase your energy level. The best source of omega-3 (LNA) fatty acids is organic flax seed oil, available in the refrigerator section of health foods stores; other sources include flax seeds and fish. Omega-6 (LA) fatty acids (especially gamma linolenic acid or GLA) are also essential to health and a healthy metabolism but are less likely to be deficient in a healthy diet. Good supplementary sources of GLA and omega-6 fatty acids are borage seed oil, black currant oil, and primrose oil.

8. ALCOHOL CAN MAKE YOU FAT. For those of you who drink alcohol, listen up. One of the greatest ways to sabotage your fat loss program is through alcohol consumption. Aside from having seven calories per gram, alcohol shifts metabolism in favor of fat deposition, burdens the liver and stimulates your appetite.

9. WATER WASHES AWAY FAT. Water is very important in helping to maintain a healthy metabolic rate. At least two quarts a day, between meals, is essential—more if you're physically very active. And water suppresses your appetite naturally.

High water intake reduces fat deposits by taking a load off the liver. The liver's main functions are detoxification and regulation of metabolism. The kidneys can get rid of toxins and spare the liver if they have sufficient water. This allows the liver to metabolize more fat. Adequate water will also decrease bloating and edema caused by fluid accumulation. Water does this by flushing out sodium and toxins. A high water intake also helps relieve constipation by keeping your stools soft. For more information on all the health benefits of water, I recommend the book, *Your Body's Many Cries for Water* by F. Batmanghelidj, MD.

10. CELLULITE CAN BE A THING OF THE PAST. Millions of people, especially women, have cellulite. In fact, about ninety percent of all women over the age of eighteen are plagued with this problem. While these may seem like hopeless odds, there is help.

Cellulite is actually a combination of fat, water, and wastes. It frequently appears on otherwise thin women. While fat is typically a generalized condition, cellulite settles predominantly on the hips, buttocks, thighs, and knees. Sometimes it even surfaces on the calves, ankles, abdomen, arms, and upper back. It most often forms in areas with poor circulation. When circulation becomes sluggish, wastes can accumulate in the connective tissues that surround the fat cells just beneath the skin. Cellular exchange slows down or stops and metabolism becomes sluggish. When cells don't receive adequate nourishment, individual cells can't function properly. Wastes continue to build up until the tissue becomes hard and lumpy beneath the surface and rippled on the surface. Cellulite takes on the characteristic appearance that has aptly earned it the nicknames 'cottage cheese' and 'orange peel' skin.

Cellulite is the result of a combination of factors. Lifestyle plays a primary role in its formation. Habits and lifestyle patterns such as stress, poor posture, improper diet, lack of exercise, poor elimination, and sluggish circulation contribute to cellulite. According to Roberta Wilson, author of *The Cellulite Control Guide*, a sound cellulite control program incorporates exercise—aerobics, weight training and stretching, daily skin brushing (to increase circulation), deep breathing, regular massages, and proper nutrition.

Good dietary guidelines for controlling cellulite including the following:

- Eat plenty of fresh vegetables and fruits and a variety of whole grains.
- Increase water intake to at least eighty ounces a day—more if you're physically very active.
- Eliminate salt.
- Avoid sugar, caffeine, alcohol, and saturated fats.
- Eat more complex carbohydrates: they provide energy and fiber necessary for proper elimination.
- Eliminate red meat. Gradually phase out other animal products and byproducts.
- Avoid preservatives, pesticides, and food additives such as food coloring and flavor.
- Make at least fifty percent of your diet living foods (not cooked).

What I'm suggesting here is what I've described in detail in Chapter Two on nutrition.

11. DO FAT BURNING SUPPLEMENTS WORK? Despite the latest wave of research into new and better ways to fight fat, I believe that the most efficient fat busters are the same old standbys: exercise and proper nutrition. But you must be consistent. Starting and then stopping your program doesn't work. Make health and fitness top priorities in your life.

12. GOOD HABITS MAKE THE DIFFERENCE. Here are some things to keep in mind to help assure success in your program.

START STRONG. People who eat a healthy breakfast generally feel less hungry throughout the day. This also stokes your metabolism.

CURB YOUR APPETITE. Drink a glass of water about fifteen minutes before a meal.

EAT WHAT YOU LIKE. Nothing makes a food program more difficult than having to eat foods that you don't like. Make wise, healthy choices from the foods you like.

SLOW DOWN. Eat slowly enough to give your body time to

release the enzymes that tell your brain when you've had all you need.

DON'T GIVE UP. Falling off your health program once or twice does not mean the effort is hopeless. Simply acknowledge that you overate, and get back on the plan.

REWARD YOURSELF. Treat yourself with a massage, a movie, a piece of clothing, or a delicious meal at your favorite restaurant for each week that you maintain your health program, achieve goals, or maintain weight.

Let's explore more closely the importance of your day-to-day choices and the need to reprogram and retrain your senses to release self-limiting beliefs and habits.

Your primary goal on this aliveness eating program is to get to the point where you are eating a minimum amount of the highest quality foods. Remember, the minimum is adequate! Euripides said, "Enough is abundance to the wise." You can put that slogan on your refrigerator door, over your mirror, and on your bathroom scale.

Although it's important to choose healthy foods, don't become a fanatic about what you eat. It's what you choose to eat on a daily basis that makes the difference, not the occasional lapse. If you were to worry about every little piece of food that went into your mouth, I believe that would be more harmful than infrequent splurges.

Learn to think in terms of whole foods. It's when you begin cutting, cooking, and preserving foods that your system gets into trouble. Whenever you are able, eat your foods whole, just the way nature made them. Remember that nature has prepared them perfectly, complete with vitamins, minerals, enzymes, amino acids, natural sugars, fibers, and water, in the right proportions for efficient use by your body. Fresh fruits and vegetables, whole grains, legumes, nuts, and seeds carefully selected and prepared to suit your particular needs and desires are ideal foods for the vibrantly alive body.

You may feel that it's too difficult to switch all at once to a new nutritional program. That's a common reaction and that's okay. You can break in gradually if you wish, switching first to the foods that appeal to you the most and gradually adding the others. It may take a while for your digestive system to become accustomed to handling these new live foods.

Your mind may have some negative programming about your eating habits that will trip you up if you aren't careful. The mind will always choose immediate gratification over long-term satisfaction. The mind doesn't care if you achieve your long-term goal for a fit, lean, healthy body. The mind wants you to feel good right now. It's important to realize that the mind isn't necessarily your friend. You must sometimes detach from it to achieve your long-term goals (see Chapter Eleven for more detailed information on goals).

Whether for food or something else, the difficulty in resisting sensory desire comes from the force of conditioning. Every time we are negatively conditioned, we lose a little of our freedom and our capacity to choose. So begin by becoming aware of what you are eating. Eating at the table, at mealtimes, and only when you are hungry helps, because you can more fully focus your attention on your food. When our attention is divided, we eat compulsively rather than from hunger. Automatic eating occurs frequently in front of the television set, or at a movie theater, parties, or sports events.

The entire process of eating needs to be given your full attention to get the maximum benefits. Be conscious of the hunger you feel before you eat; how the food looks and smells as you prepare it, serve it, and eat it; how the table setting looks; how the food tastes; the texture of the food; your chewing; your breathing; and how you feel while you are eating. Finally, after all this, be aware of and grateful for the feelings of lightness and high energy derived from the meal and the easy elimination of the food after it's digested. It's embracing this attitude about meals that enables you to appreciate simple, wholesome foods, and to eat less, feeling completely satisfied. Paying attention helps to develop the capacity to enjoy the simplest foods and to be truly healthy.

Stop eating just before you feel really full. In this way you are reprogramming your subconscious and are taking control rather than letting your habits control you. Stopping short of satiety helps you savor your food and helps you to be free and in charge of your choices.

You begin the retraining of your senses by eliminating things that injure the body. None of us would drive into a service station and fill the gas tank with oil. For the car to run efficiently, we must use a particular type of gas, lubricant, coolant, and so on. When it comes to our bodies, we are often not so careful. We put in all kinds of things that nutritionists and plain common sense tell us impair the body's smooth functioning, just because they taste pleasant. We need to reestablish that the determinants of what we eat should be our body's needs, not merely the appeal of the senses. I have found meditating for a few minutes before each meal is a powerful tool that fosters choosing foods that promote health and harmony.

Pythagoras said, "Choose what is best; habit will soon render it agreeable and easy." It does seem that our taste buds change and adapt when we alter our eating habits, and the whole wheat bread that tasted heavy and grainy a few months ago may taste chewy and flavorful this month. Feeling better and looking marvelous will soon compensate for the loss of dubious taste thrills of the past, such as fried chicken, white bread, ice cream, and potato chips. You'll find yourself looking forward to more healthful pleasures—the taste of ripe papaya, luscious strawberries, blueberries, ripe pineapple, sweet juicy grapes, a crisp garden salad, brown rice with steamed vegetables, and baked potatoes smothered in sautéed onions, broccoli, and mushrooms.

13. SELF MOTIVATION IS THE KEY TO SUCCESS. To stay motivated, make a commitment, get your priorities straight, and set realistic goals.

Make a commitment and follow through on what you say you're going to do. Lose weight because you want to, not to please someone else. You must be internally motivated to lose weight and create a fit, lean body—it's what you want to do.

Be realistic. Don't set yourself up for failure by trying to improve your lifestyle if you're distracted by other major problems. It takes a lot of mental and physical energy to change habits. If you're having marital or financial problems or if you're unhappy with other major aspects of your life, you may be less likely to follow through on your good intentions. Timing is critical. I'm not saying to abandon your health program if you're under stress. Just modify it and start with easy-to-achieve goals like drinking more water, eating more fruit, or simply walking daily.

What are your fitness goals? Write them out, both short and long term. Don't set a weight goal that conforms to unrealistic social ideals for thinness. Instead, try achieving the comfortable weight you maintained easily as a young adult. If you've always been overweight, the weight at which levels of triglycerides, blood sugar, blood pressure, and energy improve may be a realistic goal.

Accept that healthful weight loss is slow and steady. Aim to lose no more than one pound a week if you're a woman, two pounds a week if you're a man. (Men's naturally higher metabolic rate makes it easier to lose weight faster.)

In addition to longer goals, set weekly or monthly goals that allow you to check off successes.

14. MODERATE DOSES OF SUNLIGHT INCREASE METABOLISM. The sun has been getting a lot of bad press lately. Actually, sunlight in moderation is very good for the body in a variety of ways. It increases your metabolism, as documented in the excellent book, *Sunlight*, by Dr. Zane Kime. Dr. Kime states, "There is conclusive evidence that exposure to sunlight produces a metabolic effect in the body very similar to that produced by physical training, and is definitely followed by a measured improvement in physical fitness." He also explains in this book how a vegan diet (vegetarian with no dairy or eggs) will greatly decrease the risk of skin cancer.

15. NOURISH YOUR SPIRIT. To be healthy, improve your metabolism, and make healthy food and exercise choices, you must first nourish your spirit. The real epidemic in our culture is spiritual heart disease—the feelings of loneliness, isolation and alienation that pervade our culture. This is addressed beautifully in the book, *Love and Intimacy: The Scientific Basis for the Healing Power of Intimacy*, by Dean Ornish, MD. Many people who suffer from spiritual malaise use food or stimulants such as drugs, caffeine, alcohol, sex, or overwork to numb the pain and get through the day.

Stretching, deep breathing, and meditation will relax your mind and you will experience a greater sense of peace and well-being. Then you'll be able to make eating and exercise decisions—and other lifestyle choices—that are life enhancing rather than self-destructive.

Dieting alone doesn't work. Dieting combined with regular aerobic exercise is better, but it won't replace the muscle tissue that's lost in aging. But when you combine strength training, aerobic exercise, and sensible eating and nourishment for your spirit, you've got an unbeatable combination for reaching and maintaining your ideal weight, improving your metabolism, creating a fit, lean body, and celebrating life.

CHAPTER FOUR

Fats, Oils, and Flax:
Telling the Killers from the Healers

Certain types of fats called essential fatty acids (EFAs) are critical to good nutrition because humans cannot make them. Failure to eat enough EFAs is a cause of hardening of the arteries, abnormal clot formation, coronary heart disease, high cholesterol, and high blood pressure.
—EDWARD N. SIGUEL, MD

You have probably heard or read that fats are literally killing us. Actually only certain types of fats injure us, while another entire set of fats keeps us healthy and vital. The facts are in: some fats are deadly and others are life savers! The high incidence of heart disease, cancer, and numerous other degenerative diseases is not caused by the amount but rather the type of fat we consume, and the profound deficiency of 'healing fats' or essential fatty acids (EFAs) in the average diet.

Degenerative diseases that involve fat metabolism have rapidly increased since the turn of the century. During the early 1900s, only one in seven people died of degenerative cardiovascular disease. Today almost half of Americans will die from arterial, vascular, and coronary heart disease. In 1900, only one in thirty people died of cancer. Today nearly one in four die from a variety of cancers.

We can help reverse these disease processes up to a point by making prudent food choices. However, there comes a time when vital organs are so severely depleted and damaged nutritionally that they cannot recover. In other words, reversal of degeneration is no longer possible and death ensues. This process is caused by extreme free radical pathology, proliferation of metastasized cells, and cell toxemia from a lifetime absorption of environmental pollutants in food, air, and water. When this state is reached, the final stages of cellular death occur.

It takes thirty years to 'feed' a heart attack or cancer, so now is the time to make some positive changes in your eating habits. You may decide to avoid the deadly or toxic fats, or add the healing EFA (or essential fatty acid) fats to your diet. It truly becomes a choice of healthy mind over diseased matter. A healthy life starts with a healthy attitude.

Even the genetic diseases that affect one in 200 Americans may be incurable but can still be mitigated and even improved with proper nutrition. Taking into account age and genetic frailties, even depression and mental health can be greatly improved with intelligent eating.

LOW-FAT DIETS WILL NOT SAVE US

The US Department of Agriculture recommends that all Americans over the age of two should decrease their fat intake to below thirty percent of daily caloric intake, and saturated fat intake to below ten percent of total calories. Although this gesture is laudatory for most Americans who consume the Standard American Diet (SAD), following that recommendation will not save you from degenerative diseases. At best it will only moderately slow their onset. At worst, contemporary lipid (fat) research reveals that a low-fat diet may actually speed the degenerative process. This is because many low-fat diets are low in health-promoting EFA fats as well as being high in damaging saturated and trans-fats.

In order to understand the difference between good and bad fats we need to know the composition of fats. The scientific name for fats and oils is lipids. Lipids are made of carbon, hydrogen, and oxygen molecules. Both plants and animals produce fats. The exquisite biochemical architecture of fats (and how they function in our bodies) is determined in large part by their molecular structure. This structure can be described as a 'caterpillar' shape. The molecules look like a series of integrated globes. The lipid molecules are broken down into degrees of chemical reactivity based on the number of chemical bonds.

Fats may be saturated or unsaturated, according to the frequency of the bonds or 'kinks' in the molecules' shapes. The bonds or kinks in the molecule also define its stability or reactivity with other molecular substances around it. The greater the number of bonds, the greater the fragility of the lipid. Unrefined polyunsaturated oils like flax seed, hemp seed, or soybean oil, contain several kinks in the polyunsaturated fatty acids. They are made up of long chain fatty acids (in chemist's shorthand, they are called C:18:2 or C:18:3 fatty acids, which typically means eighteen carbon lengths long, with either two or three bonds in the fatty acid chain).

The inherent fragility of the bond makes them chemically very reactive, acting as an oxygen magnet in the body at the cellular level. The ability of this highly reactive bond to absorb free single oxygen molecules into the permeable cells of the body is what gives these oils their dramatic energy producing properties prized by athletes and sought by people healing from heart disease and cancer. This unique chemical property of essential fatty acids is behind the anti-carcinogenic prowess of unrefined polyunsaturated oils. As explained by Udo Erasmus in *Fats That Heal, Fats That Kill,* cancerous cells hate oxygen and typically behave anaerobically. Increasing our consumption of unrefined super polyunsaturated fats makes us more cancer resistant and energetic, and makes our heart muscle, veins, arteries and skin more supple.

Saturated fats are short and straight (C:4:0), without any kinks, so they are able to stack densely together. They are relatively non-reactive and remain solid at room temperature, unlike all other classes of natural fats. Saturated fats are most typically found in animal products. Lard and butter are almost completely saturated animal fats. Coconut and palm oil, on the other hand, are saturated vegetable fats. Saturated fats are also much more stable than unsaturated or super-unsaturated fats and go rancid less easily because of the short carbon chain length. This is why the mass market food industry prefers to use saturated fats over

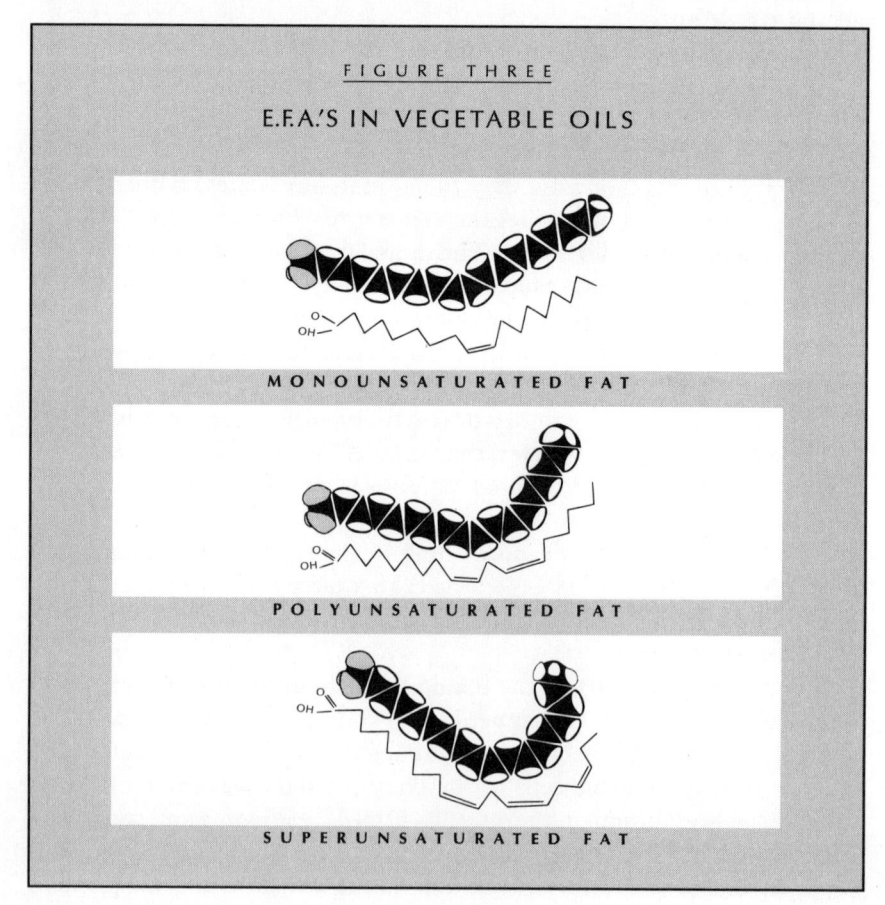

FIGURE THREE

E.F.A.'S IN VEGETABLE OILS

MONOUNSATURATED FAT

POLYUNSATURATED FAT

SUPERUNSATURATED FAT

less stable polyunsaturated fats. The shelf life of foods with saturated fats is much longer, but they are far less healthy.

Unsaturated fats have bonds or kinks everywhere there is a double bond (see Figure 3). This unsaturated spot or kink keeps the individual fatty acid chains or 'caterpillars' from stacking and compressing neatly together. This property explains why unsaturated oils are liquid at room temperature. Unsaturated fats can be monounsaturated (like olive oil), which means it has one double bond or kink in its molecular structure; polyunsaturated (like corn or safflower oil), which means it usually has two double bonds or kinks; and superunsaturated (like flax seed and fish oils), which have three or more double bonds or kinks. The superunsaturated oils are 'firecracker' reactive in the presence of atmospheric oxygen, and a single bond oil like coconut oil is 'molasses slow' in the presence of atmospheric oxygen. That is why coconut oil has ten to twenty times as long a natural shelf life as flax seed oil—and why flax seed oil needs to be refrigerated while coconut oil stores well at room temperature or higher.

Whether a fat is health promoting or disease producing is dramatically affected by how it is processed, stored, and used in the diet.

HYDROGENATION, MARGARINE, AND DEADLY TRANS-FATS

Have you noticed that the mass market food industry has recently decreased the amount of animal fat in their products to make their products seem more healthy? Don't let that fool you. They have simply replaced them with something even more deadly—*hydrogenated* (or partially hydrogenated) vegetable oils.

Hydrogenated fats are highly processed industrial oils made by fusing hydrogen atoms into the fats' molecular structure, thereby disrupting the natural double or triple bonds that shape the molecule. This results in a highly uniform, totally dead (and deadly) food!

Fats from oilseed plant sources are naturally shaped in what is called a cis-isomer molecular structure, which means that it is shaped like a horse-shoe—curved with a steep rounded angle at the midpoint. This gives the molecule a springy quality and is what makes the cells more flexible, because the fatty acids in the cis-isomer configuration are very supple. This structure creates a fluid bend and makes this oil more biologically appropriate for human consumption. By heating natural fatty acids at temperatures of 500 degrees F. in large industrial vats for prolonged periods, and the addition of nickel powder catalysts to stimulate the chemical polymerization or plasticizing of the fatty acids with bubbling hydrogen gas, a 180 degree twist occurs in the molecules' shape, and injures the natural bond of the fat drastically. It dramatically changes its formerly beneficial biochemical properties. The synthetic or man-made version is called a trans-isomer, and consequently this 'hardened' oil is called a *trans-fat*. It lacks the fluid kinks, which changes its physical properties from a liquid to a solid.

Trans-fats disrupt the body's metabolism, in part, by *altering the permeability of many cells in our body*. This syndrome is called 'leaky gut' and is indicative of many autoimmune disorders. Being unnaturally made solid, trans-fats harden like lard when a cell membrane absorbs too many, causing the cell's permeability and biochemical structure to change. Altered permeability of the cells allows many viruses, toxins, and parasites to invade more easily and prevents metabolic removal from the cell.

Dietary scientists have known this critical fact for twenty years yet haven't been overly concerned because they assume that the Standard American Diet contains only three to four percent of calories as trans-fats. According to Dr. Mary Enig, a respected trans-fat biochemist at the University of Maryland, the actual amount may be four times higher. Animal studies have shown gross cell abnormalities with just a little over four percent of calories from trans-fat sources.

Human studies have shown increased elevations in the 'bad' LDL cholesterol in only three weeks of eating a diet high in trans-fats. The amount of trans-fats in most Americans' diets is rising rapidly due to greater reliance on industrially processed food.

Reducing or eliminating trans-fats from the diet will increase the likelihood that the cell's fluid membranes will be able to transport and metabolize excess sugars, fats, and toxins. Regular cellular 'housekeeping' helps to keep our blood clean and prevents arterial degeneration and atherosclerosis.

Three recent studies clearly show the deadly effects of trans-fats. More than 85,000 female nurses were studied for eight years by researchers at the prestigious Harvard Medical School in Massachusetts. They tracked the correlation between trans-fat intake and heart disease. The women with the highest trans-fat intake had a fifty percent higher rate of heart attacks and coronary artery disease than those with more balanced diets.

A second study on fats and health was conducted at the Agricultural University in the Netherlands. Three groups of men and women with normal cholesterol were studied. Their diets were identical except for the type of fat consumed; the fats being tracked were saturated, trans-fat, and polyunsaturated fats. After three weeks the saturated and trans-fat groups had elevated cholesterol levels. Their LDL cholesterol (the bad, artery-clogging kind) rose while the 'good' HDL cholesterol levels fell. Trans-fats increased cholesterol to the same degree as saturated fats. This adverse effect didn't occur in the polyunsaturated group.

A third study conducted in Germany demonstrated the ill affects of saturated and trans-fats on premature infants. The higher the level of trans-fats in the newborn's blood, the lower the birth weight and opportunity of survival.

Trans-fats like partially hydrogenated soybean, safflower, or even coconut oils are generally solid at room temperature and melt to some degree at body temperature. Natural cis-fats like unrefined, non-hydrogenated flax seed, safflower, sunflower, and canola oils remain liquid at room temperature and also at body temperature. When consumed, trans-fats remain sticky and are likely to clog our arteries. Our blood platelets and other blood cells also become sticky because the trans-fats become incorporated in the blood cell membranes.

Trans-fats also interfere with prostaglandin production (hormone-like regulators in the blood) because they tend to thicken the blood, causing added pressure on the cardiovascular system while at the same time weakening the very arterial walls that carry our blood supply. This weakness is caused by the lower quality of a trans-fat absorbed in the cells throughout the body which are stiffer, making the arterial walls more prone to damage through thrombosis.

Trans-fat intake promotes ulcers, hypertension, and many immune system dysfunctions. Trans-fats exacerbate already low essential fatty acid (EFA) levels, because they compete with the EFAs for absorption by the cells. They do this by clogging up the enzyme reactions that transform EFAs into highly unsaturated fatty acid derivatives. These highly unsaturated fatty acids are necessary for normal function of the brain, sense organs, testes and adrenals.

The detrimental effects of trans-fats include:
- decreased testosterone production and increased abnormal sperm formation (as demonstrated in animals)
- complications during pregnancy
- correlation to low birth weight babies
- decreased quality of breast milk
- promotion of diabetes
- taxation of the liver's ability to process toxins and stress on the gallbladder
- alteration of the size, number and composition of human fat cells
- alteration of immune functions, promotion of cancer

MALEFIC MARGARINE AND OTHER MENU MISADVENTURES

Although trans-fats are usually man-made, some trans-fats do occur naturally in animal products, up to about twelve percent. Butter contains from two to twelve percent trans-fat—not a plus for sure, but the trans-fat in butter seems to be in a form that the body can break down and excrete. Margarine, on the other hand, is made from oils that were fluid at room temperature (including oils like canola, corn, cottonseed, soybean, and safflower) but which have been 'traumatized' as described above in order to make them solid. Depending on its type, margarine contains as much as fifty percent trans-fat. When you use margarine, the hardened fat is virtually pure saturated fat with a remnant percentage of trans-fat. In combination, these synthetic molecules are a deadly mixture over a dietary life span.

The detrimental effects of margarine are so well documented that the Dutch government banned the sale of margarines containing trans-fats. The head of Harvard School of Medicine, Dr. Walter Willett, says that over 30,000 American lives are needlessly lost each year to heart disease due to the harmful effects of margarine.

Both butter and margarine should be eliminated from your diet. I recommend instead a canola-oil product called *Spectrum Spread*, available in health food stores. It has a similar taste to butter, stays solid enough to be spreadable, but is fluid in the body. Its has no trans-fats (not hydrogenated), is low in saturated fat (made from expeller-pressed canola oil), low in sodium, and is made from chemical-free canola oil.

The main sources of synthetic trans-fats are margarine, shortening, and processed animal products, and any partially hydrogenated high-heat, cooked fats and oils like deep fried foods (see figure 4). Most supermarket breads, cookies, crackers, chips, and packaged foods are loaded with partially hydrogenated oils, a primary source of trans-fats. Trans-fat content does not appear on food labels because trans-fats are not officially classed by the FDA as saturated fat, so label reading becomes more difficult for health-minded consumers. Just remember to avoid all products with hydrogenated and partially hydrogenated oils as an ingredient.

We know the detrimental effects of trans-fats on our cardiovascular system, immune system, reproductive system, hormonal systems, metabolism, liver function, and cell membranes. So why would we ever consume any margarines, shortenings, partially hydrogenated oil, or any refined oils that are so obviously bad? (By the way, over eighty percent of the margarine companies are owned by tobacco companies, as reported by the Center for Science in the Public Interest in their *Survey of Margarine & Hard Yellow Fats*, 1993.)

Fortunately, trans-fats are not found in the plant world: they do not occur in fruits, vegetables, nuts, or seeds.

AVERAGE TRANS-FAT COMPOSITION OF FOODS

(Number in Parentheses Shows the Range)

Margarines
    Stick   31% (10 to 48%)
    Tub   17% (5 to 44%)
    Low Fat   (up to 18%)
Butter (Milk Fat)   15%
Vegetable Shortening   20% (up to 37%)
Salad Oils   (0 to 14%)
French Fries   (up to 37%)
Candy Bars   (up to 39%)
Bakery Products   (up to 34%)

THE FREE RADICAL THREAT

While trans-fats are definitely injurious to our well-being, healthy oils can also be turned into toxic substances called free radicals by damage from air, heat, and light. Many of the oils available in stores are damaged by processing. Unfortunately, the potentially healthiest oils (unrefined cold pressed organic oils) are particularly susceptible to damage because these are the most biologically active. The more polyunsaturated the fat, the more likely it is to form free radicals if not properly protected.

Free radicals are unstable oxygen molecules that can disrupt cellular functioning, encourage tumor formation, and accelerate the aging process. Free radicals have also been implicated in damage to arterial walls. Damage to arterial walls is probably the first step in arteriosclerosis and atheroma formation (a condition characterized by the deposit of fat in the inner linings of the arterial walls). The free radical causes an injury to the arterial wall cells and a cholesterol-laden plaque forms, acting like a bandage over the injury. Free radicals oxidize cholesterol and triglycerides to a more deadly artery-clogging form. The combination tends to form stiff, hard arteries with reduced blood flow, exacerbating hypertension and other coronary-related diseases. If this happens often enough, arteries will restrict blood flow and close off, causing strokes, heart attacks, and vascular disease.

FIGURE FOUR
TRANS- AND SATURATED FATS IN FOODS

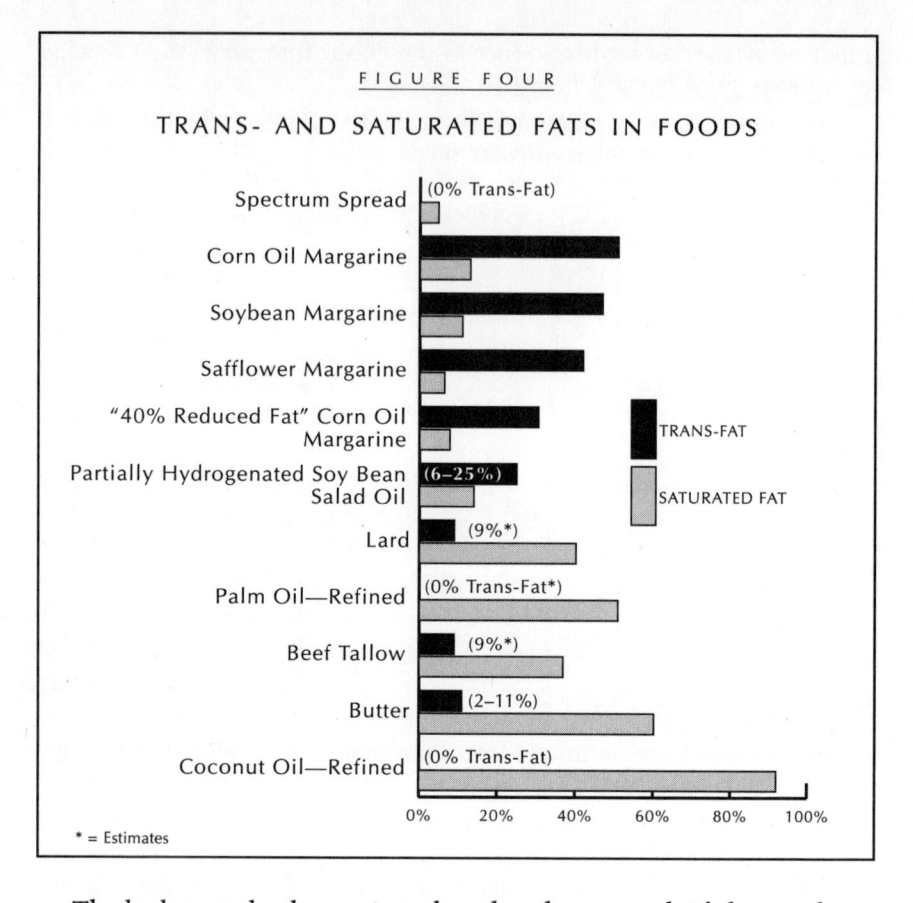

Food	Trans-Fat	Saturated Fat
Spectrum Spread	(0% Trans-Fat)	
Corn Oil Margarine		
Soybean Margarine		
Safflower Margarine		
"40% Reduced Fat" Corn Oil Margarine		
Partially Hydrogenated Soy Bean Salad Oil	(6–25%)	
Lard	(9%*)	
Palm Oil—Refined	(0% Trans-Fat*)	
Beef Tallow	(9%*)	
Butter	(2–11%)	
Coconut Oil—Refined	(0% Trans-Fat)	

* = Estimates

The body can slowly repair and unclog these vessels if chronic damage by free radicals is stopped or slowed down. Fortunately, free radicals can be neutralized by free radical scavengers (antioxidants) such as vitamin E, beta-carotene, vitamin C, selenium, and hundreds of other antioxidants found in unrefined oils (especially low temperature, expeller-pressed wheat germ oil), fresh vegetables, fruits, whole grains, legumes, and raw nuts and seeds.

Animal products are high in free radicals and almost totally deficient in antioxidants as the higher ordered species tend to suffer from the same biological stresses that humans do.

HEALTH-PROMOTING OILS: ESSENTIAL FATTY ACIDS

There are just two essential fatty acids: linoleic acid (LA) and alpha-linolenic acid (LNA). LA is also called omega-6 and LNA is also called omega-3. Consuming both in balance in our diets is very important to maintain long-term health. It is estimated that about sixty percent of the population gets too much LA while ninety-five percent gets too little LNA.

LA is found in high proportions in vegetable oils like safflower oil (seventy-five percent LA) and sunflower oil (sixty-five percent LA). Consuming large amounts of refined polyunsaturated oils rich in processed LA fatty acids has been linked to increases in some types of cancer. Excess refined LA consumption without the proper balancing ratio of LNA oils tends to suppress immune function. So getting more of the LNAs and less of the LAs is the best plan for better health and longevity.

Most American diets are sadly deficient in LNA. LNA tends to be processed out of most fresh food. It is found in very high proportions in flax seed oil, which is by far the richest source found in nature. Flax seed oil is about 50 to 55 percent LNA, about five to ten times higher than most other available nut or seed oils. Other significant vegetarian sources of LNA include canola oil at ten percent, soybean oil at five to seven percent, and walnut oil at three to eleven percent. Many dark green leafy vegetables have a micropercentage of LNA, but not enough for good health.

Gamma-linoleic acid (GLA) is another important super unsaturated fatty acid identical to LNA except for the position of one of its double bonds. Because of their similar molecular structure their health benefits are similar, although GLA is faster acting than LNA in alleviating some conditions like premenstrual syndrome (PMS) in females. GLA is a great supplement for a stressed body or anyone over forty. People with liver problems, inflammatory diseases, and PMS will experience tremendous benefits from GLA included with a sound nutritional program.

Dr. Zane Kime claims that skin cancer is promoted by a poor diet, particularly one high in refined oils and animal products. Recent research has tied skin cancer to a diet too high in refined LA fatty acids and substantially deficient in LNA fatty acids.

Another physician, Dr. Edward N. Siguel, author of *Essential Fatty Acids in Health and Disease*, states that cardiovascular disease and cancer can be prevented in many cases by controlling the balance of EFAs in our diet. Siguel claims that EFA deficiency is the genesis of heart attacks. Siguel also states that progressive EFA deficiency is the main contributing factor in heart failure in those who, over a twenty-five or more year span, chose diets too high in trans-fat and saturated fat at the expense of the LNAs and LAs.

I personally prefer to stay away from most oils or use them only very sparingly (such as extra virgin cold pressed olive oil), with the exception of flax, and hemp oils made by the Spectrum Naturals

Company. Essential fatty acids are widely distributed in whole plant foods, even in dark leafy vegetables, which don't seem oily at all. Pumpkin seeds and walnuts are especially well-endowed with essential fatty acids.

'REFINED' MEANS NOT-SO-FINE

Refining an oil takes away its natural flavors and compromises many of the nutrients, such as phospholipid (helps emulsify fat in the body), lecithin (makes oils easier to digest), carotene (anti-cancer compounds), tocopherols (antioxidants, free radical scavengers), and EFAs (essential fatty acids, which assist in cellular integrity).

Olive oil is high in monounsaturated and polyunsaturated fatty acids that protect our body's cells from mutation, but only if it is marked as either virgin or extra virgin olive oil. 'Extra virgin' simply implies that it is the first oil pressed out of the olive, as opposed to later pressings. But because the liquid constituents of olives are typically twenty percent oil and twenty-five percent water, what forms is a paste. The oil residue must be centrifuged or decanted to release the oil from the water. The oil separation process is called extra virgin, simply another marketing gimmick to differentiate an oil. Therefore, virgin or extra virgin olive oils are the only mass marketed oils that have not been heated above 150 degrees C (302 degrees F). Oils heated higher than this not only lose their nutritional benefits, but also become nutritionally damaging.

Refined oils are heated to much higher temperatures. In the refining process, poisonous solvents (such as hexane, a cousin to gasoline) may be used to extract the oil left behind after pressing. In addition, phosphoric acid (an extremely caustic chemical) may be used to degum the oil, which removes several health-promoting substances such as lecithin, chlorophyll, and several trace minerals. The oils may then be bleached and deodorized with other solvent chemicals and heated up to 270 degrees C (518 degrees F) for thirty to sixty minutes. Fully refined olive oil loses over 100 volatile compounds that give olive oil its unique flavor and aroma. It is the lowest grade of olive oil. The final product of all this is a mutated oil stripped of all its healthy components and the nutritional integrity of the EFAs. All refined oils are severely damaged.

Beware of the term 'pure' olive oil on the label! 'Pure' olive oil is a fully refined solvent-extracted low-grade oil.

I recommend choosing organic oils whenever possible. Oils from Spectrum Naturals, which are available in health food stores, are top quality. Organic oils are pesticide-free and unrefined and make a better overall choice for healthier eating. The bottom line on buying healthy oils is to get organically grown, cold or mechanically pressed oils that are protected from light, air, and heat.

COOKING: GO LOW AND SLOW

Cooking is an art and like all good art, it requires time and attention to become a masterpiece. High cooking temperatures destroy the healthy properties of biologically intact oils. The more unsaturated the bonds of the oil and the higher the ratio of essential fatty acids (EFAs), the greater the polymerization (or plasticizing) of the oil. When your frying pan is used on the high heat setting, it becomes a mini-refinery. If you start burning the oil (smoking it or having it pop and fizzle with smoke emerging), you have a free-radical factory in your frying pan.

High temperatures create ketones, aldehydes, and tri-terpine alcohol—which all break down to products that can become carcinogens. In addition there are deadly dienes, trienes (you'll be hearing more about these in the coming years), and other destructive compounds created, plus dozens of other post-oxidation products which can be just as detrimental as trans-fat. Oils that have undergone thermal conversion at 215 degrees C (410 degrees F) for fifteen minutes or more have been implicated in the formation of atherosclerosis when fed to lab animals in research experiments. High heat cooking becomes an unhealthy culinary practice when we abuse a delicate oil.

Our bodies can cope with an occasional dose of a toxic substance like a trans-fat. But over a period of ten, twenty, or thirty years these toxic and unnatural substances accumulate and interfere with the normal biological chemistry of our bodies. These corrupted materials create corrupted organs and muscles. Cells lose their DNA reproductive integrity, leading to degenerative disease and rapid aging.

I do not recommend frying, not only because of the fat damage, but also because it can turn proteins into carcinogens such as acrolein. Frying also destroys much of the nutritional value of all foods. Udo Erasmus recommends that if you really insist upon frying foods, use naturally occurring saturated fats like those of the least processed tropical oil (coconut). There are new varieties of high-oleic oils (super-canola), hybrids which also take heat quite well.

If you must fry, use these oils in limited amounts. Although refined saturated fats are very unhealthy, they are at the same time much less reactive and form fewer toxic fats when heated at high temperatures. Damage occurs rapidly to unsaturated fats and even more rapidly to essential fatty acids (EFAs), which tolerate heat quite poorly.

Most fast food and other restaurants deep-fry foods in hydrogenated vegetable oils that have been kept at high temperatures, often for days.

Instead of frying, I like to take traditional stir-fry vegetables and steam them for a few minutes. I then add flax seed oil that has had garlic pressed into it and allow the vegetables to marinate for about fifteen minutes. Another healthier way is to stir-fry with small amounts of water, adding a little oil later on. Keeping some water in with the oil keeps the temperature down to 100 degrees C (212 degrees F), which is a non-destructive temperature. Food will retain more nutrients and taste better using this innovative method. For good results, I recommend organic canola or virgin olive oil for this lower temperature method.

The simple technique of boiling food in water doesn't damage even the most sensitive EFA-rich oils. Baking, on the other hand, does damage sensitive oils on the outside of baked goods such as the crust of bread. However, the majority of the oil in the center of the loaf does not get destroyed, because the center of a cooked loaf of bread or cake is essentially steamed by the baking action. If you don't use non-stick pans, then use tropical oils (coconut) or try lecithin to prevent sticking. The small amount recommended should not harmfully affect your overall dietary intake.

The more saturated or damaged oils you consume, the more antioxidants you need in your diet to neutralize the production of excess free radicals that are formed by consuming these oils (see Chapter Two on nutrition). If you eat a lot of commercial cookies, crackers, baked goods, candies, or sweets like chocolate, you need to increase consumption of both EFAs and antioxidants. Antioxidants are especially found in vitamin E oil (from wheat germ), vitamin C, vitamin A, beta-carotene, and selenium.

Hundreds of independent research studies have shown the disease producing effects of animal fats, trans-fats and too many refined LA fatty acids. Research has also demonstrated the disease fighting effects of the unrefined LNA fatty acids.

Fats and oils are a sharp, double-edged sword in your nutritional arsenal, valuable but requiring careful handling. It is well worth your while to understand them. You now have the basic knowledge to improve your health. It is up to you to choose health one tablespoon at a time.

FLAX SEED: NATURE'S MIRACLE MEDICINE

With its rich satin brown hues, smooth and almond shaped, the tiny flax seed is a surprise miracle factory of healing substances. Often referred to as 'nutritional gold,' flax seed is rapidly becoming a wonder grain of health. It has the potential to heal and prevent cardiovascular disease, cancer, diabetes, and many other degenerative conditions, as well as to improve skin and vitality.

Its history is as rich as its medicinal benefits. For more than 7,000 years, flax seed (also known industrially as linseed) has been consumed by humankind. The main foods mentioned in the Bible are flax, wheat, barley, corn, wine, and manna—flax being referred to most often. It is one of the oldest known cultivated plants and certainly one of the most useful. Not only is the seed a first-class food, but flax fiber makes a first class cloth—linen.

According to archaeological authorities, flax fiber was used by Stone Age people for constructing ropes and fish nets, and the flax seed was used for food. Flax was cultivated in Babylon in 5000 BC. As early as around 3000 BC ancient Egyptians used it to make linen mummy wrappings; the oil was used as a cosmetic and applied to wall paintings for the tombs and temples. Greek and Roman writings dating back to 650 BC reveal some of the healing properties attributed to flax. In the fifth century BC, Hippocrates wrote about using flax to relieve inflamed mucous membranes and for relieving abdominal pains and diarrhea. Flax was also historically used in hot compresses to treat both external and internal ailments. Ancient East Indian scriptures state that a yogi must eat flax daily in order to reach the highest state of contentment and joy. More recently, Mahatma Gandhi observed: "Whenever flax seed becomes a regular food item among the people, there will be better health." In Vedic medicine, flax is considered a 'cooling' oil, reducing inflammation.

Until recently, in the West you were more likely to find flax derivatives in house paint, linoleum floors, and bed linens than on your dinner plate. The English word 'linoleum' from the combined words 'linseed' and 'oleum' (meaning 'oil-of-the-linseed') illustrates its use as a polymerized vegetable veneer when applied to and cured upon coarse linen fabric or jute cloth. This invention made up the popular linoleum tile material found in many early American kitchens. The word 'linen' comes from the Dutch and German root word meaning fiber or stem of the flax plant. As a result when we say linens we really mean cloth made from flax. The world's finest linens still come from Ireland and Belgium where exquisite linen lace is handmade.

Today edible flax seed is being rediscovered for its abundant healing properties. Flax seed and its healing oil are being hailed as the latest cure in the fight against cancer and coronary heart disease by plant biochemists and health researchers.

What makes this plant so healthy? During the last decade research scientists have uncovered components of the flax seed which offer extraordinary nutritional advantages. A real powerhouse, this seed packs a quadruple whammy: a high dose of LNA (omega-3) fatty acids, a healthy fat which helps lower cholesterol; a proper ratio of LNA to LA (omega-6) fatty acids; fiber, especially cholesterol-lowering soluble fiber; and lignans, a kind of fiber that is looking more and more like a potent blocker of some kinds of cancer. All this and it tastes good, too. It's hard to believe that flax is full of fat and still good for you.

Let's look more closely at flax and its highly regarded nutritional components. Flax is an annual plant with small green leaves and delicate blue flowers. Its Latin name is *Linum usitatissimum*, meaning 'the most useful.' This miracle grain is truly one of the most nutritionally complete foods ever studied. Flax seed is a top quality food because it contains most of what makes a complete diet. According to Udo Erasmus, the components of flax are used to treat many ailments which wouldn't occur if flax seed were a regular part of the diet.

WHAT FLAX SEED OFFERS

PROTEIN: Flax seeds contain high-quality, easily digestible protein with all the amino acids (the building blocks of protein) essential to health. This means that it is a complete protein. These essential amino acids are leucine, isoleucine, lysine, valine, threonine, methionine, phenylalanine, and tryptophan. Flax seed also contains histidine and arginine, which are amino acids essential for infants. When all of the essential amino acids are supplied, our body can manufacture from them the other dozen amino acids required to make proteins. Complete proteins are essential for building muscles, blood, skin, hair, nails, and internal organs, including the heart and the brain.

COMPLEX CARBOHYDRATES: Flax seed provides instant calories for energy and assists in digestion and regulation of protein and fat metabolism.

FIBER: Flax seed is an excellent source of both soluble and insoluble fiber and keeps the digestive tract from becoming clogged with mucus. Fiber helps to keep everything moving, maintains healthy intestinal flora and helps to keep the colon clean. It also helps to keep cholesterol and bile acids from being re-absorbed into the body though the intestinal walls. When foods progress into the small intestine, the gall bladder secretes bile acids to assist in breaking down fats in the foods. Bile is actually produced in the liver and concentrates in the gall bladder as a dietary fat emulsifier. Bile is rich in enzymes that break apart triglycerides. A healthy person's bile excretion will absorb ninety-five percent of fat consumed. However, as liver and gallbladder efficiency are taxed from too much fat, wear and tear on these organs takes place. Fiber from flax helps in binding excess fats and allowing their excretion into the large intestine and ultimate expulsion from the body, according to Elson Haas, MD, in *Staying Healthy with Nutrition*.

MUCILAGE: Structurally, mucilage resembles hemicellulose (the most popular source is oat bran), but it is not classed as such due to its unique location in the seed portion of the plant. It is generally found within the inner layer (endosperm) of the plant seeds, where it retains water to prevent the seed from drying. Mucilage is a thick gum found in many plants, especially flax seed (twelve to fifteen percent of volume), which makes flax seed one of the best natural laxatives available. Like the pectin found in apples, mucilage in flax is important in maintaining bowel regularity. Due to the presence of essential fatty acids in the mucilage, it tends to soothe and protect the delicate stomach and intestinal linings and keeps the contents moving progressively along.

One of the most highly respected natural healers, Bernard Jensen, DC, reveals that many degenerative diseases start in the colon through the toxic effects of constipation and poor peristaltic action of the colon muscle. When flax seed (oil and ground meal) is taken with fluids, the mucilage assists in alleviating constipation, increasing stool bulk and softness, and speeding up transit time (hastens the movement of stool out of the body). All this helps prevent toxic buildup in our bowel. As a result, the stools smell less foul, breath freshens, and there is less stress on the liver and eliminative organs, including the kidneys and skin. You can chew flax seed, although sometimes the small seeds can get stuck in your teeth. I prefer the oil and ground meal.

Flax mucilage also has the ability to buffer excess acid in sensitive stomachs and helps to stabilize blood glucose due to its absorptive properties. Insulin production is thus more stabilized as the pancreas is not force-cycled through dramatic highs and lows of excess sugars in the diet and the resulting overage/shortage of blood saturated/starved glucose levels between snacks or meals. Sufficient quality fiber from foods such as flax retards the cycles of sugar highs and lows frequently associated with such progressive diseases as hypoglycemia and late-onset adult diabetes, both of which have a defective glucose metabolic factor.

MINERALS: Flax seed contains most known major and trace minerals—phosphorous, magnesium, potassium, calcium, sulfur, sodium, chlorine, zinc, and iron and adequate trace amounts of manganese, silicon, copper, fluorine, nickel, cobalt, iodine, molybdenum, and chromium.

VITAMINS: Flax seed contains fat-soluble vitamins E and carotene, and water-soluble vitamins B_1, B_2, and C. The tocopherol compounds found in vitamin E act as antioxidants in the body (see Chapter Two on nutrition), protecting other molecules and cell components from damaging reactions with oxygen. Vitamin E is an antioxidant substance which works as a synergistic ally with vitamin A and vitamin C and as a regulator of cell respiration. Flax is particularly high in minerals and vitamin co-factors.

LIGNINS AND LIGNANS: Unlike many other plant fibers, flax seed is high in lignan and lignin. Lignin is an insoluble fiber which our bodies convert to several kinds of lignans. Flax seed is the richest known source of lignans, containing 100 times as much as the next best source—wheat bran. While all vegetables provide lignin precursors to some degree, flax provides much more, about 800 micrograms per gram, as compared to only eight micrograms per gram in common fiber such as bran. Lignans have only recently attracted the attention of researchers. They have been found to be useful in treating viral, bacterial and fungal infections as well as cancer. In fact, high levels of lignans in the bowel are associated with reduced rates of colon and breast cancer.

The lignans formed from flax are pseudo-estrogens that block estrogen receptors in the body. The molecular shape of the lignans is such that they bind with the estrogen receptors in the body, thus 'smoothing out' the hormonal and metabolic effect of estrogen release in the body. Over-production of estrogen can stimulate colon and other forms of cancer. Thirty to fifty percent of all malignant colon tumors contain numerous estrogen receptors. It is also significant to note that the rates of colon cancer tend to correlate with those of breast cancer, and that both seem to be high in people with low-fiber diets.

Studies reveal that lignans resemble estrogens and attach to estrogen receptors in the body, but do not have the tumor-stimulating effect of hormonal estrogen. Hormonally induced syndromes, like hot flashes or elevated body temperature, are slightly mitigated by these lignans and lignins. Further, research shows that lignans derived from flax also work to reduce levels of unbound estrogens in the blood, which explains how they can also help prevent breast cancer. Perhaps the presence of lignans, derived from plant fiber, may be one of the main reasons why vegetarians have substantially lower cancer rates than meat eaters.

ESSENTIAL FATTY ACIDS (EFAS): EFAs are part of every cell in our bodies, where they play important roles in maintaining the structure of the cells and in producing energy. Our glands need EFAs to carry out the minute secretion of hormones and other biological regulating substances. In our muscles, EFAs help the cells to recover from use and abuse. In addition to fulfilling these basic roles, the EFAs are critical to infants' prenatal and postnatal development, especially brain development, and for growth spurts throughout childhood.

Our bodies do a remarkable job of creating most of the nutrients we need from the resident cell materials on hand, except in some cases. The nutrients our bodies can't synthesize are called the essential nutrients, and these we must make sure are adequately supplied in our diets. Of the forty-five essential nutrients, two are fatty acids: called LNA (alpha-linolenic acid or omega-3) and LA (linoleic acid or omega-6). Besides being an excellent source of the essential LNA fatty acids, flax seed also contains important trace nutrients such as phospholipids, phytosterols, and beta-sitosterin. These naturally occurring compounds assist in the digestion of fats and are just beginning to be recognized for their immune-enhancing properties.

THE MODERN DIET AND LNA DEFICIENCY

In the past 100 years, modern food processing developments have drastically reduced the nutrient value, including the LNA content, of many of the foods we eat. In his book *The Omega-3 Phenomenon,* Dr. Donald O. Rudin explains that modern food processing and food selection opportunities severely distort the availability of many essential nutrients—especially limiting the LNA essential fatty acids. Whenever high heat and caustic agents are used to sterilize food, the incidence of peculiarly twentieth-century diseases such as cancer, heart disease, and arthritis will skyrocket. Heart disease and many cancers are linked to distortions of dietary fats. Dr. Rudin calls LNA "the nutritional missing link" and attributes its profound absence in most foods to the cause of many degenerative conditions.

For the body to stay healthy, we must have a proper balance of LNA and LA fatty acids in our diets. When your body is homeostatic (balanced in health), you receive pain messages only when you've experienced real injury or when blood clots form at the initial phase of wound healing. Without such homeostatic balance, the LAs (when consumed to excess and in absence of LNAs) can produce pain messages in the brain for no reason or form an unwanted clot spontaneously.

Most Americans who eat highly refined and processed foods, such as regular patrons of fast food restaurants, get excess amounts of refined LAs and insufficient amounts of unrefined LNA fatty acids. The hamburger cooks and fish fryers of fast food restaurants usually cook with highly refined, unstable polyunsaturated oils such as corn, sunflower, safflower, and soy oils. These oils are very highly concentrated with LA fatty acids and deadly trans-fats. The physiology of fast food consumers remains in a perpetual state of fatty acid imbalance. Consequently, they are more predisposed to degenerative diseases such as heart attacks, cancer, arthritis, stroke, kidney impairment, liver disease, auto-immune disorders, and skin disorders.

According to Udo Erasmus, a highly regarded lipid (fat) scientist, North Americans typically consume only about twenty-five percent of the quantity of LNAs needed for optimal health. He suggests an intake of LNAs equivalent to about two percent of total calories, or about fourteen grams per day. Flax seed is by far the most potent natural source of LNAs.

COMPARISON OF LNA SOURCES

Percentage of LNA Fatty Acid by Total Weight of Seeds

Flax seed	57%
Chia seed	30%
Hemp seed oil	15%
Pumpkin seed	15%
Canola oil	10%
Soy bean oil	8%
Walnut	5%
Fresh leafy vegetables (average serving)	0.009%

Fish oils have been touted for the 'heart saving' LNA fatty acids found in the flesh of deep-sea fish such as salmon and mackerel. But what are these animals doing with so much plant-derived essential fatty acids in their fat? They obtain them from the algae and plankton that comprise the foundation of the ocean's food chain. Unfortunately, research shows that along with a concentration of LNA, fish also concentrate in their bodies traces of pesticides, heavy metals, and other industrial pollutants such as PCBs. According to Ralph Nader and other respected environmental activists, our deep-sea waters are now polluted, and the fish store the pollutants in their livers and fatty tissues. Organic flax seed contains no such toxic residues.

THE PROVEN BENEFITS OF LNA

In the last ten years many scientific studies have been released on flax seed and its oil. At a recent conference held at the Flax Institute of the United States in Fargo, North Dakota, scientists focused attention on flax seed and its role in healing and preventing numerous degenerative diseases. It was reported that LNA deficiencies contribute to many conditions and may be the ultimate cause of many widespread degenerative diseases. At this same conference, a report from Canada's Department of Health and Welfare (comparable to US Food & Drug Administration) dispelled any fears about flax seed's possible toxicity.

Research and clinical experience demonstrate the following benefits from regular consumption of flax seed:

CANCERS. For over thirty-five years, German lipid researcher Johanna Budwig has been using flax seed oil successfully in cancer therapy. She has more than 1,000 documented cases of successful cancer treatment with flax seed oil as the main treatment. In his New York City clinic, Dr. Max Gerson used fresh flax seed oil as the principal cancer fighting agent. Nobel humanitarian Dr. Albert Schweitzer wrote of Dr. Gerson: "I see in Dr. Max Gerson one of the world's most eminent medical geniuses."

More recent research shows that LNAs kill human cancer cells in tissue culture without harming the normal cells. Breast, lung, and prostate cancer cell lines were studied. Research evidence suggests that lignans may fight off chemicals responsible for initiating tumors and block estrogen receptors, which may reduce colon cancer risk. According to Dr. James Duke of the US Department of Agriculture, flax seed contains twenty-seven identifiable cancer preventive compounds. Additional studies show that LNAs inhibit tumor formation (smaller tumors, less metastasis, longer survival time). The National Cancer Institute is currently researching flax seed for its potential ability to prevent cancer.

HEART DISEASE. Dr. Gerson also treated heart patients with flax, using fresh organic flax seed oil for its cholesterol-lowering ability. LNAs lowered blood cholesterol and triglyceride levels an average of twenty-five percent, and this treatment lowered the triglyceride levels of some patients as much as sixty-five percent.

One of the unique features of flax seed oil is that it contains a substance which resembles prostaglandins, which may well be part of its potent therapeutic value. The prostaglandins regulate blood pressure and arterial function, and have an important role in calcium and energy metabolism. No other vegetable oil examined so far matches this property of flax seed oil.

At the Department of Clinical Chemistry in Denmark, Professor H. O. Bang conducted studies on cardiovascular stress in populations with diets high in animal fat. Interestingly, populations like those of the Greenland Eskimos, who consumed diets high in LNAs derived from ocean fish and northern cetaceans (whales and sea mammals), had only three cases of heart trouble among a population of 2,400 people over four years of study. Two of those cases involved people over seventy-eight years old, and the other case was complicated with rheumatic fever.

It's interesting that some studies have suggested that high fat intake is a cancer risk, but Greenland Eskimos have a high total fat intake and relatively low rates of cancer. They also have a very low incidence of ischemic heart disease (the leading cause of death in the industrialized world), attributed to their diet, which contains high levels of LNAs. This suggests that the prevention of cancer and heart disease is less related to the quantity of dietary fat and more related to the quality of fat.

Further studies showed that when Greenland Eskimos moved to Denmark and adopted the Danish diet, which includes significant saturated fat, they experienced a higher heart attack rate, even though the total caloric fat content of their diet decreased. Although the Eskimo people did not consume flax, they did consume large amounts of LNA fatty acids present in northern species of fish and sea mammals like seals and walrus. Professor Bang concluded that the relative deficiency of essential fatty acids common in Western diets plays an important part in the causation of atherosclerosis, diabetes, hypertension, and certain forms of malignant diseases.

It was further revealed that Greenland Eskimos of all age groups and both sexes had levels of total cholesterol and 'bad' LDL cholesterol that were significantly lower, and levels of 'good' HDL cholesterol that were higher, than when they lived among Danes. In other words, even though the Eskimo diet is higher in fat, their intake of LNAs was much higher and their blood lipid (fat) levels were healthier.

Similarly, the blood regulating capabilities of LNAs prevent spontaneous blood clots caused by an excess of LA fatty acids. This has implications for preventing strokes, if used at an early enough stage in a remedial lifestyle change that includes both exercise and improved diet.

DIABETES. Late-onset adult diabetes is suspected to originate partially from a deficiency of LNAs and an excess of saturated and trans-fats in the diet. Although this syndrome can take as long as thirty years to emerge as a full blown disease, reversal of symptoms can occur with positive changes in the diet and proper supplementation of LNAs from flax seed oil. A concurrent lack of vitamins and minerals makes the disease worse. LNAs may also lower the insulin requirement of diabetics.

INFLAMMATORY TISSUE CONDITIONS. LNA fatty acids decrease inflammatory conditions of all types—a confirmation of ancient Vedic medicine mentioned above that considers flax a 'cooling' agent. Inflammatory conditions are the diseases that end in 'itis,' including bursitis, tendinitis, tonsillitis, gastritis, ileitis, colitis, meningitis, arthritis, phlebitis, prostatitis, nephritis, splenitis, hepatitis, pancreatitis, and otitis, as well as lupus. Many of these inflammatory conditions may be eased by use of LNAs.

SKIN CONDITIONS. Pedigree show animals are fed linseed oil, made from flax seed, to keep their coats glossy. Along the same lines, recent research has shown that skin conditions in humans, such as psoriasis and eczema, have improved dramatically when flax seed and flax seed oil was added to the diet. These skin conditions are exacerbated by lack of LNAs in the diet. You will see that your skin gets smoother, softer, and velvety from taking flax seed oil regularly in your diet. It's also helpful for treating dry skin, dandruff, and sun-sensitive skin.

SEXUAL DISORDERS. Dr. Budwig has found flax seed oil to be a natural aphrodisiac. The most common physical cause of impotency in men and non-orgasmic response in women is blockage of blood flow in the arteries of the pelvis. Decrease of blood flow prevents full expansion (erection) of the penis and/or the clitoris. Thus ejaculation and/or orgasm cannot occur. The solution is to unblock narrowed arteries in general, and the consumption of flax seed oil will help. Flax seed oil is quickly gaining a reputation as one of the best aphrodisiacs for the new millennium.

CALMNESS UNDER STRESS. Many people find increased calmness to be the most profound effect of using fresh flax seed oil. It brings on a feeling of calmness often within a few hours. This may be partly due to that fact that, under stress, LNA fatty acids appear to slow down the over-production of stressing biochemicals like arachidonic acid.

The 'fight or flight' stress response is mitigated by the LNAs, which compete against the arachidonic acid cascade that happens when we are chronically stressed. Arachidonic acid in our blood thickens the blood platelets in anticipation of wounding and bleeding, which is an ancient natural defense mechanism. The LNA fatty acids keep these in check.

WATER RETENTION. The LNA and LA fatty acids in flax seed oil help the kidneys excrete sodium and water. Water retention (edema) accompanies swollen ankles, some forms of obesity, PMS, and all stages of cancer and cardiovascular disease.

VITALITY AND ATHLETIC ABILITY. One of the most noticeable signs of improved health from the use of flax seed oil is progressive and increased vitality and energy. Athletes notice that their fatigued muscles recover from exercise more quickly. LNAs also increase stamina. Flax does have a cooling effect on inflammatory conditions, but it also generates a healing 'heat energy' in the body due to the fact that the fatty acids are burned up for energy production. Its vital energy is enormous and is attributed to the triple bonds in the flax molecules which make them very receptive to other biochemicals, speeding up biochemical processes like metabolism. In simple terms, flax increases metabolic rate and the efficiency of cellular energy production. It stimulates respiratory and cellular oxidation, producing energy that we experience as warmth. For athletes, or anyone wishing to reduce fat and create a fit, lean body, this is great news! Adding flax seed to your diet will enhance all life processes, because all our life processes depend on energy production.

OTHER CONDITIONS. LNAs are necessary for visual function (retina), adrenal function (stress), and sperm formation. They often improve symptoms of multiple sclerosis (MS). In fact, when LNA consumption is high, MS is rare. According to *Fats That Heal: Fats That Kill*, flax seed oil can also be helpful in cystic fibrosis (LNA helps loosen viscous secretions and relieves breathing difficulties); some cases of sterility and miscarriage; some glandular malfunctions; some behavioral problems (schizophrenia, depression, bipolar disorder); allergies; addictions (to drugs or alcohol); and some deviant behaviors.

WHEN TO EXPECT BENEFITS FROM LNA SUPPLEMENTS

Some remarkable facts are brought forth in the excellent book by Dr. Donald Rudin and Clara Felix, *The Omega-3 Phenomenon*, not only about clinical results from ingesting a significant daily level of LNA, but also the length of time usually required before results are noticed. This landmark book reveals the scientific evidence from Dr. Rudin's research with forty-four patients over a period of several years, showing how the critical LNA fatty oils profoundly affect a broad range of contemporary health problems, including those of the heart and arteries,

Fats, Oils, and Flax

the brain, the emotions and general body functions. The general consensus from clinicians and researchers indicates that about fourteen grams of combined LNA fatty acid and LA fatty acid per day is optimum. This equates to 8.5 grams of LNA per 100 pounds of body weight and 4.5 grams of LA per 100 pounds of body weight per day. Ideally this should be consumed in equal portions before each meal. Thus a pre-meal ratio would ideally be about 4.7 grams per 100 pounds. This is about one teaspoon before meals.

The following charts, excerpted from *The Omega-3 Phenomenon*, show typical periods of time in which human subjects of the pilot study noted beneficial effects of the LNA flax seed supplements. You'll see that a long wait is not always necessary before results are visible.

TIME AFTER TAKING OIL SUPPLEMENT	REACTION
2 hours	Mood improved, feeling of calm • Depression relieved
2–7 days	Skin smoother, with less flaking and scaling • Backs of hands and fingers smoother
2–14 days	Fewer hallucinations • Relief for disturbed mental patients • Relief from feelings of anxiety
2–6 weeks	Osteoarthritis relieved, with easier movements and less inflammation and pain • Bursitis and other soft-tissue inflammations reduced • Tinnitus and noises in the ears subside • Dandruff and flaking of the scalp less noticeable • Dry skin alleviated
2–4 months	Rheumatoid pain diminished • "Easy bruising" reduced • Choking spasms subside • Fewer muscular spasms • No nighttime leg cramps • Relief from ocular spasms • Relief from itching and burning sensations • Improved skin color • Reduced sun sensitivity
3–6 months	Diminished food allergies • Healing of chronic infections • Disappearance of rough, bumpy skin on upper arms • Improved alcohol tolerance • Improved cold tolerance • Lessening of fatigue • Overall increased calm and feeling of well-being on a more consistent basis as supplementation is maintained and fully incorporated into diet.

As you can see from this table, the response time can vary from hours to months. Improvement in some cases can continue for up to one to two years before leveling off. Allergies often require a long time for improvement. Nothing is guaranteed, because each person's makeup is so individual. Persistent emotional or physical problems may improve only after several months, if at all.

Here's another summary of the benefits of LNA supplementation from *The Omega-3 Phenomenon*.

BENEFITS OF THE OMEGA PROGRAM

BIOCHEMICAL EFFECT	CLINICAL RESULT
Normalizes the body's fatty acids	Smoother skin, shiny hair, soft hands • Increased stamina, vitality, agility, and a zest for life
Normalizes and rebalances prostaglandin	Smoother muscle action • Improvement of many other functions
Reduces appetite provocation	Eliminates binging or addictive need for food
Stabilizes insulin and blood sugar levels	Keeps stamina high for long periods
Strengthens the immune system	Avoids or overcomes food allergies • Fights off some diseases more effectively
Increases fiber and aerobic bacteria	Promotes proper function of the digestive tract to avoid gas, constipation, and other disorders
Normalizes blood fats and lowers cholesterol	Stronger cardiovascular system • Clear thinking
Corrects the body's thermogenic system (ability to burn off calories)	Burns off fat • Increases cold weather resistance • Increases comfort
Brings enjoyment of total good health	Improved quality of life

THE DELICATE FLAX SEED OIL

Producing an oil from flax seed without damaging or destroying the vital LNA is no simple task. Udo Erasmus summarized the challenge in this way, "As essential as linoleic (LA) and alpha-linolenic acids (LNA) are to our health, they are also very temperamental and easily destroyed by light, air, and heat. For this reason, care must be taken in processing, packaging, and storing oils containing EFAs."

It was the knowledge that extraordinary precautions were necessary to produce an oil rich in LNA fatty acids that inspired the Spectrum Naturals company to develop a revolutionary new oil extraction technology. They call it the SpectraVac process because it presses the oils in an inert gas environment and in a vacuum, eliminating the destructive effects of atmospheric oxygen, high heat, and toxic chemicals. Spectrum Naturals uses this process to make Veg Omega-3 Organic Flax Oil and other nutritional supplement oils. This unique oil removal process eliminates the damaging consequences of light, air, and heat.

Spectrum Naturals uses in-line refrigeration between the seed press and oil storage and settling vessels (which are also refrigerated). This extra step provides the oil maximum protection from damaging heat. (Some other flax seed brands are refrigerated only at the retail outlet.) Spectrum Naturals also ships the fragile oil by refrigerated truck and requires retailers likewise to keep it under refrigeration. The bottles are opaque black to keep light out. No one can protect as well as Mother Nature, but Spectrum Naturals takes every step they can to try to measure up. Spectrum Naturals has done such an excellent job of establishing methods for nutritional oil handling that the Natural Products Quality Assurance Association has used its standards in measuring natural oils manufacturing in the organic and natural foods industry.

Make sure your keep the oil in your refrigerator and use it up within six weeks or it will turn rancid. I keep mine in the freezer as it remains a liquid and lasts longer—up to three months.

I think Udo Erasmus said it best: "The fresh oil of the very useful flax seed is the very best oil there is, in every way. It looks good: a rich, deep golden color like fresh liquid sunshine—which by the way, it is. The aroma is a gentle, pleasant, nutty bouquet. It has a variety of flavors. It varies depending on where it is grown to being robust and slightly bitter to light and nutty. Its texture is so light that it is hard to believe that it is oil at all. We usually associate oil with a 'heavy', 'oily' texture. Not so for flax."

I include it in blender drinks, as the oil in salad dressings, and sprinkle it on steamed vegetables, potatoes, and brown rice.

FORTIFIED FLAX MEAL

Another beneficial way I get LNAs into my diet is by eating flax seed meal. Keep in mind that if you swallow flax seeds whole, your body will not get the nutrients they contain, because they are protected by a tough seed coat. In fact, after the seeds go through you, you could actually plant them and they would still grow. If you eat them whole, they must be chewed and chewed and chewed. To break the seed coat and make the nutrients available for digestion, you can either grind the flax seeds yourself or get flax seed meal at your health food store.

I use Fortified Flax from the Omega-Life company (see Resource Directory), which is a whole unrefined organic flax seed meal that is fortified and stabilized in a unique grinding process. Zinc, iron, niacin (B_3), B_6 and B_{12} are added to the product to keep it fresher and to help in the digestion and assimilation of nutrients. This meal provides all the advantages of flax seed oil and none of the disadvantages like quick rancidity and free radical or trans-fat acid formation. Fortified Flax is sealed in an oxygen-barrier liner so no refrigeration is necessary until opening (although you may refrigerate or freeze it before opening to extend its freshness).

In a study conducted under the care of Milwaukee Wellness Clinic, it was found that in only three weeks of taking two tablespoons daily of Fortified Flax, serum triglyceride levels dropped almost fifty percent in subjects with above normal levels. In her book *Seven Weeks to Sobriety*, founder and director of the Minneapolis Recovery Center, Dr. Joan Matthews Larson, suggests two tablespoons of Fortified Flax and meganutrients as part of a daily regime for recovering alcoholics. Dr. Larson has had a seventy-five percent success rate.

Dr. Herbert Pierson, formerly with the National Cancer Institute, has researched flax and found anti-cancer compounds in it. On an appearance on the "CBS This Morning" television show, he demonstrated the breakfast drink he makes for his family consisting of Fortified Flax, fruit juice, and other ingredients. In her book, *Is This Your Child?*, Dr. Doris Rapp suggests Fortified Flax for children with allergies.

Further research also shows that the use of this type of freshly ground flax seed can also improve digestion, prevent and reverse contipation, stabilize blood glucose levels, improve cardiovascular health, hibit tumor formation, and bring about other benefits.

Make sure you take this ground flax seed with plenty of fluid, because its mucilage absorbs five times its own weight of water. In addition to taking one tablespoon of Spectrum Naturals Flax Seed Oil, I use from one to three tablespoons of Fortified Flax meal per day. I mix it in juice or water, blend it in smoothies, or sprinkle it on cereal, cooked grains, salads, and soup. I also add it to my homemade breads. I prefer, however, to use the oil and meal raw, without heating them.

Nature has provided us with everything we need to be radiantly healthy and free from disease. This is especially true when it comes to this marvelous plant, flax. Our ancestors knew instinctively that flax is nourishing, soothing, and healing. Their intuitive wisdom is now being confirmed by modern scientific analysis.

CHAPTER FIVE

Chlorophyll and Greens: The Great Cleansers

Chlorophyll, or 'solar energy,' should become a welcome addition to the menu of those wishing to attain and maintain radiant health. Its uses are as many and varied as the people who use and swear by it.
—PAUL DESOUZA

All life on this planet is derived either directly or indirectly from the sunlight that falls on chlorophyll. Chlorophyll is the green pigment found in plants, algae, and fresh dark green vegetables. Chlorophyll in all its forms has been receiving a lot of media attention of late. Some of the best sources of nutrients that prevent disease and support health are found in plants that are a rich green color—and one of the reasons is the color itself. If you've ever noticed parts of the broccoli in your refrigerator turning yellow with age, you are witnessing the fading of this green pigment. Green plants have been revered throughout history as effective tissue cleansers as well as effective agents in the treatment of many chronic disorders.

Chlorophyll got its name in 1818 from the Greek words *chloros* (green) and *phyllum* (leaf). There is a blue-black 'chlorophyll-a' as well as the more familiar dark green 'chlorophyll-b.' Both of these chlorophylls are formed in the leaves' chloroplasts—little organized units of special cells, where stacks of chlorophyll molecules are stored up until used.

In 1915, Dr. Richard Willstatter won a Nobel prize for discovering the chemical structure of chlorophyll, a network of carbon, hydrogen, nitrogen, and oxygen atoms surrounding a single magnesium atom. Fifteen years later, Dr. Hans Fisher won a Nobel prize for unraveling the chemical structure of hemoglobin, and was surprised to find out it was almost the same as chlorophyll. Hemoglobin is the pigment that gives red blood cells their red color, just as chlorophyll is the pigment that gives plants their green color. When Dr. Fisher separated the heme from the protein molecule to which it was attached, the main difference between it and chlorophyll was a single iron atom at its center instead of a magnesium atom, as in the chlorophyll molecule.

Heme and chlorophyll are fascinating in both their differences and similarities. Both are pigments that carry out their functions in cells, both are vital to the life of the organism to which they belong, both work with carbon dioxide and oxygen, and both have structural similarities.

Among their differences, heme has iron at its center, whereas chlorophyll has magnesium; heme takes in oxygen and gives off carbon dioxide, while chlorophyll takes in carbon dioxide and gives off oxygen. The iron in blood contributes to the vitality level of the person, while magnesium, as found in chlorophyll, is a relaxant that also acts as a catalyst in the use of protein, carbohydrates, fats, calcium, and phosphorus.

Dr. Fisher, excited by the similarity in structure between chlorophyll and heme, immediately began research on possible medical uses for chlorophyll. He was not alone. In laboratories and hospitals throughout the United States, excited researchers and doctors had already begun to investigate the 'life blood' of plants.

HEALING THE BODY WITH CHLOROPHYLL

Not surprisingly, chlorophyll is known to have revitalizing, rejuvenating, and detoxifying effects. Foods high in chlorophyll help oxygenate the body, thereby offsetting the deleterious effects of living in an environment polluted with smog and carbon monoxide. Many decades of research have revealed an abundance of other noteworthy benefits.

One of the first in-depth medical tests on chlorophyll was reported in the July 1930 issue of *The American Journal of Surgery*. Doctors at Temple University's department of experimental pathology used chlorophyll packs, ointments, and solutions to treat over 1,200 patients whose ailments ranged from the common cold to a burst appendix with spreading peritonitis. Chlorophyll diluted with sterile water was used to clean out deep surgical wounds, some of them badly infected. Ulcerated varicose veins, osteomyelitis, brain ulcers, and shallow open wounds were cleansed with the chlorophyll solution or covered with a chlorophyll salve. Diseases of the mouth, such as trench mouth and advanced pyorrhea, were also treated.

The results were spectacular. The doctors who tested the chlorophyll hailed it as an important and effective therapy. Over 1,000 cases of respiratory infections, sinusitis, and head colds were treated under the supervision of Dr. Robert Ridpath and Dr. T. Carroll Davis. They reported, "There is not a single case in which improvement or cure has not taken place." Chlorophyll packs placed on sinuses gave great relief. Head colds were described as being cleared up in twenty-four hours.

Temple University researchers found that chlorophyll did not kill germs in test tube experiments, but rather that it increased the resistance of cells and inhibited the growth of bacteria.

In another study, Drs. Smith and Livingston demonstrated that chlorophyll caused an "almost immediate growth response" of fibroblasts—the cells the body uses to repair wounds. In the treatment of a variety of types of skin ulcers, chlorophyll was found to have a stimulating effect on the supportive tissues, promoting rapid healing.

Similarly, chlorophyll is effective as an external ointment for reducing or removing bad odors from poorly healing wounds. When doctors replaced the chlorophyll ointment with a placebo, the wounds began to reassert their disagreeable odor as well as poor healing. This is because chlorophyll is both wound-healing and inhibiting to bacteria. With all the oxygen contained in chlorophyll, it is easy to see why oxygen-hating microbes would suffer when bathed in this plant juice.

As a topical ointment, chlorophyll has also been shown to be effective in the treatment of inflammation that occurs in the skin after radiation treatments for cancer and other conditions. French scientists have shown that chlorophyll can reduce tissue damage caused by radiotherapy. Radiation burns have been repaired by plants that contain significant amounts of chlorophyll, suggesting that this substance may be the common active constituent.

A CLEANSER FOR ALL KINDS OF THINGS

The common skin disease known as athlete's foot is really the result of fungus infection. The fungi are carried between the toes of the feet and remain dormant until the feet become moist or cracks appear in the skin. When this happens, the fungus enters the outer layer of tissue and establishes a place in which to increase its size.

Because fungi live on organic matter, they are not only hardy, but extremely difficult to abolish. That's why athlete's foot has taxed the ingenuity of many doctors. Although there are many salves, solutions and other patented remedies purported to be successful in treating athlete's foot, nothing compares with chlorophyll. In this natural product, we have a healing agent as well as a bacteriostatic and so it is possible to correct the cause and the effect at the same time.

A podiatrist I know recommends the following: After washing and drying the feet thoroughly, put them in an enamel basin containing a diluted solution of ten parts warm water and one part liquid chlorophyll. Be sure to cover the toes entirely for at least thirty minutes, then dry them well. This treatment should be followed daily for two weeks, then two or three times weekly for two weeks longer to be certain all fungi are destroyed. In obstinate cases, rolls of cotton soaked in full strength liquid chlorophyll, or a chlorophyll ointment, may be put between the toes. Chlorophyll stops the offensive odor as well as the underlying condition.

Chlorophyll has also been shown to be helpful in the treatment of pancreatitis. Pancreatitis is an inflammation of the pancreas that can be very painful and life threatening. It may be caused by excess consumption of alcohol, gallstones, poor nutrition, excessive calcium in the blood, and excessive blood fat. Chlorophyll-a derivatives (from blue-black colored sources) inhibit proteases, which are enzymes that break down proteins. Protease enzymes support inflammation and are in large part responsible for the harmful effects of pancreatitis.

Chlorophyll has a long history of being effective at deodorizing bad smells. You may be aware of chlorophyll-containing gum for bad breath, and some kitty litter contains chlorophyll. It is also found in mouthwash and toothpaste to help control bad breath, and it's in some skin lotions. Chlorophyll has also been used and documented to act as an underarm deodorant. It is well known among workers in nursing homes, geriatric hospitals, and mental institutions that chlorophyll is an important aid in the control of odors from incontinent patients.

In 1990, the Food and Drug Administration determined that the clinical use of chlorophyll taken internally was both safe and effective for reducing body odors. This is especially so for people who have had surgeries such as ileostomies, where the more difficult elimination of bowel or bladder wastes can lead to problem odors.

As documented by research, many diseases are aggravated by poor bowel health. Although not very precise as a diagnostic method, smelling a person's breath is one way of determining if a person is suffering from bowel toxicity. Chlorophyll helps clear bowel toxicity within a few days.

One colon-related ailment is chronic constipation, one of those problems that seem to afflict many people as they grow older. In addition to infrequent and hard stools, constipation may cause bad breath and headaches and has been associated with the development of pancreatitis, hypoglycemia, and even breast and colon cancer. It has been shown that chlorophyll helps relieve chronic constipation problems and also relieves intestinal gas in terms of amount and odor.

The detoxifying and stimulating effect of chlorophyll on the bowel produces an interesting result at times. Many people will release more gases than usual for three to seven days after beginning to use it. Probably the harmful intestinal bacteria are being fermented and destroyed. After this initial adjustment period, the bowel functions better, and the gas problems disappear.

The deodorant properties of water-soluble chlorophyll are dependent on the acid-base (pH) balance of the material that needs to be neutralized.

Chlorophyll exhibits deodorant actions on neutral or alkaline material with an optimum pH between eight and 10.5. Chlorophyll also exhibits antibacterial properties on neutral or alkaline material. Bowel toxicity and constipation are associated with a stool pH of greater than seven, with the worst cases having a stool pH of nine. Chlorophyll functions best in treating colons that are suffering from anaerobic bacterial overgrowth syndromes, which are usually associated with a stool pH of greater than seven. Anyone can test their stool by buying pH litmus paper, which is available at drugstores, and observing the color changes on the paper.

Many impressive studies too numerous to mention here have noted chlorophyll's ability to nourish the intestines and to have a very soothing or healing effect on the mucous linings. It has also been used beneficially in the detoxification of all the organs, particularly the liver. It can help to wash drug deposits from the body, purify the blood, and counteract acids and toxins in the body.

Besides its tonic effects at improving tissue oxygenation and removing unpleasant internal odors, chlorophyll has been considered as an effective means of removing heavy metal buildup. In her book *Are You Radioactive? How To Protect Yourself,* Linda Clark states that chlorophyll can bind with several toxins, including heavy metals, and help eliminate them. Research done during the last few years has found that chlorophyll can help offset the damaging effects of the environment, radiation, and x-rays.

Physicians and dentists have used chlorophyll for years to successfully treat oral diseases, kidney stones, and acute infections of the upper respiratory tract and sinuses. In addition, nutritionists and researchers believe that it may also play an important role in the prevention of cancer. Chlorophyll has also been shown to increase the effectiveness of penicillin by as much as thirty-five percent.

CHLOROPHYLL'S BOOST TO IMMUNE FUNCTIONS

Let's not forget chlorophyll's increasing popularity due to its use as an immune-building food supplement. Immunology is fast becoming one of the most exciting and potentially rewarding areas of modern medicine. Immunology is the study of the immune system: the body's mechanisms that fight off foreign invaders, whether they be bacteria, viruses, chemicals, or foreign proteins. The body's defenses have a unique way of inactivating or detoxifying each of these types of substances. Chlorophyll has been found to stimulate all the different organs and components of the immune system.

One of the key components of the immune system is macrophage cells, which are active against cancer, foreign proteins, and chemicals. Macrophages are large cells located in the abdominal cavity, the blood (monocytes), joints (synovial lining cells), bone marrow, and connective tissue. In a process is called phagocytosis, they clean the blood, body fluids, and cavities of harmful substances.

One way to fight cancer is to stimulate macrophage production and activity. This macrophage stimulation causes increased cancer cell destruction and the removal of harmful cancer debris from the blood by this phagocytic activity. Interferon is a natural secretion of the body, a protein substance produced by virus-invaded cells that prevents reproduction of the virus. Interferon is thought to be a stimulator of macrophages. Numerous studies show chlorophyll increases the levels of interferon in the body and thereby stimulates the immune system.

Chlorophyll is water soluble and easy to digest. Interestingly, it is also rich in the fat-soluble vitamin K, which is necessary for blood clotting. Because of this and other benefits, chlorophyll has been used for women with heavy menstrual bleeding as well as for anemia by holistic doctors, herbalists, and other health professionals. According to Dr. Amanda Crawford, a member of Britain's National Institute of Medical Herbalists, vitamin K also helps form a compound in the urine that inhibits growth of calcium oxalate crystals (common kidney stones) and may be helpful in the prevention of this very painful condition.

When the diet is lacking in a sufficient amount of fruits and vegetables, the body tends to become more acidic, and thus a fertile environment for many diseases and ailments. To assist the body's pH balance, chlorophyll can help neutralize the acidifying and stimulating effect of excess protein, sugars, and starch. Like vegetables, fruit, and nongluten grains such as millet, chlorophyll is alkalinizing and cleansing.

TO SUM UP CHLOROPHYLL'S BENEFITS

In general, the healthy action of chlorophyll is subtle, yet remarkable. Here's a brief summary of the healing power of chlorophyll.

- Strengthens immunity—especially of the surface or 'mucus' immune system. This is the first line of bodily defense and functions best against allergens, airborne microbes, and chemical pollutants.
- Protects the body from and helps neutralize a range of chemical environmental pollutants including low level radiation.

- Acts as a major detoxifier of metabolic waste products in blood. In a 'micro' sense, chlorophyll benefits the body much as green plants benefit our 'macro' environment.
- Stimulates circulation, metabolism and cellular respiration. This attribute has a tremendous application in the recovery phase of debilitating illness and in weight loss.
- Helps prevent Candida, Epstein-Barr virus, Cytomegalovirus, and chronic fatigue syndrome.
- Acts as an internal deodorant/topical antiseptic. Liquid chlorophyll can be used as mouthwash and as a cleanser for cuts, abrasions and minor burns. Liquid chlorophyll concentrate also reduces urinary and bowel odors.
- Establishes a healthy intestinal ecosystem by promoting the growth of probiotic (friendly) intestinal bacteria.

There is no toxicity associated with chlorophyll; cramps or mild diarrhea may occur with large quantities, but will disappear by reducing or stopping its intake. A large dose of chlorophyll may turn the stool green, especially if you haven't been in the habit of eating many green foods. This is not harmful and can even be helpful if you are trying to determine your digestive 'transit time' (how fast or slowly food moves through the body). Transit time gives some information about how well the digestive process is functioning: too fast, and we can't absorb all our nutrients; too slow, and bacterial changes in a stagnant colon may lead to other health risks. A healthy transit time is between twelve and seventeen hours.

How do you take chlorophyll? Eat green plants! Alternatively, you may choose liquids, capsules, or tablets of chlorophyll, available in your health food store. I use the liquid chlorophyll and other chlorophyll products by the DeSouza company (see Resource Directory) because of their superb quality.

LIQUID CHLOROPHYLL

In 1935, Paul DeSouza investigated, studied, and began the manufacture of chlorophyll products—offering only those products meeting his high standards. DeSouza was one of the pioneer health enthusiasts and avant-garde exponents of the natural, organic farming methods that are in wide use today.

As a young man of twenty-seven, DeSouza moved to California and discovered that the fertile farmlands were being destroyed by chemical

Chlorophyll and Greens

fertilizers and pesticides which drained the essential minerals from the soil. He searched the world to find an area where the farming methods had not left a depleted, desecrated land as a result of over-production and chemical destruction, and to his amazement he found the answer in Israel. The ancient knowledge of the Hebrews included the wonderful secrets of soil renewal.

He was a true pioneer in this field and continued to share his vision of "good ground to grow good food." He knew that if the Hebrew agriculturists could renew their lands and keep the thin, poor soil of the desert always productive for more than 6,000 years, it could be done with the rich, formerly fertile lands of California. The science used today in organic farms came from the great Jewish tradition to DeSouza, who carried the knowledge to organic and ecologically aware commercial farmers. DeSouza Liquid Chlorophyll is an essential part of my health program (see Resource Directory).

GREEN AND LEAFY VEGETABLES

Green and leafy vegetables should become a part of your daily diet. They add vitamins, minerals, usable calcium, and beta-carotene needed for the immune system. They also help ward off diseases such as cancer. Leafy greens are excellent for the gall bladder, spleen, heart, and blood, and are a good brain food. Most greens can be cooked or eaten raw in salads or fresh juices (see Chapter Six on juices).

To clean them, soak in a sink of cold water for a few minutes and swirl around, then drain the water. Pat dry. Tear the leaves into small pieces, trim the ends of the stems, and chop when necessary. All leafy greens contain chlorophyll, iron, magnesium, calcium, manganese, vitamin C, potassium, vitamin A, and a bonus of the essential fatty acids, with no cholesterol. The vegetables with the darkest, most intense colors tend to contain the highest level of nutrients.

For dressing on a salad of greens, I usually combine one of Spectrum Natural's delicious vinegars (my favorites are raspberry, mango, peach, garlic, and Italian herb) with their organic flax seed oil and some herbs. It's fresh, easy to make, flavorful, and healthy.

Here is a brief listing of some of my favorite leafy greens I eat on a regular basis.

ARUGULA: This green from the mustard family is peppery and tart, and mixes well with other greens. It is also known as roquette. It adds pizzazz to any raw salad, is high in vitamins A and C, niacin, iron, and phosphorus, and is good for normalizing body acid with its high alkalinity.

BEET GREENS: Best used in juices, they are very high in nutrients, especially iron and calcium. These greens can be used in cooking also. They are known for their benefit in blood disorders, liver function, and the flow of bile.

BELGIAN ENDIVE: Good in a salad with raspberry or mango vinaigrette dressing. I also use the leaves for dipping in place of crackers or chips. It has pale yellow or white leaves. It is similar to chicory in healing qualities and nutrient content.

BUTTERHEAD LETTUCE: Also known as Boston Bibb, this is a very tender leaf, with an almost buttery taste. Makes a good salad when used with spinach, endive, or watercress. Lettuce is said to calm the nerves.

CHICORY: A bitter green with curly leaves; the young leaves are best in salads. High in vitamins C and A, and calcium and iron. Aids in liver function and blood disorders. Try radicchio, often called red-leaf chicory, good in salads.

COLLARDS: A member of the cabbage family. Use only the leaves; they tend to be tough, so steam them for five to eight minutes. Collards can be used in salads as a substitute for cabbage and are also great for juicing. Because of its high nutrition content, no leafy green is more valuable in the body for disorders of the colon, respiratory system, lymphatic system, and skeletal system.

DANDELION GREENS: The young leaves have a tangy taste. They are good for gall bladder disorders, rheumatism, gout, eczema, and skin disorders. Dandelion is also an excellent liver rejuvenator. They cook the same as any leafy green. Rich in calcium, potassium, and vitamins A and C. These are also excellent to add to juices.

ESCAROLE AND ENDIVE: From the chicory family. The leaves are very dark green, with a slightly bitter taste. These make a good salad with a warm citrus-flavored dressing, and can also be steamed. Both are rich in vitamin A, calcium, minerals, B-vitamins, iron and potassium. They're good for most infections, liver function, and internal cleansing.

KALE: This is the king of calcium. Use only the leaves of this plant. It tastes like cabbage. I often add the juice of kale to carrot and other juices. It's very high in usable calcium and is excellent for prevention and care of osteoporosis.

MUSTARD AND TURNIP: These greens have a zippy taste with flavors varying from mild to hot. They are good sautéed with a little garlic, or steamed. They can also be used in juices. They're high in calcium and vitamin C. Good for infections, colon disorders, colds, flu, and elimination of kidney stones due to excess uric acid.

PARSLEY: All types of this plant are rich in vitamin A, B-complex,

C, minerals, potassium, and manganese. Parsley contains mucilage, starch, opinol, and volatile oil. It is very crisp and tangy. This green has an 'odor eating' quality that helps restore fresh breath after a meal with such foods as garlic and onion. Add to fresh juices or chop to add to salads. Good for digestive disorders, also an excellent diuretic. Try cilantro, a Chinese and Mexican parsley, essential in many Chinese, Spanish, Mexican, and Thai dishes.

ROMAINE LETTUCE: This is a wonderful, crunchy green that is highest in nutrients of all types of lettuce. Great in salads. I always keep lots on hand for salads and juicing. This lettuce is not good for cooking. Being high in chlorophyll, it is a good blood purifier.

SORREL: This green has a pleasantly sour and slightly lemon flavor. It is easily perishable and best bought fresh or grown in your garden. Try sorrel in salads or as a seasoning in soups and casseroles. Sorrel is a powerful antioxidant with the same healing properties of kale.

SPINACH: Its tender bright green leaves are most beneficial when eaten raw. Because of the oxalic acid content, some of the calcium becomes unavailable to the body. Spinach contains many valuable nutrients and is high in iron.

SWISS CHARD: From the beet family, this green has a mild taste and is good with walnuts and pine nuts added to a salad. It has the highest content of sodium of all greens. Chlorophyll and calcium-rich, Swiss chard is a natural cleanser and helps strengthen bones.

WATERCRESS: This green has young, tender leaves, which should be picked before the plant flowers. The spicy-flavored green goes well with romaine and butterhead lettuce. It's higher in nutrient content than most greens and is excellent for vitamin deficiencies and illnesses of all types. Good added to fresh juices, too.

CHLORELLA

This chapter wouldn't be complete without information on a superlative super-food called chlorella. The chlorella algae is a single-celled plant which grows larger by maturing and developing its own food, rather than by adding new cells as do most other plants. It is the richest source of chlorophyll on Earth, and particularly valuable for its ability to balance the body chemistry and raise the level of health of the entire body.

Chlorella is noted for its ability to detoxify pollutants in the body and can remove heavy metals such as lead, mercury, and cadmium. It also provides many vitamins and minerals. In addition, it is a complete protein because it supplies more than nineteen amino acids, including all eight essential amino acids, and the important nucleic acids DNA and

RNA, which help repair and rejuvenate the body.

For decades, scientists and nutritionists have known about the marvelous nutritional value of chlorella. But for many years, one seemingly insurmountable problem remained—the outer cell wall of chlorella was thick and impenetrable. All previous attempts to break down that wall with heat or chemicals negatively affected its nutritional content. In 1981, Sun Chlorella of Japan scored a significant nutritional breakthrough. It developed a patented process using the Dyno-Mill. There are many chlorella products on the market, but the only digestible chlorella is Sun Chlorella. It has twice the digestibility rate of other chlorella products.

I have been taking Sun Chlorella tablets for over ten years and am a big fan of this wonderful, nutrient-dense, whole food. It's available in health food stores. For more information, please refer to the Resource Directory.

CHAPTER SIX

Juices: Radiant Health in a Glass

Vegetable and fruit juices are packed with concentrated nutrients, and simply by drinking a few glasses of delicious juice every day, you supply your body with many of the essential elements that contribute to its strength and general well-being.
—JAY KORDICH

For centuries, juices from fruits and vegetables have been used to help heal disease and build up the body's natural immunities. It is known that:

- CABBAGE, BROCCOLI, GARLIC, ONIONS, LEEKS, and CITRUS FRUIT are loaded with antioxidants, which suppress the growth of deadly cancer cells.
- APPLES contain sorbitol, a gentle laxative.
- GRAPES and BLUEBERRIES are filled with polyphenols, which kill viruses.
- CABBAGE is famous for its ulcer-healing properties.
- CANTALOUPE and GARLIC are blood-thinners, which can help prevent heart attacks and strokes.
- The juices of GREEN VEGETABLES as well as DARK ORANGE VEGETABLES act as antidotes to the cancer process (a process that continues for years after exposure to carcinogens).
- CHERRIES are a remedy for gout.
- PINEAPPLE juice is rich in anti-inflammatory agents to soothe sore throats.
- LEMON helps digestion by stimulating the flow of saliva and digestive juices.
- GINGER relieves motion sickness.

Sounds incredible, doesn't it? I agree with Bernard Jensen, ND, who said in his book, *Vibrant Health from Your Kitchen*: "The power and effectiveness of foods in healing and in keeping people well is sometimes astonishing."

Why not eat the whole fruit or vegetable instead of juicing it? Solid food requires hours of digestive activity before its nourishment is finally available to the cells and tissues of the body. Juices are easy and quick to prepare and drink, supply an abundance of nutrients, increase the servings of fruits and vegetables in your diet, and are absolutely delicious.

I do not advocate a total liquid diet, because the fibers found in solid foods are important, too. While fibers have virtually no nourishing value, they act as an intestinal broom pushed by the peristaltic activity of the intestines. Nevertheless, juices are one of the main ingredients of health.

EAT IT RAW!

According to the American Cancer Society, the National Cancer Institute, and the National Research Council, Americans do not eat enough fresh fruits and vegetables to prevent disease. Yet these foods have been proven to have powerful protective effects for the body.

Many health professionals are now saying that we need to eat at least seven servings of vegetables and at least two servings of fruit each day. It has also been proven that fifty to seventy-five percent of our diet should be raw food if we are to enjoy optimal health and abundant energy. Authors of *Raw Energy*, Leslie and Susannah Kenton, state that a "vast quantity of evidence...exists showing that the high-raw diet—a way of eating in which seventy-five percent of your foods are taken raw—cannot only reverse the bodily degeneration which accompanies long-term illness, but retard the rate at which you age, bring you seemingly boundless energy and even make you feel better emotionally." I know personally that this is true because for years I have eaten a diet which is at least seventy-five percent raw.

While cooked foods sustain life, they do not necessarily have the power to regenerate the cells that furnish the life force to our body, writes Diane Olive in her excellent book, *Think Before You Eat*. On the contrary, continuous consumption of cooked and processed foods results in progressive degeneration of cells and tissues. You can eat three or four big meals a day, yet your body may be starved for vital nutrients and enzymes. Very few people in our urban Western culture eat three-quarters raw food.

The addition of fresh fruit and vegetable juices will not only add more raw foods to your diet, but also increase the number of servings of fruits and vegetables you get daily. This will help your body to heal itself and be healthy. I have been an avid juicer for twenty-five years and know it's one of the main reasons I'm radiantly healthy with an abundance of energy. I've also done extensive research on the healing powers of juicing and juice fasts.

Usually you just can't eat enough raw fruits and vegetables in a day to nourish your body properly. I don't think I could stomach eating five pounds of carrots. But it's easy to drink their nutritional equivalent in a delicious, nutritious glass of carrot juice. That's why juicing is such an important and easy addition to a busy lifestyle.

Let's take a closer look at why fresh fruit and vegetable juices are so beneficial. Fresh juices are powerhouses of nutrients that revitalize and regenerate your entire body and mind. Juices made fresh and taken immediately send forth cleansing catalysts that penetrate the innermost recesses of your body and help dislodge toxins from your cells. At the same time, the abundant nutrients help repair your vital tissues and organs and give you more energy and health.

Fresh fruit and vegetable juices are an excellent way to get vitamins, minerals, purified water, proteins, carbohydrates, and chlorophyll. Fresh raw juices are also full of enzymes. Enzymes are organic catalysts that increase the rate at which foods are broken down and absorbed by the body. Enzymes are found in plant foods such as fruits and vegetables, but are destroyed by the heat of cooking. This is one of the reasons why fresh raw produce should constitute at least half of your diet.

Another benefit is that it takes little energy to digest juice, so you feel the benefits more quickly than when eating the whole food. It can take many hours to process whole foods, especially when fat is present. But fresh fruit and vegetable juices, which are already separated from the fiber, are easy to digest. Within moments after you consume a glass of your favorite raw juice, the nutrients and enzymes go to work to create internal rejuvenation. For this reason, you often feel an instant 'lift' when drinking a glass of fresh orange juice, as opposed to eating a whole orange.

The juice nutrients speed up the biological process of detoxifying the dead and decaying cells and washing them away. The juice nutrients then accelerate the building of new cells. When the toxic waste products that have been blocking cellular oxygenation and nourishment are washed out, the juices stimulate metabolic and cell-rebuilding functions.

The extracted liquid portion of fruits or vegetables is a highly concentrated source of super cleaning without compare. Vegetable juices are dynamic sources of alkaline reserve. This helps establish the important acid-alkaline balance in your bloodstream. In addition, abundant supplies of minerals in the juices restore the biochemical and amino acid balance in your bloodstream, cells, tissues, and organs.

And here's a special benefit of juices: minerals provide needed oxygen and nourishment and accelerate the detoxification. With ordinary foods, mineral deficiency often precedes oxygen loss, which chokes and starves your cells and allows waste buildup.

THREE CATEGORIES OF JUICES

GREEN JUICES or 'GREEN DRINKS.' Green juices stimulate cells and rejuvenate the body. They also build red blood cells. Green juices contain chlorophyll, which heals and cleanses the body. 'Green drinks' can also be made by adding liquid chlorophyll to the juice. Green juices are made from spinach, lettuce, wheatgrass, celery, cabbage, dandelion greens, alfalfa sprouts, and other similar leafy greens and vegetables.

VEGETABLE JUICES. Fresh vegetables are restorers and builders. They help remove excesses of protein, fat, and acid wastes from the body. Vegetable juices help build the immune system, guard against illness, and are excellent sources of alkaline reserve. Both vegetable and green juices are extensively used in fasting and as nutritional supplements because of their high vitamin and mineral content. But they don't travel well because they oxidize quickly, which breaks down the protective enzymes and vitamins, so they should be taken immediately after juicing.

FRUIT JUICES. Fruit juices are cleansers. They provide a quicker pick-me-up than vegetable juice because they are almost immediately absorbed, where vegetable juices are absorbed within an hour if taken on an empty stomach. Fruit juices also remain stable for a longer period of time and 'travel' better than vegetable juices. The juices of different fruits are wonderful combined. I usually have some type of fruit juice combination each morning and another one before lunch as a snack. Since fruit juices have a high sugar content and ferment rapidly in the stomach, I recommend they be diluted with an equal amount of water. People with diabetes or hypoglycemia should be sure to take food with fruit juices.

JUICING MADE EASY

It's easy to make fresh juices. All you need is high-quality produce and a good juicer. Many different kinds of juicers are available, and I have tried all of them (for information about different juicers, see HealthForce in the Resource Directory). When shopping for a juicer, look for one that is very practical and efficient, and easy to use and clean. Your juicer should be strong enough to juice skins and all—including pineapples, watermelons, and cantaloupes—and vegetables such as cauliflower and broccoli, which may look like they're not very juicy. Not so. Their juices are excellent when combined with carrot juice. You're wasting your money and valuable nutrients if you purchase a juicer that's not designed to juice skins: many of the most important nutrients are in the skins and rinds. However, if you are not able to purchase organically grown, unsprayed produce, I suggest you peel the produce before juicing.

There's one exception to juicing the skins. It's best to peel oranges and grapefruits before juicing, even if they are organically grown, because their skins contain a toxic substance that should not be consumed in large quantities, and because these skins are somewhat bitter. Leave on the white pithy part of the peel, though, because it contains valuable bioflavonoids and vitamin C. Tropical fruits like kiwi and papaya should also be peeled if they have been grown in foreign countries where the use of carcinogenic sprays is still legal. The skins of all other fruits and vegetables, including lemons and limes, may be left on if certified grown in the United States. However, if the produce has been waxed, I recommend removing the peel.

When you aren't able to get organic produce, and the produce is not the type that can be peeled, make sure you wash it thoroughly. Here's a formula for helping remove toxic surface sprays from your non-organic produce: fill your kitchen sink with cold water; add four tablespoons of salt and the juice of half a fresh lemon (this makes a diluted form of hydrochloric acid); soak fruits and vegetables five to ten minutes (leafy greens two to three minutes and berries one to two minutes); rinse well after soaking and use. There are also a variety of produce washes available at health food stores. I use SunSmile Fruit and Vegetable Rinse (see Resource Directory).

Never wash or hull strawberries until just before use. They lose their freshness quite rapidly after washing. Leafy greens store better if spun dry after washing. Store greens in resealable bags. Celery stores best in long plastic produce bags with a little water added to the bottom of the bag. For greater freshness, leave the stalks attached until ready to use. Do not juice celery leaves—they add a bitter taste to the drink.

Make sure you drink your juice right after juicing. Researchers at Stanford University found that in only one minute after the juice is extracted, the therapeutic qualities begin to dissipate. Orange juice, if not consumed within five minutes, loses half of its vitamin C content; if it sits for an hour, it loses all of its vitamin C. Always try to drink your juice when it's fresh. If you want to take juice to work with you, moisten the inside of a stainless steel thermos with water and put it in the freezer overnight. Before going to work, make your juice and put it directly into the cold thermos, filling the thermos to the brim. Juice will stay fresher (less oxidation and vitamin loss) for up to eight hours this way.

Contrary to popular belief, you can get protein from juices. In the cellulose matter of greens lies the finest protein in the world. The strongest creatures on the planet are strictly vegetarian: horses, gorillas, and elephants. The only protein that nurtures these creatures is in green plants. Studies reveal that the most disease-free humans are vegans (vegetarians who eat no animal products including dairy or eggs). Humans have the same protein sources available from vegetables, including juices. You may be surprised to learn that one large glass of carrot juice has at least five grams of protein, which is equal to the protein of two eggs.

In general, I do not recommend combining fruit and vegetable juices on a regular basis, with the exception of apple juice. While there's really no known scientific basis for restrictions on food combining, some people with impaired digestion, multiple food allergies, or severe fatigue benefit from avoiding combinations of fruit and vegetables. If you experience no adverse symptoms (such as gas or stomach aches) from combining fruit and vegetable juices, let your taste buds be your guide, and make the combinations you like best.

At least once a month I do a one to three day juice-only diet (refer to the book, *3 Days to Vitality* by Pamela Serure for more information on how to do this), and a few times a year I do a several day juice fast. Dr. Elson Haas, a dear friend whose medical practice is in San Rafael, California, uses juice fasts as a form of medical therapy. In the twenty-five years he has been in practice, Dr. Haas has regularly fasted on juice, as have thousands of his patients. He told me: "I did my first ten-day juice cleanse in 1975 and the experience changed my life and health. I realized the importance of diet and fasting in preventing disease and maintaining health. I cleared my allergies and back pains, normalized my weight, and felt a new level of vitality and creativity." Dr. Haas finds juice therapy very helpful with colds and flus, recurrent infections, allergies, skin disorders, and gastrointestinal problems, as well as other congestive or chronic disorders.

Every day, I have at least one glass, and often two or three glasses, of fresh juices. I recommend one or more glasses in addition to meals as an excellent nutritional supplement. Drink as much vegetable juice as fruit juice to avoid getting too much fruit sugar (see contraindications at the end of the chapter).

MAKE JUICING A HABIT

- Set a time each day to juice. Be sure to stock up on produce.
- Produce should be fresh, seasonal, and free of decay. If you notice any signs of deterioration, just cut away that portion and discard.

- Wash all fruits and vegetables before juicing.
- In general, don't hesitate to include stems and leaves along with the fruits and vegetables. However, carrot and rhubarb greens contain toxic substances and should be removed.
- All pits from peaches, plums, and other fruits must be removed before juicing. In general, seeds (from lemons, limes, melons, and grapes) may be juiced. Apple seeds should not be juiced because they contain small amounts of cyanide.
- Cut up the produce in slices or chunks that fit the size of your juicer.
- Don't get in a rut of having the same juices or combinations day after day. Select a variety of fruits and vegetables and different combinations. This will delight your taste buds and assure a bounty of nutrients to boost your immune system and keep you healthy.
- Strong-tasting vegetable juices such as spinach, beet, and parsley are high in compounds that should be consumed in small quantities. You can dilute these with milder-tasting juices or water. Vegetables like rutabaga, onions, turnips, and broccoli should also be juiced in small amounts; for example, 1/4 turnip would be sufficient per glass. Foods that have a high water content like carrots, cabbage, apples, and grapes should be your base.
- Always sip your fresh juices slowly—don't gulp them down.
- Add raw foods and juices gradually to your current diet. Begin slowly so your body can adjust to a new way of eating.

PRODUCE SUGGESTIONS AND HEALTH BENEFITS

ALFALFA (sprouts) contains vitamins A, B, C, E, K, and U in addition to B_{12}, magnesium, essential fatty acids, selenium, enzymes, and much more. It is also one of the richest sources of chlorophyll. It is high in nutrients because alfalfa roots go deep, as far as 130 feet into the earth. It contains natural fluoride that prevents tooth decay and is used in the treatment of arthritis, mineral deficiencies, and many illnesses. Taken with lettuce juice, it also stimulates hair growth.

APPLES are a very nutritious fruit filled with vitamins C and A, lots of potassium, and modest amounts of B vitamins. They also contain pectin and malic acid. This juice is good for the gall bladder and is known for its cleansing and healing effects on internal inflammation. Apples can help lower blood cholesterol, aid liver function, rid the body of toxins, and lessen the effects of X-rays. Apples are also rich in sorbitol, a natural form of sugar and a gentle laxative. Five apples make one large glass.

ASPARAGUS contains high amounts of vitamins A, B-complex and C, as well as potassium, manganese, and iron. It contains rutin, which contributes to a strong capillary system, and asparagine, which stimulates the kidneys (a natural diuretic). Cancer clinics around the world use three tablespoons of pureed asparagus a day in their therapies. The high amounts of carotene, vitamin C, and selenium make this vegetable excellent for cancer treatment.

BEETS provide one of the very best juices for the liver, gall bladder, red corpuscles, anemia, cancer, blood cleansing, and stimulation of the lymph glands. Beets are rich in magnesium, beta-carotene, vitamins C and E, potassium, folic acid, and the antioxidant gluathione. Juice the tips, too. Be sure to dilute the juice with pure water or other juices such as carrot and celery since it is very potent.

BERRIES of all kinds are delicious as well as nutritious, including blackberries, blueberries, boysenberries, raspberries, and strawberries. They have vitamin C and potassium and are good blood purifiers. Blueberry juice can help prevent recurrent urinary tract infections. This fruit is also a source of polyphenols, an antioxidant that has been shown to kill viruses.

BROCCOLI is a cruciferous vegetable high in cancer antidotes like indoles, glucosinolates, and dithiolthiones. It also contains carotenoids (vitamin A). It blocks cell mutations that foreshadow cancer, possibly due to the abundance of chlorophyll. Studies have shown that people who ate more broccoli, broccoli sprouts, cabbage, and Brussels sprouts had a lower risk of colon and rectal cancer. Other studies revealed that women who ate more broccoli were less prone to cancer of the cervix.

BRUSSELS SPROUTS are also a cruciferous vegetable and very important to health. Countries where Brussels sprouts are frequently consumed have a low incidence of gastrointestinal cancer. Researchers have found there are specific substances in Brussels sprouts that retard cancer. These include chlorophyll, dithiolthiones, carotenoids, indoles, and glucosinolates.

CABBAGE is another cruciferous vegetable. It is used in the treatment of colon cancer. The juice heals inflammation of the colon and stomach, and is effective for heartburn. It's also famous for its ulcer-healing capabilities, but should be used only in conjunction with a doctor's prescribed therapy for ulcer treatment. In addition, cabbage has helped eczema, seborrhea, and skin infections. It stabilizes chemical reactions in the body and makes a good poultice for leg ulcers. It's high in calcium, vitamin C, sulfur, vitamin A, and other vitamins. Prepare it fresh and drink immediately, as the vitamins are destroyed very rapidly by air and cooking.

CANTALOUPE has a blood-thinning effect that can help prevent heart attacks and strokes. It's an excellent source of beta-carotene. This is one of my favorite juices and I have a few glasses each week.

CARROTS are an excellent source of beta-carotene. Foods rich in beta-carotene are powerful antioxidants and protect against cancer, boost the immune system, and help the body heal itself. Carrot juice also aids in colitis, constipation, all forms of arthritis, and skin disorders. In addition, the juice helps to improve eyesight, stimulate appetite, and is good for heart disease. Yellowish coloration of the skin may occur when large amounts are consumed. This coloration is harmless and will fade when consumption is reduced. I drink carrot juice daily, usually in combination with other juices such as beet, celery, parsley, ginger, and apple.

CAULIFLOWER is another cruciferous vegetable, rich in vitamin C, potassium, indoles, and essential sulfur compounds. It's been found to reduce the risk of cancer, particularly of the colon, rectum, and stomach, and possibly the prostate and bladder.

CELERY contains vitamins A, B-complex, and C, as well as choline, magnesium, manganese, iron, iodine, and calcium. It's also rich in pectin. The juice helps regulate the nervous system and chemical imbalance by having a calming effect. It is also helpful in diseases of inflammation, including arthritis. It's good for reducing water retention, for weight loss, and for stimulating the sexual drive. It's excellent added to other vegetable juices. Celery is a good brain tonic, enhances memory, is good for dizziness, headache, and arthritis. Celery juice can be diluted with water and used as a sports drink to replace fluid and mineral loss due to sweating. It contains the same ulcer-healing factors found in cabbage juice.

CHARD is high in vitamins A and C, potassium, calcium, and iron. It is used to build energy and as a diuretic and laxative. When the juice of chard is mixed with carrot juice, it helps control urinary tract infections, hemorrhoids, constipation, and skin diseases.

CHERRY is a traditional remedy for the pain of gout. I love this juice even though it takes extra time to remove all of the cherry pits before juicing.

COLLARDS are a close cousin to kale and an excellent source of calcium and vitamins A and C. Collards improve the nervous, respiratory, skeletal and urinary systems, and aid in osteoporosis, arthritis, and colon disorders.

CRANBERRY JUICE is commonly known to help prevent recurrent urinary tract infections when consumed on a regular basis. I usually combine it with grape and apple juices for a natural sweetener.

CUCUMBER promotes urination and is good for the spleen, stomach and large intestine. It's also good for acne and as a blood cleanser.

DANDELION is most often known as a weed, but it's rich in many minerals like calcium, magnesium, potassium, phosphorus, sulfur, silicon, iron, and chlorophyll. Dandelion greens are good for liver disorders and help cleanse the blood. It also promotes the flow of bile in the liver, removes wastes from the bloodstream and liver, and has a healing effect on the kidneys and all infections.

GARLIC is a treasure trove of healing compounds. It acts as a natural antibiotic and blood thinner and can reduce cholesterol levels. Juice a clove and add it to your favorite vegetable mix.

GINGER ROOT has anti-inflammatory properties and will also protect the stomach from irritation caused by nonsteroidal anti-inflammatory drugs. Migraines and motion sickness can also be relieved by ginger juice. A good digestive aid, ginger thins the blood, lowers blood cholesterol, and reduces fever. It's also good as a tonic, for colds, cough, asthma, and relief of vomiting. Ginger contains a substance called gingerol, which may prevent so-called 'little strokes.' I often combine its juice with a carrot and apple combination or an apple, lemon, and wheatgrass combination. A small amount goes a long way—use only a one-quarter to one-half-inch slice per drink.

GRAPEFRUIT is an excellent source of vitamin C. The juice aids digestion and utilization of foods, helps reduce inflammation, and is good in weight loss programs. I have grapefruit juice almost every morning, either alone or combined with orange, pineapple, or tangerine juices.

GRAPE JUICE has long been recommended for healing and cleansing. It's an excellent source of natural sugars, minerals, and vitamins. It's good for edema and cancer, and it combats toxins. It's also a good source of the antioxidant polyphenols.

KALE is one of the best cancer-fighting vegetables. It's the richest of all leafy greens in carotenoids, which are powerful anti-cancer agents. Kale is rich in vitamins A and C, riboflavin, niacin, calcium, magnesium, iron, sulfur, potassium, phosphorus, sodium, and chlorophyll. This member of the cruciferous family is also excellent for arthritis, osteoporosis, and bone loss disorders.

LEMON is a good source of vitamin C and the juice makes an excellent blood purifier. Upon rising each morning, I drink the juice of one-half lemon in a large glass of very warm water. It helps detoxify the entire body and promotes healing. Lemon juice is a traditional appetite stimulant. Place one tablespoon of fresh, unsweetened lemon juice in a glass of water and drink half an hour before meals. This remedy stimulates the flow of saliva and digestive juices.

MELONS make delicious juices. Besides cantaloupe, I also juice casabas, honeydews, and watermelon when in season.

ORANGES are high in vitamin C. One of the most commonly used fruits in America, they also have beta-carotene, which helps fight infections and protects against cancer by supporting the immune system.

PAPAYA is a delicious fruit high in beta-carotene and vitamin C. It is best known for its digestive support, as it contains the enzyme papain. It's also good for inflammation, heartburn, ulcers, back pain, and any disorder involving the digestive system. Chymopapain, contained in papaya, softens tight muscles, which is the reason it is the main ingredient in meat tenderizers. It also has been found helpful in pain relief.

PARSLEY is a powerhouse of nutrients, which is why I juice it daily and combine it with other juices such as carrot, bell pepper, cucumber, and celery. It is very concentrated so you only need small amounts. It helps maintain the thyroid and adrenal functions, is a natural diuretic and aids in digestion.

PARSNIPS are rich in potassium, and sweet and delicious. They're one of my favorite vegetables. Though they contain more fiber than most vegetables, they are still juiceable. They help to keep the digestive tract free of cancer-causing substances, and they are also helpful in colon disorders, constipation, heart problems, and for reducing high blood pressure.

PEPPERS (red, yellow, orange, and green) are also known as bell or sweet peppers and contain more vitamin C than citrus fruits. Because of this, they are good for all types of illnesses.

PINEAPPLE is a wonderful fruit containing bromelain, a digestive enzyme. Bromelain also has an anti-inflammatory action in the body. Swish the raw juice around the site of a tooth extraction to reduce swelling, or eat a homemade frozen pineapple juice Popsicle to soothe a sore throat. I enjoy this juice by itself or combined with grapefruit, especially after a strenuous weight workout in the gym.

SPINACH is an excellent blood cleansing tonic, healing the intestinal tract, hemorrhoids, anemia, and vitamin deficiencies. This juice is rich in all mineral and organic substances. However, those who have liver disease, kidney stones, or arthritis should not drink this juice—the oxalic acid content may prohibit the absorption of the calcium found in the spinach.

TOMATOES are high in lycopene, another type of carotene, which possibly gives the tomato its cancer-protecting qualities. A study of 14,000 American and 3,000 Norwegian men showed that eating tomatoes more than fourteen times a month cut the chances of lung cancer. Other studies have shown tomatoes to be a protection against acute appendicitis and other digestive disorders. The juice also aids in cleansing the body of toxins. Fresh, vine-ripened tomatoes are the best.

TURNIPS produce a juice with twice the amount of vitamin C as oranges or tomatoes. If you have arthritis, you might want to omit oranges and tomatoes from your diet (especially when heated, they have been found to exacerbate inflammation in some people) and use turnips to provide yourself with a source rich in the vitamin C you need. Use the tops, too. Turnip juice is good for the elimination of uric acid and kidney stones derived from uric acid. This is good for people who want to lose weight and for gout sufferers. I like it best when mixed with cabbage and carrot juice.

WATERCRESS is rich in many nutrients, including potassium, calcium, sulfur, sodium, chlorine, magnesium, phosphorus, iron, and iodine. It also contains vitamins A, B-complex, C, and D. Watercress is a powerful intestinal cleanser, and blood cleanser and builder. I like to combine it with the juices of carrot, green pepper, dandelion, and cucumber for hair, nails, skin, bones, collagen formation, and muscle, and to combat vitamin deficiencies.

WHEAT GRASS JUICE is high in chlorophyll and will stop the development of unfriendly bacteria. It is actually akin to human red blood cells and is excellent as a blood purifier. Wheat grass juice is great for energy and body building. However, it's so potent that it can have a nauseating effect in the beginning if you take too much of it. Start off with an ounce and gradually build up. I usually have it combined with my carrot juice unless I need a powerful energy boost, in which case I'll take two to three ounces by itself.

Important Nutrients in Juices

NUTRIENT	JUICE
Beta-carotene	Carrot, cantaloupe, papaya
Folic acid	Orange, kale, broccoli
Vitamin B_6	Kale, spinach, turnip greens
Vitamin C	Peppers, citrus fruit, cabbage
Vitamin E	Asparagus, spinach
Vitamin K	Broccoli, collard greens, kale

Calcium	Kale, collard greens, sweet pepper
Magnesium	Brussels sprouts, cabbage, turnip greens
Potassium	Celery, cantaloupe, tomato
Selenium	Apple, turnip, garlic
Zinc	Carrot, ginger, green peas

There are several terrific books available about juicing. Here are a few of my favorites:

The Juiceman's Power of Juicing by Jay Kordich
Juicing for Life by Cherie Calbom and Maureen Keane
Heinerman's Encyclopedia of Healing Juices by John Heinerman
Fresh Vegetable and Fruit Juices by N.W. Walker
The Joy of Juicing Recipe Guide by Gary and Shelly Null
The Complete Book of Juicing by Michael Murray
Juicing for Good Health by Maureen B. Keane

There are a very few contraindications to juice therapy. Never drink juices from vegetables or fruits to which you are allergic or sensitive. If you react to sugar (either hypo- or hyperglycemic), dilute high sugar content juices, such as carrot and beet, with other low sugar juices such as celery. You also might want to dilute fruit juices with an equal amount of water. Consider stabilizing blood sugar with juices of Jerusalem artichokes and green beans. Avoid juice fasts if you are pregnant or lactating. For diabetics, close supervision is required.

Juicing has made a world of difference in my health, and I know it will make a big difference for you, too.

CHAPTER SEVEN

Exercise for Your Life!

Even the best diet combined with the most potent vitamins will never tune up your muscles the way good exercise will.
—COVERT BAILEY

I live in Los Angeles, the fitness capital of the world. We're so body-conscious, the first thing you might be asked when you meet someone is, "Have you got a good trainer and gym?" I wouldn't be surprised to start seeing ads in the personal columns that read: "Fit, trim, female bodybuilder who bench presses 150 pounds and has a cholesterol level of 150 looking for a tan, strong, toned man who has completed at least a dozen triathlons and has a triglycercide level of 75."

More and more people are beginning to see that beyond the fashionable aspects of fitness are many reasons why it's desirable to stay in good shape. Fitness is a key to enjoying life—it can unlock the energy, stamina, and positive outlook that make each day a pleasure. Ask almost anyone about exercise and they'll say it's good for you. Ask most doctors and they'll say it's one of the main ingredients of health. Along with good eating habits, adequate rest and relaxation, and enough sleep, exercise is an important facet of a total program for well-being. It is one of the common sense ways to take responsibility for your own health and life.

EXERCISE YOUR WAY TO VITALITY

Let's take a closer look at the latest research on all the beneficial effects of exercise on your health—physically, emotionally and spiritually.

MENTAL HEALTH: Exercise physiologists and medical researchers are now discovering that our sense of happiness and well-being is greatly influenced by the presence of certain chemicals and hormones in the bloodstream. Vigorous exercise stimulates the production of two chemicals that are known to lift the spirit, norepinephrine and enkephalin.

A British medical team headed by Dr. Malcolm Carruthers spent four years studying the effect of norepinephrine on 200 people. Their conclusion: "We believe that most people could ban the blues with a simple, vigorous ten-minute exercise session three times a week. Ten minutes of exercise will double the body's level of this essential neurotransmitter, and the effect is long-lasting. Norepinephrine would seem from our research to be the chemical key to happiness."

FATIGUE: Inactivity leads to fatigue. According to Dr. Lawrence Lamb, consultant to the President's Council on Physical Fitness and Sports, part of the reason for this has to do with the way we store adrenaline. Lamb reports, "Activity uses up adrenaline. If it isn't used, adrenaline saps energy and decreases the efficiency of the heart." The downward spiral of energy you feel at the end of the workday will only be worsened if you come home and collapse in an easy chair. "Exercise will get the metabolic machinery out of inertia," says Lamb, "and you'll be refreshed and ready to go."

STRESS: Only when we are in harmony with ourselves physically and mentally can we experience the beauty within and around us and fully share with others. According to the medical profession, eighty to ninety percent of today's illnesses are stress-related. Each one of us can choose to live productive, energetic lives, based on an inner strength and calmness. Stress does not need to be a way of life. Physical exercise is commonly regarded as an effective means of reducing stress and tension. A single dose of exercise works better than tranquilizers as a muscle relaxant among persons with symptoms of anxiety and tension, without the undesirable side effects.

In a classic study of tense and anxious people, Herbert de Vries, Ph.D., former director of the Exercise Physiology Laboratory at the University of Southern California, administered a 400-milligram dose of meprobamate, the main ingredient in many tranquilizers, to a group of patients. On another day he had these same patients take a walk vigorous enough to raise their heart rates to more than one hundred beats per minute. Using an EMG (electromyogram) machine to measure the patients' tension levels as shown by the amount of electrical activity in their muscles, de Vries found that after exercise the electrical activity was twenty percent less than the patients' normal rate. This means that the body was less tense. By contrast, the same patients showed little difference after the dose of meprobamate.

HEART HEALTH: Regular exercise is one important way to help reduce heart attack risk. It improves blood circulation throughout the body. The lungs, heart, other organs, and muscles work together more effectively. Exercise also improves your body's ability to use oxygen and provide the energy needed for physical activity.

Exercise raises HDL (a lipoprotein associated with decreased probability of developing atherosclerosis) and, in some people, also lowers both LDL (a lipoprotein associated with increased probability of developing atherosclerosis) and triglycerides. It can also lower your blood pressure.

OSTEOPOROSIS: This is a condition characterized by decreased bone density. It is never too early or too late to build bone mass. Strength training may be the best exercise for cutting the risk of osteoporosis. Researchers indicate that after the mid-thirties, one percent of our bone mineral mass dissolves each year.

Strength training (weight lifting) workouts tug on the bones, exerting pressure—much more pressure—than non-weight-bearing exercises such as cycling or swimming or even moderate weight-bearing exercises like walking or jogging. That tugging action triggers bone mineralization, stimulating the flow of bone-hardening calcium into the skeleton.

Scientists from the US Department of Agriculture and Tufts University in Boston ran a one-year strength-training test on ten postmenopausal women (average age sixty-seven years old), six of whom worked out, with the other four used as controls. Exercises included double leg press, leg extension, lat (for latissimus dorsi or upper back) pull-down, back extension, and abdominal flexion. At the end of the year, body weight and fat mass had not changed in either group. However, while bone density of the lumbar spine of the control group had decreased by 3.7 percent, it had increased by 6.3 percent in the high-intensity strength-training group.

CANCER: Investigations during the past decade at the Harvard School of Public Health and Center for Population Studies showed that risk of cancer was lower in athletic women. Regular, long-term, vigorous exercise established a lifestyle that lowered the risk of breast cancer and cancers of the reproductive system. The study of several thousand women, both athletic and sedentary, found that the less-active women were nearly twice as likely to suffer from breast cancer and almost three times as likely to suffer from cancer of the reproductive system. The incidence of benign tumors of the breast and reproductive system was also significantly lower in athletic women.

The study points up the importance of starting vigorous exercise at an early age. The great majority of the active women in the study started exercising in high school or earlier. Prevention is clearly a long-term effect. Lead investigator, Rose E. Frisch, Ph.D., said the best time to start exercising is about the age of nine, and to keep it up. Those who began exercising young also avoided fatty foods in favor of those foods that supported their activities, namely fresh fruits and vegetables.

Research shows that women who do not exercise tend to become obese, with increased levels of toxic forms of estrogen. After menopause, this condition is an established breast-cancer risk factor. Studies at the

Norris Comprehensive Cancer Center of the University of Southern California showed that women under age forty who exercised at least four hours a week could cut their risk of the disease up to sixty percent. Those under forty who exercised one to three hours a week lessened their risk by up to thirty percent.

STRENGTH AND ENDURANCE: Even into the ages of eighty and ninety, resistance training (weights) can help or prevent deterioration of muscles and bones and increase energy and strength. A few years ago, Dr. Maria Fiatarone of Penn State and Dr. William Evans at the Tufts USDA Nutrition Research Center on Aging engaged ten nursing home residents, all between the ages of eighty-six and ninety-six, and asked them to sit on exercise benches and lift weights, extending one leg at a time, three times a week. At the end of just eight weeks, the men and women tripled their muscle strength. The absolute weight lifted increased from about fifteen pounds on each leg to forty-three pounds. The researchers found similar results with a twelve-week program of resistance training for sixty- and seventy-year-old men. Muscle strength of all twelve men doubled and tripled. Muscle mass grew by ten to fifteen percent.

Just recently, Dr. Fiatarone and associates were able to show just how important these muscle-building efforts were for enjoyment of everyday living. The scientists recruited one hundred frail nursing home residents between the ages of seventy-two and ninety-eight and placed fifty of them in a strength-training program; the other fifty, the control group, remained sedentary. Over a ten-week period, muscle strength among the fifty exercisers more than doubled, which resulted, the researchers discovered, in a thirty percent increase in spontaneous physical activity. "The exercise intervention," wrote the researchers, "significantly improved habitual gait velocity (speed of walking), stair climbing ability, and the overall level of physical activity." As reported in the *New England Journal of Medicine*, several participants who had been limited to using a walker graduated to the use of only a cane.

WEIGHT CONTROL: Food fuels the furnace of metabolism and exercise fans its fire. Exercise that causes sweating and heavy breathing is sugar-burning exercise. However, overweight people need fat-burning exercise, which requires slow, sustained activity such as walking. Thirty to sixty minutes of vigorous walking every day will help people lose weight. In addition, lifting weights helps increase lean muscle mass. Sufficient muscle mass is desirable because it burns calories, whereas fat stores calories. As a person loses muscle due to inactivity, he or she loses the ability to use calories effectively and usually gains fat and weight even when eating fewer calories. The lack of consistent exercise (both aerobics and weight training) may be the most important factor in explaining why so many of us are overweight.

LONGEVITY: There is no guarantee that exercise will add years to your life, but there's compelling evidence that it might. A study done by Dr. Ralph Paffenbarger, a noted medical researcher at Stanford University, showed that those participants who expended 2,000 calories a week in vigorous exercise such as brisk walking and cross-country skiing lived two years longer than those who did not.

SEX AND LIBIDO: If none of the above interests you, maybe this one will. Exercise makes you sexy. A physically fit body is brimming with sex appeal, and exercise unleashes the libido. A recent comprehensive survey showed that exercise increased the sexual confidence of most women; a third of them made love more often, and nearly half of them had an enhanced capacity to be sexually aroused. Studies also show that exercise is a potent stimulus to hormone production in both men and women, chemically increasing desire by stepping up the levels of such hormones as testosterone and prolactin. It is a scientific fact that exercise can dramatically improve your sex life, at any age.

SPIRITUAL HEALTH: Exercise is also very important for spiritual health. A well-exercised and fit body can relax and meditate better. I know my meditations are deeper when I'm exercising every day.

INDIVIDUALIZE YOUR EXERCISE PROGRAM

There are several different considerations in setting up an exercise program in which your time is used efficiently and for maximum results.

Aerobic Exercise

FREQUENCY: Four to six times per week.

INTENSITY: To find your training rate, subtract your age from 220 and then take sixty percent and eighty percent of this number. This is the target range for your pulse. At the halfway point and at the end of your routine, take your pulse for six seconds and add a zero to the number. You will soon recognize your aerobic training intensity without continually taking your pulse.

DURATION: Twenty to sixty minutes of continuous aerobic activity.

METHOD: Any aerobic activity using the large muscle groups (back and legs) performed continuously in a rhythmic manner is suitable. Fast walking is highly recommended for people of all ages since walking provides all the benefits of aerobic training with a minimum of impact stress on weight-bearing joints like hips, knees, and ankles.

Resistance Training

Whether with cables, barbells, dumbbells, or machines, or even free-hand movements such as push-ups and sit-ups, this type of training is an essential accompaniment to aerobic activities in terms of its effects on body composition and appearance, as well as on cardiovascular, musculoskeletal, and psychological health and well-being. In addition to developing muscular strength and endurance, one of the unique benefits of resistance exercise is that it helps develop and maintain lean body mass, the majority of which consists of muscle tissue. The importance of muscle is that it burns more calories—far more—than other tissues in the body (see Chapter Three on body weight). When you increase muscle mass, you increase the number of calories your body is using every moment of the day, not just during exercise, but also at work, at play, and even when sleeping.

The American College of Sports Medicine recommends at least two sessions a week in which the major muscle groups of the body are exercised to fatigue. A sample program might consist of the following:

Exercise	Sets	Reps
Leg Press or Squat	1-3	10-15
Back/Trunk Extension	1-3	10-12
Lat Pull-Down	1-3	10-12
Chest Press	1-3	10-12
Bent-Over or Machine Row	1-3	10-12
Overhead Shoulder Press	1-3	10-12
Biceps Curl	1-2	10-12
Triceps Extension	1-2	10-12
Abdominal Curl	1-3	15-20
Calf Raise	1-2	15-20

You should strength train at least two, and better yet three, times a week. Allow at least one day between sessions. An ideal system would be to take two days off between training sessions. If all this seems foreign to you, consult a fitness trainer and ask for help setting up a program geared to your specific needs.

Perform at least one set (which consists of a series of continuous repetitions) of each exercise and work up to three sets, time and energy permitting. Use enough weight to cause fatigue in the muscles at the end of each set. When you've finished the set, it should be difficult to perform more repetitions. Rest up to two to three minutes as needed between sets.

Remember, as with aerobic exercise, the goal is to enjoy yourself, not kill yourself. Try to make progress in the amount of weight you lift, but remember that the most important thing is to be consistent. Listen to your body and keep the weights and pace within comfortable limits. Learn as much as you can about strength training and body building. Many fitness magazines are now available on most newsstands. And don't forget to always use good exercise form. You will progress if you just stick to it and don't overdo it.

WALK YOUR WAY TO RADIANT HEALTH

Walking is one of the most convenient ways to exercise, but should be done correctly to get the most benefit. The following tips can help make a walking program beneficial and enjoyable.

- Be aware of your posture. Make sure your shoulders are directly over your hips and your hips are moving front to back, not side to side.
- Keep your head up and your chin parallel to the ground.
- Bend your arms at a ninety-degree angle to help propel you forward.
- Wear comfortable shoes with good support. Make sure they are suitable for the type and amount of walking you will be doing.
- Keep up a good pace by rotating your hips front to back while pushing off with one foot and pulling the other forward.
- Warm up slowly and establish a pace that is brisk, but not exhausting or painful.
- Make sure your weight rolls through your entire foot, from your heel through to your toes. Be light on your feet.
- Easy does it. Start by walking twenty minutes a day and progressively increase the time.
- Hand weights probably won't help your walk. Increase your workload by walking uphill, in sand, or against the wind.
- Drink at least eight eight-ounce glasses of water a day. Drink a large glass of water about fifteen minutes before you start your walk.

Two formulas are used to compute the percentage of maximum heart rate at which one should work to improve aerobic capacity. One method involves multiplying your estimated maximum heart rate (obtained by subtracting your age from 220) times a percentage (from around sixty to eighty percent) that's related to your fitness goals and condition. For example, if you're thirty years old, your estimated maximum heart rate would be 190 beats per minute (220-30=190). Multiplying 190 by sixty percent (or 0.6) equals 114; 190 times eighty percent (0.9) equals 171.

The older, less conditioned, or more obese you are, the better it is to start off easier. Work at the low end of your target heart range and keep up the activity for longer periods. As your condition improves, you can up the intensity so that you're working harder, perhaps seventy to eighty percent (0.7-0.8 times maximum heart rate, which would be 133 to 152 beats per minute).

How do you know what your exercise heart rate is? To take your heart rate, place your index and middle finger just to the side of your windpipe with a slight pressure toward the back of your neck until you feel the pulse in your carotid artery. Count the beats over a ten-second period and multiply by six (or you can count for fifteen seconds and multiply by four) to get your heart rate. Take it about five to seven minutes into your exercise and every ten to fifteen minutes thereafter until you learn what the appropriate intensity feels like.

Constantly trying to increase your exercise intensity will help burn more calories as well as increase your aerobic power, but what matters in the long run is consistency. When in doubt, always be conservative and go easier rather than harder. The real key is to work at activities that you like and at a pace or intensity that you're comfortable with. You should finish each exercise session feeling exhilarated—not exhausted—and looking forward to your next session.

As an alternative to measuring your exercise heart rate (I recommend that you do so for safety, effectiveness, and to enhance your body awareness), you can use the talk test. If you can carry on a conversation without significant difficulty while exercising aerobically, you're working at a level that's well within your capacity.

See the chart below to help you locate your target heart rate easily and quickly.

I love to walk for exercise and, whenever possible, I find beautiful places in nature to do it. I live a couple of minutes from the magnificent Santa Monica mountains and often go there to delight in the scenery while I work out.

Although I enjoy working out at the gym, I think many people get into a rut of only working out indoors. We can feed our bodies and souls more effectively by getting out into nature. In nature, you find renewal and inspiration and pure air to breathe. Walt Whitman said, "Now I know the secret of making the best persons. It is to grow in the open air and sleep and eat with the earth."

There are numerous activities I do outdoors, such as jogging, skating, hiking, cycling, walking, and kayaking. I also do my stretching and yoga at the beach after skating or cycling on the bike path in Santa Monica. In

FIGURE FIVE
MONITORING YOUR PULSE

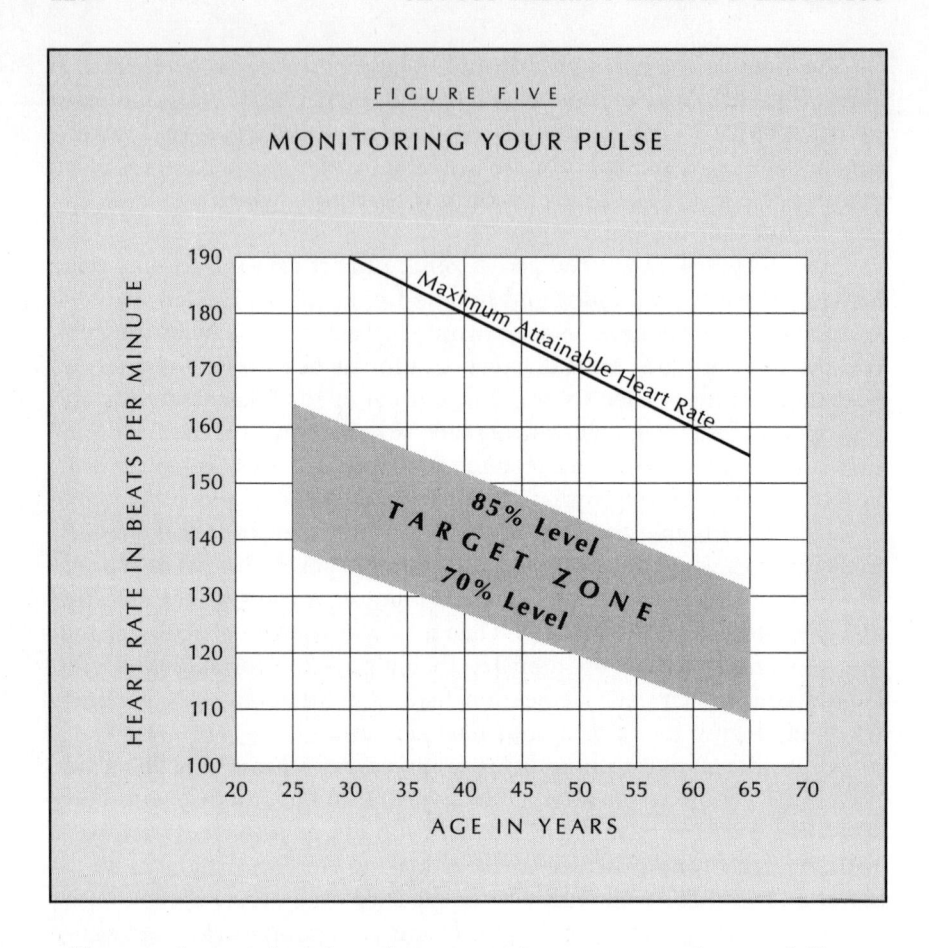

Heart rate chart showing Maximum Attainable Heart Rate and Target Zone (70% Level to 85% Level) plotted against Age in Years (20–70), with heart rate in beats per minute (100–190) on the vertical axis.

addition, I love to kayak and swim in the ocean. Combining different activities (cross-training) assures I'll never get bored and helps me to stay motivated to exercise regularly.

HOW TO DEVELOP IMPRESSIVE ABDOMINALS

As a fitness instructor at UCLA and a personal fitness trainer for more than twenty years, I get asked lots of questions about fitness. One of the most-asked questions is, "Why aren't my sit-ups helping me lose fat around my waist?" Some people mistakenly think they can burn fat around their waists by doing exercises involving muscles in that area, such as sit-ups and side bends. Unfortunately, sit-ups will not reduce observable fat around the waist. Exercises aimed at any single muscle group do not burn enough calories to noticeably reduce fat in that area. Spot reducing doesn't work.

To get rid of undesirable fat through exercise, your body as a whole must burn excess calories by involving as many muscle groups as possible. This means doing exercises like walking, jogging, hiking, rowing, cycling, skating, jumping rope, aerobic dance, or circuit training. Plus, you must do them consistently over a period of time. Fat then comes off from all over the body, not just from the areas being worked.

Like other muscles, your abs (abdominals) thrive on variety and change. And in terms of toning and tightening, they seem to respond best when constantly thrown new stresses.

Have you ever heard someone complain that they've been doing 200 crunches every day for the past six months with no results? Or have you noticed how a new ab routine you could barely finish the first time became pretty easy after a few sessions? That's because muscles adapt to the stress placed upon them pretty quickly. In the case of your abdominals, since you're only lifting your body weight, you can't really increase the load. Once this happens, they aren't being challenged anymore and you stop making improvements in strength and tone. So what do you do? Get out of the rut. Change your routine. Sneak up on your abs and they'll respond. Give them a wake-up call. With your abdominals in a perpetual state of surprise, they're always exerting more effort. And because these following exercises work the muscles in your torso from a variety of angles, you recruit different muscle fibers from each of the abdominal muscles.

I've used these six exercises for abdominal strengthening in my UCLA fitness classes for years. They are among the best. They will not place any stress on your back. You should do them in the order listed so you work your lower abdominal muscles before the uppers. If you tire the upper abdomen first, fatigue will limit the amount of lower abdominal work you can do.

KNEE LIFT REVERSE CRUNCH. Lie on your back, feet up in the air and knees bent at a 90-degree angle so they're directly over your hips. Place your hands behind your head in the basic position. (Don't lace your fingers together or pull on your neck; instead, you put your thumbs behind your ears, fingertips just touching. Lengthen your neck. You should be able to see your elbows out of the corners of your eyes.) Keeping your upper body still and flat on the floor, contract your abdominals and lift your buttocks upward one to two inches, allowing your knees to move slightly toward your chest, then lift your upper torso until your shoulder blades clear the floor. Hold a moment, return to the start, and repeat to fatigue. (By fatigue I mean until your muscles are exhausted and it's difficult to do another repetition. A specific muscle fatigue is a different fatigue from a general over-all body fatigue or tiredness.) Your hands function as a cradle to prevent your lower back from arching. Your lower back should remain flat against the floor throughout the exercise.

BASIC CRUNCH. Lie on your back, knees bent, feet on the floor, with heels a comfortable distance from your buttocks. Align your spine in the neutral position. (Rotate your hips backward and pull your abs inward so your lower back is in contact with the floor. Not only will this neutral position protect your lower back, but it will make the exercises more challenging and effective.) Place your hands behind your head in basic position. Curl your upper body upward in one smooth movement until your shoulder blades clear the floor, exhaling as you lift. Hold a moment, return to the start, and continue until fatigued.

ROTATION CRUNCH. Lie as in the basic crunch. Bend your right leg and place the heel on your left thigh (your right knee will point out to the side). Put your left hand behind your head and your right arm at your side on the floor. Curl your upper body upward and then, leading with your left shoulder, rotate your torso toward your right knee. Return to the start and do several reps until fatigued, then change sides.

CONTINUOUS ROTATION CRUNCH. Lie on your back as you did in the basic crunch. Curl your upper body up until your shoulder blades are off the floor and then, leading with your right shoulder, rotate your torso toward your left knee. Without rolling down, rotate your torso toward your right knee, leading with your left shoulder. Continue your reps without stopping or rolling down until fatigued. (One rotation left and right equals one repetition.)

DOUBLE ARM CRUNCH. Lie on your back with feet in the air, knees bent and directly above hips, so that your calves are parallel to the floor. Extend both arms straight behind your head close to your ears, fingers interlaced. Lift your arms, head, neck, and shoulders up and off the floor in a smooth motion. Hold a moment at the top, lower to the start and do several reps.

OPEN KNEE CRUNCH. Lie on your back with your feet in the air, knees bent and directly over hips. Place your hands behind your head in basic position. Cross your ankles and turn your knees out to the sides. Curl your upper body upward and forward until your shoulder blades clear the floor. Hold a moment, lower to the start and repeat to complete reps.

When doing these abdominal exercises, exhale when you lift, inhale as you lower. Don't just go through the motions. Think about what you're doing! Research has shown that if you visualize each contraction you may use more muscle fibers. Always work your abs slowly and with control. Don't bounce up off the floor between repetitions. You're moving at the right speed if you feel a contraction through your abdominals on the way up and on the way down. Also, when you exercise, be sure to wear comfortable clothing that allows you freedom of movement as well as evaporation of perspiration.

HOW TO ATTAIN OPTIMUM FLEXIBILITY

Take time to stretch every day. A flexible body, especially for an active person, greatly reduces the chance of injury because muscles that restrict the natural range of motion in the joints are susceptible to pulls, tears, and stress injuries.

For the less athletic, flexibility can provide relief from everyday muscle tension and stiffness, and is also crucial for proper posture.

When we lack flexibility, our bodies compensate in ways that create poor posture, resulting in mechanical imbalances in the back, hip, and neck. These imbalances pull the body out of line, causing stress, strain, and even worse posture. Inflexible joints and weak muscles in the shoulder and chest can cause rounded shoulders, which can lead to kyphosis (humpbacked spine), a sunken chest and impaired respiratory capacity.

Tight calf muscles can place undue stress on the foot, leading to a variety of orthopedic problems, including painful Achilles tendinitis.

Tight hip-flexor muscles, hamstrings, and back muscles can rotate the pelvis forward, resulting in excessive curvature of the lower back, chronic lower back pain, and sciatica.

Drooping your head forward may produce dizziness and chronic strain on the muscles along the back of the neck, resulting in neck and shoulder pain.

The preferred method for enhancing flexibility (which can increase a muscle's length) is through a stretching or yoga program. Muscles exert force by pulling, not pushing. Most muscles attach to bones and cross over one or more joints. When the muscles contract and shorten, they cause a limb or body part to move in a particular direction. The external opposing force can be applied by gravity, by the contraction of an opposite muscle, or by a stretching partner.

The approach to increasing flexibility in a progressive stretching program is related to the overload principle used to build muscle strength. To increase muscle strength, you must regularly contract the muscle against progressively more resistance with a slightly greater force than that to which it is accustomed. In time the muscle responds to the overload by becoming stronger. Similarly, to increase flexibility, you must regularly stretch the muscle slightly beyond its normal length. It will adapt to this overload by increasing its length, thereby rewarding you with a greater range of joint motion. To increase a muscle's length, you must regularly pull it about ten percent beyond its normal length: that is the point where your muscles feel stretched enough to be slightly uncomfortable but not enough to cause pain. Typically, you should hold this position for thirty seconds, relax, and then repeat the stretch three to four times. Studies show that you should stretch three to seven days a week, holding the stretch for at least thirty seconds, to increase your flexibility.

For six weeks, fifty-seven men and women with tight hamstrings (back of the thigh) stretched that muscle for different periods. Groups held stretches either fifteen, thirty, or sixty seconds, or didn't stretch at all. Only when the muscle was stretched for thirty seconds or more did it respond by lengthening, thereby allowing more range of motion. Anything less than that was just going through the motions. As reported in the September 1994 issue of *Physical Therapy*, the surprise was that more wasn't better—the minute-long stretch was only about as effective as the half-minute hold. This is the first study to test which stretch offered the most benefits over a long period of time.

It's worth tacking those thirty seconds of stretching onto your walking, cycling or other exercise routine, says study leader William D. Bandy, Ph.D., PT, associate professor of physical therapy at the University of Central Arkansas. Tight hamstrings may force your quadriceps muscles (front of the thigh) to work harder, and that may set you up for knee problems. In addition, tight muscles can be injured by sudden overstretching.

Dr. Bandy feels that people should try to include stretching in their everyday lives. The best time to stretch is whenever you're really going to do it. I teach my fitness clients and students to stretch during commercials while they're watching television. That's a thirty-second to one-minute period or longer. If I were to ask them to warm up, run, and come back and stretch, I don't think they'd do it.

I enjoy doing some type of stretching every day. My rule of thumb is to stretch half the time I've engaged in an aerobic or weight workout. For example, if I cycled, jogged, or did a weight workout for thirty minutes, I would devote fifteen minutes to stretching. I usually do five minutes of stretching before the aerobic workout and the remainder after the workout. When lifting weights, I stretch before, during the workout—in between sets—and after the workout is over. Besides elongating your muscles and increasing flexibility, stretching is also a wonderful way to breathe deeply and just relax.

An excellent book for stretching is *Stretching* by Bob Anderson. If you'd like to start stretching today and want some ideas, here are five important stretches. I do these before and after my aerobic or weight workouts.

GENERAL FLEXIBILITY AND UPPER THIGHS. Sitting with soles of the feet together, grasp ankles and pull toward groin area. Then place hands on the inside of your knees and push them out and down toward floor until you feel a stretch. Hold ten to thirty seconds and repeat.

QUADRICEPS. While standing, bend one knee and grasp ankle behind you. Pull ankle toward buttocks until you feel a stretch. Hold ten to thirty seconds. Repeat. Alternate legs. Variation: use a towel to help you stretch if you cannot easily reach your feet.

HAMSTRING. Sit on the floor with one leg straight, the other leg bent with heel against upper part of the other inner thigh. Lean over straight leg and grasp calf or ankle, wherever your extended arms reach, pulling chin towards your knee. Keep knee straight and soft (don't lock knee). Hold ten to thirty seconds. Repeat. Alternate legs.

CALF. Stand facing a wall. Using hands against the wall for balance, lower hips by bending knees toward ground and wall until you feel a stretch in lower calf. Do not allow heels to come off the floor. Hold ten to thirty seconds, relax. Repeat. Alternate legs.

LOWER BACK. Lie on back. Raise one knee to chest, keeping opposite leg slightly bent. Grasp with hands and pull in towards chest. Hold the stretch for thirty to sixty seconds. Relax and repeat with opposite leg, then both legs together. End by curling your head up toward your knees.

HOW TO STAY MOTIVATED

Every person who exercises regularly, whether an athlete or not, will have to cope with lack of motivation, boredom, or burnout at one time or another. Here are a few helpful tips that can keep you motivated to stick to your routine.

MAKE A COMMITMENT. Once you decide to make exercise a part of your life, take precautions that will keep you on the right track. Arrange your personal circumstances so your lifestyle supports your commitment. Make time for exercise. Seek the support of others, but realize the prime reason to exercise must come from within yourself.

DEFINE YOUR FITNESS GOALS. Write down realistic short term and long term goals. Your goals provide a path for a specific direction and let you know how you are doing.

REPETITION. Repetition is the key to mastery. It takes twenty-one days for the mind and body to create a new habit. During this time, remind yourself that for at least twenty-one consecutive days you'll stick to your new exercise program. It also helps to share your goals with a friend.

REAFFIRM YOUR FITNESS GOALS DAILY. Post your goals where you can see them every day. In addition to a concise list of goals, make a list of your plans for achieving them.

VISUALIZE YOUR FITNESS GOALS. Visualizing your fitness goals as already completed will increase your motivation, keep you on course, and hasten your success.

KEEP TRACK OF YOUR DAILY PROGRESS. Plan your workouts in advance and keep track of your progress in a diary or on a calendar. Seeing your daily accomplishments is encouraging and increases self-esteem.

BE REALISTIC. Don't set yourself up to fail. If you've just started a walking program and are now up to two miles nonstop, don't make it one of your goals to run a marathon at the end of the month.

EXERCISE WITH SOMEONE ELSE. Working out is easier when you have someone to give you support. Many times I've been grateful for friends who got me through workouts I might have skipped if I were working out alone.

USE AFFIRMATIONS. Affirmations greatly enhance motivation. They can be mental, verbal, written, or recorded on a cassette for later listening. Keep affirmations positive and in the present.

REWARD YOURSELF. You've kept your agreement, you've worked out hard, you've been consistent, and you're seeing positive results. Reward yourself. Rewards increase motivation and create positive associations toward your exercise program.

It's always prudent to check with your doctor if you are middle-aged or older, have not been physically active, and plan a relatively vigorous exercise program.

Like eating habits, exercise is a lifetime commitment. And if you stop exercising, the beneficial effects are rapidly lost; it requires consistent reinforcement.

Will exercise add years to your life? Maybe, maybe not. But you can expect it to improve the quality of your life in the years you have. Being fit will improve your vigor and make you feel good, physically, emotionally, and mentally. It gives you a psychological lift and strengthens your sense of accomplishment. The discipline associated with exercise also makes you feel good about yourself. So get started now. The only things you have to lose are some pounds, sleepless nights, and fatigue. Go for it!

CHAPTER EIGHT

Sweating Your Way to Radiant Health

For thousands of years, cultures throughout the world have enjoyed the therapeutic benefits of saunas, from the elaborate bath/sauna/exercise complexes of the Romans, to the simple but effective sweat lodge structures of the Scandinavians and Native Americans. These cultures recognized the many therapeutic benefits of the sauna, fully enjoying these benefits in a community setting.

In Finland, the sauna is an historic tradition. According to Paavo Airola in his book *Health Secrets From Europe*, for over a thousand years the sauna has been an important part of Finnish life and Finnish culture, cherished by every Finnish man, woman, and child. The sauna is credited for much of the rugged vitality and endurance—the *sisu*—of the Finnish people. In a country of approximately five million people, there are an estimated 700,000 saunas—one for every seven people! Airola writes, "Most Finnish saunas are in separate buildings specially constructed for this purpose. Every farm has its own sauna, usually built on the shore of a lake or river. Most family houses in the city have saunas built on the lot, usually in the back yard."

In Finland, business meetings between strangers are often conducted in the soothing surroundings of the sauna, and it has been suggested that the combination of high heat and nakedness enabled the Finns to successfully negotiate the international trade minefields between East and West during the Cold War. There is a saying in Finland that one must behave in the sauna just as in church. They consider taking saunas very sacred. What can we learn from the Finns about the benefits of saunas?

THE HEALTH BENEFITS OF SWEATING

Sweating is not only an important part of our physical well-being, but in these modern times of water and airborne pollution, toxic chemicals, heavy metals, and poor dietary and exercise habits, the therapeutic internal cleansing of regular sweating is critical to maintain a healthy body and mind.

The hot, dry air of the sauna is therapeutically different from the steam room sauna. The dry sauna causes profuse sweating, with the air itself absorbing the sweat. But the water-saturated air of the steam room doesn't readily accept the sweat released by the body. The steam room makes you feel hotter because your sweat doesn't evaporate and carry away the heat. This raises a question: Is it better to be warm on the inside or sweaty on the outside?

That depends on what you want from either system. When exposed to heat of any kind, blood vessels in the skin dilate to allow more blood to flow to the surface. This activates the millions of sweat glands that cover the body. The fluid in the blood hydrates the sweat glands, which pour the water into the skin's surface. As the water evaporates from the skin, it draws heat from the body. It's nature's cooling system.

Either the sauna or the steam room can be used to relax and unwind, but the dry sauna clearly has more therapeutic benefits. The dry sauna has an advantage over a steam room by helping to rid the body of more toxic metals picked up from our environments. Of course, the kidneys take out many of these toxins, but a daily sweat can help reduce the body's accumulation of lead, mercury, and nickel in addition to cadmium, sodium, sulfuric acid, and cholesterol.

The sauna is also more beneficial over the steam room if weight loss is desired, because of the energy expenditure. Compared to the steam room, the sauna places a greater demand on the body in terms of using up calories and therefore assists in fat loss. The heart has to work harder to send more blood to the capillaries under the skin. The energy required for that process is derived from the conversion of fat and carbohydrates to calories. In addition, the sweat glands must work to produce sweat, which also requires energy and more calories. Many studies show that a person can burn up to 300 calories during a sauna session, the equivalent of a two- to three-mile jog or an hour of moderate weight training.

From sweating, you can lose up to a quart of water during a twenty-minute sauna. Without replacement, such a high water loss can lead to disruption of normal heart rhythms, and cause fatigue and nausea. Therefore, I recommend drinking fresh fruit juice or water before, during, and after the sauna. Any attempt to lose weight by depriving your body of replacement fluid is extremely risky and can land you in the hospital. I also suggest eating plenty of leafy greens and a variety of other vegetables to replace essential minerals such as iron, zinc, copper, and magnesium that are lost in sweat.

SAUNAS ARE BODY-FRIENDLY

Sweating by overheating the body in a dry sauna also produces these effects:

- Speeds up metabolic processes of vital organs and inhibits the growth of pathogenic bacteria or virus. The vital organs and glands, including endocrine and sex glands, are stimulated to increased activity.

- Creates a 'fever' reaction that kills potentially dangerous viruses and bacteria and increases the number of leukocytes in the blood, thereby strengthening the immune system—important for fighting colds, flu, and cancer and bolstering resistance to infections. Sweating increases and accelerates the body's own healing and restorative capacity.
- Places demands upon the cardiovascular system, making the heart pump harder and producing a drop in diastolic blood pressure.
- Stimulates vasodilation of peripheral vessels, which relieves pain and speeds healing of sprains, strains, bursitis, peripheral vascular diseases, arthritis, and muscle pain.
- Promotes relaxation, thereby lending a feeling of well-being.

There is a great health benefit of fever. Nobel Prize winner Dr. Andre Lwoff, a French virologist, believes that high temperature during infection helps combat the growth of virus. "Fever should not be brought down with drugs," he said.

Two medical doctors, Werner Zable and Josef Issels, have this to say about fever: "Artificially induced fever has the greatest potential in the treatment of many diseases including cancer."

A German physical education professor named Dr. Ernst has found that there are no cancer patients among marathon runners. He conducted a study of marathon runners who logged about twenty miles a day. Analyzing their sweat, he found it contained cadmium, lead, and nickel. Ernst concluded that these athletes excreted these potential cancer-causing elements from their bodies by perspiring. He and other scientists conclude that it is necessary to sweat profusely at least once a day to maintain good health.

Usually only the most active of athletes achieve sweat through heavy exercise on a daily basis, the deep, prolonged, therapeutic type that will flush out toxins and heavy metals. Unfortunately, most people do not exercise enough or spend time in saunas to sweat frequently to eliminate these accumulated toxins. And yet we now know to maintain a healthy body and mind, everyone needs to eliminate and flush out these accumulated poisons regularly. Those who are unable to exercise heavily for whatever reason have an even greater need to create a regular sweat. Deep sweating through daily saunas is the best method of doing this.

When saunas are used regularly, studies have shown such benefits as improvement of blood circulation, restored youthfulness, toxin and heavy metal reduction, weight control, cellulite reduction, skin cleansing and rejuvenation, allergy reduction, rash reduction, and muscle and joint pain reduction.

THE BEST SAUNA FOR HOME OR OFFICE

My personal preference among saunas is the radiant heat infrared sauna made by a company called *Health Mate*. This is the same sauna used by many doctors, physical therapists, and professional athletes. Using safe and UL approved radiant heat infrared technology, similar to that used by doctors and physical therapists to treat muscle injury and strains, and hospitals to warm newborn babies, has greater therapeutic results than the high temperature saunas. I have used my Health Mate sauna for ten years and consider it an essential part of my holistic health regimen. They're designed to fit into any home or office and come in a variety of sizes and beautiful woods. Mine includes a stereo system with speakers, radio, and tape player. I usually listen to motivational tapes in the sauna.

Unlike the old technology saunas with their high air temperature, which some people find uncomfortable because of the choking sensation, radiant heat infrared saunas warm the body muscle directly, only warming the air to a comfortable level, allowing for fresh air ventilation so that you never get that feeling of suffocation.

Because a person is able to use this type of sauna for a longer time, one is able to reap greater benefits than through the use of regular saunas. Body temperature will rise slightly, and the body will react in the normal manner by raising the heart rate to a mild aerobic range, increasing blood flow, opening up the capillaries for greater blood flow to sluggish areas, opening up the pores, and creating the deep sweat that flushes out the toxins.

On a cautionary note, certain people need to approach saunas slowly and cautiously. Folks over age sixty are in a high-risk group for undiagnosed heart disease. The sauna is no place to find out. See your doctor before using the sauna. So should those who are on regular medication, obese, pregnant, or have thyroid, kidney or respiratory problems, diabetes, or high blood pressure.

Sweating has been proven to be one of the healthiest things a body can do. Nothing beats the feeling of overall well-being or the health benefits you get after you've worked up a good sweat, and the easiest key to a good sweat is a sauna. (For more information on the portable Health Mate sauna, see the Resource Directory.)

CHAPTER NINE

Massage: The Healing Touch

Treat yourself to a massage. It can be equivalent to a long nap, in terms of refreshment; it not only gives you energy, it calms your nerves, releases stress and makes you glow with a feeling of well-being.
—ALEXANDRA STODDARD

One of the earliest and most basic forms of healing, massage has been used successfully throughout history as a means of restoring and maintaining well-being. Skin is the human body's largest organ. It accounts for nineteen percent of our body weight and covers about nineteen square feet. From the ancient Greek gymnasia and Roman baths to modern day spas and health clubs, massage has been recognized for its health enhancing effects. This age-old healing practice has experienced a great resurgence in popularity in the last quarter century. Today, massage is a flourishing art form.

Athletes, dancers, over-stressed executives, and weary housewives or househusbands have all discovered its pleasure and benefits. From infancy to old age, massage has been found to enhance general health and well-being. Because it is used for health promotion as well as for its curative aspect, it can truthfully be said, "If you have a body, you can benefit from therapeutic massage." Once experienced, massage often becomes a regular part of maintaining wellness. Therapeutic massage is truly one of the most pleasurable and healthy treatments life has to offer.

As a result of its acceptance both as a healing tool and relaxation vehicle, many schools have been founded which emphasize various techniques. Therapeutic massage has many applications and variations. Many of the therapeutic effects of massage recognized by personal and clinical experience over the years have been supported by scientific research. In addition to the commonly known benefits of relaxation and stress relief, new applications for therapeutic massage are surfacing in areas related to mental and emotional well-being, infant care, aging, athletics, and other special situations. Exciting new discoveries link touch, and therapeutic massage, to improved immune system functioning.

PROVEN EFFECTIVE

Why include massage as part of your life? Consider the numerous benefits. Therapeutic massage reduces stress and tension, improves circulation, aids in removing cellulite, relieves muscle spasms, and helps to rid the body of toxins and extra retained fluids. It also helps improve the skin. Of course, it feels fantastic, but the therapeutic benefits of massage have largely been relegated to intuition and ancient wisdom until recently. Science is now confirming what we knew in our hearts—massage is good medicine. Dr. Diana J. Wilkie, an associate professor at the University of Washington School of Nursing, is a nationally recognized pain researcher. Together with her colleagues, Wilkie has documented the intensity of pain (as well as the pulse and respiratory rates) of hospice residents with cancer, before and after they received massage therapy. Wilkie's group found that massage therapy provided immediate relaxation as well as pain relief. Their study results will be used to help plan a larger study of massage therapy as a means of relieving cancer pain and stress. As a result of her study and exemplary contribution, Wilkie has recently become the first recipient of the National Hospice Foundation Research Award.

The University of Miami's School of Medicine opened what they call "the first institution in the world for basic and applied research on the sense of touch"—The Touch Research Institute (TRI). More than fifty TRI studies have shown massage to have positive effects on conditions from colic to hyperactivity to diabetes to migraines—in fact, on every malady TRI has studied thus far. Their projects have included researching the impact of massage on the immune functioning of AIDS and cancer patients, the effects of touch on patients with addictions, and the effects of touch on physical and emotional development. Psychologist Tiffany Field directs a staff of twenty-eight students, volunteers, and massage therapists, and collaborates with researchers at several universities, including Miami, Duke, and Harvard.

The Institute reports some impressive initial results.

- Premature "crack babies," each given three fifteen-minute massages a day for ten days, suffered fewer complications, displayed markedly more mature motor behavior, and gained an astounding twenty-eight percent in weight by the end of the test period.
- Abused children living in a shelter became more sociable and active with regular massage.
- Preschoolers were more focused when given massages.
- Adult office workers were more alert when given regular massages.
- HIV positive males who received five massages a week for a month showed improved immune function and significantly reduced anxiety and stress.

Field worries that Americans aren't getting enough touch, especially with growing concerns about sexual harassment and abuse in school and workplaces. Even in preschools, touch has become taboo. (The National Education Association, which represents two million teachers, sums the matter up in a slogan: teach, don't touch.) "The implications for children involve significant effects on their growth, development and emotional well-being," observes Field. She says America is suffering from an epidemic of skin hunger and talks about a "dose of touch" as if it were a vitamin.

At the TRI preschool, teachers encourage positive touch. They dole out unlimited hugs, back rubs, and shoulder pats. Massages are as much a part of the curriculum as story time. According to the August 1997 issue of *Life Magazine*, most of the forty children (from six months to five years old) get a daily fifteen-minute rubdown. This leaves them more alert, more responsive, and able to sleep more deeply. TRI research set up another study in which volunteers over age sixty were given three weeks of massage and then were trained to massage toddlers at the preschool. Giving massages proved even more beneficial than getting them. The elders exhibited less depression, lower stress hormones, and less loneliness. They had fewer doctor visits, drank less coffee, and made more social phone calls.

Massage is clearly therapeutic.

MASSAGE IN YOUR FITNESS OR SPORTS PROGRAM

Many sports and fitness enthusiasts include regular therapeutic massage as part of their conditioning programs. There is a growing awareness that a complete workout includes not only the exercise itself, but also caring for the wear-and-tear and minor injuries that naturally occur with strenuous movement. The physiological and psychological benefits of massage make it an ideal complement to a total conditioning program.

Anyone who routinely stretches their physical limits through movement such as running, cycling, hiking, swimming, dancing, tennis and other racquet sports, strength training, and aerobics can benefit from regular massage. In fact, anyone who experiences regular physical stress like mothers with small children, carpenters, gardeners, or those who use their bodies strenuously in their work, will find relief with therapeutic massage.

Massage is beneficial when starting a conditioning program because it helps you get into good shape faster, and with less stiffness and soreness. It helps you recover faster from heavy workouts and relieves conditions which may cause injury. Did you know that a muscle which as been worked to its maximum will recover only twenty percent after a thirty-five minute rest, but will recover 100 percent after a five minute massage? Needless to say, massage is especially effective for athletes when given before and after strenuous workouts or competition. And it can be something to look forward to after a workout—a healthy reward.

Regular exercise increases vigor and promotes a general sense of well-being. If done in moderation, exercise can help relieve the effects of stress, and has been linked to decrease in psychological depression. The fun of sports and physical activity is a healthy pleasure and greatly improves the quality of life. Regular exercise produces positive physical results, like increased muscular strength and endurance, more efficient heart and respiratory functioning, and greater flexibility.

These positive physical changes occur as the body gradually adapts to the greater demands put on it by regular exercise. Conditioning has been described as a process of pushing the physical limits ('tearing down'), recovery, and then building up to meet the new demands. Recovery is often overlooked, but is essential for the rebuilding phases, and to realizing the benefits of a conditioning program.

The 'tearing down' phase of the adaptation process often involves stiffness and soreness, especially when the amount of movement is significantly increased from what the body has been used to in the past. Referring to post-exercise soreness, people often comment about finding muscles "I didn't even know I had."

Delayed muscle soreness (twenty-four to forty-eight hours after exercise) may be caused by any of a number of different factors. Some possible causes are minor muscle or connective tissue damage, local muscle spasms that reduce blood flow, or a buildup of waste products (metabolites) from energy production.

Trigger points or stress points may also cause muscle soreness and decreased flexibility. These points are specific spots in muscle and tendons which cause pain when pressed, and which may radiate pain to a larger area. They are not bruises, but are thought by some to be small areas of spasm. Trigger points may be caused by sudden trauma (like falling or being hit), or may develop over time from the stress and strain of heavy physical exertion or from repeated use of a particular muscle.

Heavily exercised muscles may also lose their capacity to relax, causing chronically tight (hypertonic) muscles and loss of flexibility. Lack of flexibility is often linked to muscle soreness, and predisposes you to injuries, especially muscle pulls and tears. Blood flow through tight muscles is poor (ischemia), which also causes pain.

Therapeutic massage helps the body recover from the stresses of strenuous exercise, and facilitates the rebuilding phase of conditioning.

The physiological benefits of massage include improved blood and lymph circulation, muscle relaxation, and general relaxation. These in turn lead to removal of waste products and better cell nutrition, normalization and greater elasticity of tissues, deactivation of trigger points, and faster healing of injuries. It all adds up to relief from soreness and stiffness, better flexibility, and less potential for future injury.

In addition to general recovery, massage may also focus on specific muscles used in a sport or fitness activity. Areas of greater stress for runners and dancers are in the legs, for swimmers in the upper body, for tennis players in the arms. These areas are more likely to be tight, lose flexibility, and develop trigger points.

Adequate recovery is also a major factor in avoiding the overtraining syndrome. Overtraining is characterized by irritability, apathy, altered appetite, increased frequency of injury, increased resting heart rate, and/or insomnia. It occurs when the body is not allowed to recover adequately between bouts of heavy exercise. Therapeutic massage helps you avoid overtraining by facilitating recovery through general relaxation, and its other physiological effects.

You may also have your own unique trouble spots, perhaps from past injuries. A massage therapist can pay special attention to these areas, monitor them for developing problems, and help keep them in good condition. An experienced massage therapist can also complement treatment received from other health care professionals for various injuries.

FOR THE COMPETITOR

During competitions, such as tournaments and races, athletes push themselves to their limits performing at maximum effort. At these times, explains chiropractor Joel Bienenfeld of Pacific Palisades, California, sports massage is used to prepare for and recover from the stresses of all-out effort.

PRE-EVENT: Pre-event sports massage is given within the four hours preceding an event to improve performance and help decrease injuries. It is normally shorter (ten to fifteen minutes) than a regular conditioning massage, and focuses on warming up the major muscles to be used and getting the athlete in a good mental state for competition. Certain massage techniques can help calm a nervous athlete, and others can be stimulating.

INTER- /INTRA-EVENT: Inter- and intra-event massage is given between events or in time-outs to help athletes recover from the preceding activity and prepare for the activity coming up. It is also brief and focuses on the major muscles stressed in the activity.

POST-EVENT: Post-event massage is given after a competition and is mainly concerned with recovery. Recovery after competition involves not only tissue normalization and repair, but also general relaxation and mental calming. A recovery session might be fifteen to ninety minutes in length.

Some tournaments and races provide sports massage for competitors, or you may want to schedule an appointment before and/or after an event with your own massage therapist. You don't have to be a professional athlete to benefit from therapeutic massage.

Traditional Western (Swedish) massage is currently the most common approach used for conditioning programs. It is frequently supplemented by other massage therapy approaches including deep tissue, trigger point work, and acupressure. Some massage therapists have special training in sports massage and greater experience working with athletes. Discuss your conditioning program with your massage therapist to choose the approach best suited for your needs.

MAKING THE MOST OF YOUR CONDITIONING MASSAGE

- Schedule your conditioning massage (thirty to ninety minutes duration) for after your workout or on a rest day.
- Cool down completely after your workout before getting a massage.
- Take a shower, sauna, steam bath, or Jacuzzi before a massage, if available. This will give a head start to the recovery and relaxing process.
- Tell the massage therapist about your current activity, work-out, and/or sport participation so she or he can tailor the massage to your unique needs. The massage therapist may want to talk to your personal trainer, aerobics teacher, or coach to confer about your situation.
- Let the massage therapist know about upcoming competitions or events. It might affect their approach to an individual session.
- Tell the massage therapist about past or recent injuries which continue to cause problems or pain. The massage therapist may want to talk to your health care provider about your injuries, either to help the healing process or to avoid further damage.
- Give the massage therapist feedback on painful areas that may need special care or attention.

- Depending on your general physical condition, your first massage may leave you slightly sore. It's like exercise—your body may have to adjust to it. As tissues become healthier, you will appreciate deeper and more vigorous massage.
- Just like your regular exercise or training schedule, plan ahead for regular massage appointments. 'Regular' means once-a-week to once-a-month.

MORE CLOSENESS AND INTIMACY

Massage is also an excellent way to become comfortable being touched by another person. This may sound elementary, but for many being touched in a nonsexual, caring fashion is not an accepted part of our daily lives.

Dr. Barbara De Angelis, world renowned relationship expert and author of several best-selling books, including *Are You the One For Me?* and *Real Moments*, feels that massage is a terrific way to foster closeness and intimacy. She says that "one of the biggest problems between couples is the lack of real intimacy. In my workshops, I teach people that every moment is an opportunity to make love, whether we express that love sexually or not. I suggest scheduling what I call 'planned intimacy'; a time when you plan to be together with someone you feel close with, without specifically planning to be sexually intimate. This is a perfect time to give and receive a massage with your partner."

Dr. De Angelis explains that massage is an ideal way to express one's love and caring for another person through the hands. To be touched lovingly, without feeling like someone is trying to excite you, can create a great deal of trust and intimacy between two people. She adds that one of the most common complaints from women about loving relationships is that they don't get enough non-sexual touching and caressing. Massage is not only a wonderful way to receive that healing touch, but also a way to teach your partner how you would like to be touched.

VARIATIONS

In massage, one person uses his or her hands to touch and manipulate either one's own body or the body of another. There are many types of massage.

ACUPRESSURE is a traditional healing treatment used in China, and consists of pressing on certain points related to all parts of the body and to different health problems. For example, the Chinese claim that a toothache can be relieved by pressing certain points underneath the eyes. Shiatsu is a more modern version of acupressure, developed in

Japan. In this form, the ball of the thumb is usually used. Kum Nye is a Tibetan form of massage only recently introduced in the West.

POLARITY THERAPY is said to be derived from yogic and spiritual practices in India. Often, the therapist's hands are held far apart while applying pressure and rocking motions to specific 'poles of energy' in the body.

TRAGER massage usually involves vibratory and shaking motions, and, like Polarity, may be performed while the recipient is clothed.

ZONE THERAPY OR FOOT/HAND REFLEXOLOGY is not really a complete massage because only the feet or hands are treated. For example, the technique claims to affect remote parts, such as the eyes, by massaging the junction between the second and third toes. Its practitioners believe that every part of the body is mapped into a specific part of the feet and hands, and that by massaging the hands or feet only, effective benefits are obtainable.

REICHIAN massage is intended to break down 'body armor,' which is said to be formed as a defense against releasing emotions and built-up tensions. Much attention is paid to breathing and verbal analysis.

PROSKAUER massage also works with breathing, and is usually light and subtle. The more advanced techniques such as deep tissue and lymph massage and Rolfing should not be attempted by people not specially trained in these methods. It is important for the massager not to work beyond his or her understanding.

Of course, the easiest way to be massaged is to pay a professional masseuse for a therapeutic massage. But it's not always necessary to pay for such a service if you have thoughtful friends who wish to share in the experience. Often, it is more enjoyable to have a friend massage you rather than a stranger, even though your friend may not be a professional therapist.

If you want to learn more about the technique of massage, check in your community for classes. You may look into your local YMCA, hospital or community centers. Often times they offer massage classes. Look in the Yellow Pages under 'Massage Schools.' You might also consider reading books and gathering information on the topic. An excellent introduction to massage and a variety of bodywork therapy is *Bodywork* by Thomas Claire (see LivingArts in the Resource Directory).

For those of you who would like some pointers so you can get started right away, consider the following.

THE MAIN INGREDIENTS FOR GOOD MASSAGE

The only good way to do massage is with oil. Your hands cannot apply pressure and at the same time move smoothly over the surface of the skin without some kind of lubricating agent. Oil fulfills this function better than anything else. The skin will absorb most of the oil and so I don't recommend petroleum products like baby oil. If you can eat it, it's probably okay to use on your skin. I personally like to use cold-pressed almond or canola oil by Spectrum Naturals which is available in health food stores.

What about a massage table? Its advantage is that it eliminates some bending and stooping as you work. This means that if you are giving a long massage, your own back is less likely to get tired. A table also makes it easy for you to change your position around the person you are massaging—from head to leg, from one side to the other side—without a break in the flow of your massage.

When looking for tables, take a number of things into account. The standard twenty-seven inch wide table is wide enough for most people although the twenty-nine inch wide ones can be more comfortable. The price of portable tables runs from as low as $250 for a twenty-four inch wide table with no head rest (face cradle) to about $750 for a wide table with good covering and a headrest. A headrest is essential for people with neck tension and/or injuries because it permits lying face down without twisting the neck. Look for a table that is strong, stable, and silent even under vigorous massage. It should not rock, wiggle, or squeak. It should be comfortable and secure to lie on, and should easily support two or three adults.

Adjustable height is another added bonus on tables. Look for those with at least a five-inch range, preferably nine or twelve. Adjustable height allows you to find your best working height by trial and error, allows people of different heights to use the same table, and gives a larger resale market.

Before buying, find out if the warranty covers both faulty materials and workmanship and for how long the builder has been in business. I keep a massage table in my home so when I get a massage, the massage therapist doesn't have to bring one.

THAT SPECIAL TOUCH

I consulted two of my favorite massage therapists, Jackie Day in Bandon, Oregon and Karen McGuire in Coos Bay, Oregon, to find out the essential points in giving a good massage. This is what I learned. A person receiving a massage enters a universe where the sense of touch alone is important. For this reason, any outside noise and bustle can be extremely disconcerting. Make the room as comfortable as possible. Dim the lights. Some people also prefer tranquil, soothing music.

The next thing to consider is warmth. Nothing destroys an otherwise good massage more quickly than coldness. The temperature in the room in which you give a massage should be about seventy degrees F. or slightly more, and be free of drafts.

It is insignificant whether you start at the top or bottom of the body. Your choices are as varied as your creativity. Your choice basically comes down to whether you wish to work across the body or to proceed up the same side. As long as you have some methodical way of covering every part of the body that is to be massaged, the massage will be complete with no obvious omissions.

Allow the person being massaged to choose whether to first lie face down or face up. It's helpful to have a clock or watch placed so that various areas of coverage can be conveniently timed. If you are giving a thirty minute massage, ask the receiver to turn over after fifteen minutes. At this halfway point, make sure that you, the massager, are relaxed. Oftentimes, there is a tendency to neglect any discomforts you might have if you are giving a good massage. During all phases of the massage, check your posture and make adjustments for any difficulties you are experiencing.

Make sure that you feel good before you work on another person. If you're run-down physically or emotionally, you should be receiving, not giving. Re-schedule the session, if possible. Otherwise, your rundown state might be transmitted to your partner.

BIRTHDAY SUIT?

What should the person wear or not wear? Jackie Day says, "I think draping is necessary most of the time, except if you know someone very well. Never assume because you are 'dressed' friends that you are also 'undressed' friends. Issues of abuse, boundaries, sexuality, being able to say what your needs are, and self-image can all arise."

She suggests to always tell a person to take off as much as they are comfortable taking off. If they are nude because you told them to take it all off, they may be unable to relax and feel safe, which are primary considerations in therapeutic massage.

Your nails need to be trimmed as short as possible and filed smooth, otherwise acupressure becomes acupuncture! Remove all jewelry. Avoid loose clothing or long hair that will trail over their body. The recipient should also remove contact lenses and jewelry.

Ask about cuts, bruises, other injuries, and recent operations in order to avoid touching these spots. Find out about which areas are the most tense. These are the areas where you can spend the most time. Ask your partner about past and present health. If in doubt, wait until after a physician has been consulted before massaging. If there are any serious medical problems such as cancer or heart disease, check with a physician before proceeding.

Be very careful with senior citizens as they tend to bruise more easily, with bruises that can sometimes last for days or even weeks. Their ability to repair damaged tissue is diminished with age. Deep tissue work is contraindicated in treating the elderly; however, gentle massage can be most beneficial. Atherosclerosis is a common condition among senior citizens so care must be taken to stay away from the carotid arteries located on each side of the neck.

Be sure to establish a communication code for pain. You'll want to apply pressure to the edge of pain, not past it. Ask the person to say 'good' when the pressure is best and don't press any harder. To help you feel relaxed while massaging, make sure your center of gravity (two inches below the navel) is directly over the area you are massaging, whenever possible. Position yourself right next to the body part you are massaging. Move your entire body, not just your hands. Let your legs—not your lower back—support and move you.

If you have never given or received a massage, you might consider first giving a massage to those areas on your own body which you can reach comfortably without straining. See what feels good to you. Do you like movements to be fast or slow, soft or hard? A good area for practicing on yourself, as well as your first attempts with another person, is the foot.

Here are some simple guidelines from Jackie Day: "Steady the left foot with your left hand. Stroke the knuckles up and down from just below the toes to the heel pad. Move your knuckles in small circles; press firmly yet gently. Be sure to cover the entire sole, including the bottom of the heel. Next go over the sole with the thumbs of both hands. Hold the foot in place with your fingers and work both thumbs at once in small circles. Again cover the entire sole. Go slowly. Be thorough. Remember those thousands of nerves connecting the foot with the rest of the body."

GETTING STARTED

Two of the best overall how-to-get-started books on massage are *The Book of Massage* by Lucinda Lidell and *The Massage Book* by George Downing. Another book that is effective in summarizing the importance of being touched for our development and well-being is Ashley Montagu's *Touching*. For massaging young ones, I recommend *Loving Hands: The*

Traditional Indian Art of Baby Massage by Frederick LeBoyer. There are also numerous new videos and books available in the LivingArts catalog (see the Resource Directory) you may want to consider.

For couples or for others sharing the same life and home, the ten-minute massage can open the door to something extraordinary: doing massage together every day for ten minutes each. When a day comes along in which you have the time and inclination, trade a full massage. Even ten minutes every day may sound hard if your life is a busy one. It is often difficult until you get in the habit of it. Yet nothing else in the world requiring so little effort will as effectively change over the course of time the mood and tempo of your entire life.

If you follow some of the simple guidelines included in this chapter, you can give a friend or family member as much joy as you will receive from the massage. What could be a nicer gift for someone you love? With loving intentions, your therapeutic touch can truly be a magical one.

CHAPTER TEN

Be More Childlike

This ability to see, experience and accept the new is one of our saving characteristics. To be fearful of tomorrow, to close ourselves to possibilities, to resist the inevitable, to advocate standing still when all else is moving forward, is to lose touch. If we accept the new with joy and wonder, we can move gracefully into each tomorrow. More often than not, the children shall lead us.
—LEO BUSCAGLIA

So many people are searching for the fountain of youth, the secret that will enable them to live a long and full life. Some follow strict diets, exercise vigorously, or swear by expensive supplements. Yet few have looked deeply enough to understand that the secret to living a life full of aliveness and fulfillment lies within. This secret is expressed in our attitude, our expression, our thoughts, and how we view ourselves and the world around us. Young children are forever my inspiration and teachers. They have much to teach us about experiencing life to the fullest.

PARTY TIME

A few years ago I decided to have a party to which I invited several neighborhood children. The party took place in my yard. The children ranged in age from three to six. Just before the party began I received an upsetting telephone call. The caller was a close friend and we were not seeing eye to eye on something important to both of us. We started out calmly but ended up with raised voices and feelings of frustration.

I went back outside to greet my young guests as they arrived. The toys, decorations, and snacks were ready and I was ready to call the whole thing off. I'm so glad I didn't. That day became one of the most significant days of my life. Within no time at all, I forgot about my telephone conversation and got involved with the children, allowing myself to become a child again.

As time went by I began to realize that children instinctively understand the secret of living fully. Their moments appear to be almost magical as they are totally fascinated by their world, unmindful of the problems of yesterday or tomorrow. Somehow children are able to let go and embrace life with passion. They are able to give themselves permission to be free, to be totally absorbed in the present, and to embrace the unfamiliar and the out of the ordinary.

I have always had a great fondness for children. While I was still living with my family during school and my first year at UCLA, the children of the neighborhood would often come to my home to see if I could come out and play. I could rarely resist. I remember with great vividness the games we would play, the hours we laughed, the endless moments when we were silly and goofy. Those times will always hold a special place in my heart. When was the last time you played hide-and-go-seek with some children, or tag, or pin the tail on the bush? I recall with warmth the hours I spent as a child riding my bike, pretending it was a magnificent white stallion. As I rode, the horse and I were like one, galloping strongly and swiftly, the wind gently embracing my face and hair.

Even today some of my best times are with children. Each year I take a group of children to Disneyland or the circus, and I can often be found at my local park, playground, or beach with some small friends, playing ball, swinging, running, feeding birds, or just laughing a lot.

I can also remember the numerous times during my life that adults have asked me why I didn't act my age. I figure that as long as I continue to hear that, I must be doing just fine.

I am reminded of something I heard Buckminster Fuller once say. "I have great hope for tomorrow. And my hope lies in the following three things: truth, youth, and love."

CHILDLIKE VERSUS CHILDISH

There is a distinct difference between being childlike and being childish. To be childish means either to be a child and act like one, which is perfectly normal, or to be an adult and act like a child in ways that indicate your growth and maturity were somehow impeded and you have been stagnating ever since.

To be childlike means to be innocent of strange, authoritarian ideas of what adulthood ought to be; to be trusting and straightforward; and to be more concerned with your experience of life than how you look to others.

It is important to understand that you do not have to give up being an adult in order to become more childlike. You do not have to become infantile or in the least bit irresponsible or unaccountable. The fully integrated person incorporates a harmonious blending of adult and child.

Within each of us is a child waiting to come forth and express itself more fully. What usually keeps us from getting back in touch with the child within is our own unwillingness to recognize and accept that child. It seems we often feel that "now that I'm grown up, I have to act my age." There is a lovely passage in Matthew 19:14 of the Bible that says, "Let the children come to me, and do not hinder them; for to such belongs the kingdom of heaven." Young children live in their own heaven, no matter what their background, the language they speak, or where they live. Their celebration of life, their passion and joy are universal.

The children at my party all had something in common that transcended words—the joy of living fully, of celebrating life and each moment. Part of living fully is laughing a lot. This means laughing not only at the everyday incongruities of life but most especially at ourselves, as children do so well.

While jogging in a park in Switzerland, I noticed several children playing a game that was new to me. Their parents and guardians were sitting quietly, not talking to each other or paying much attention to the children. The kids were having a fantastic time laughing, running, touching, being silly, and just enjoying each other's company. It looked like so much fun. After watching for a few minutes, I felt compelled to join them. Through hand signals I asked if I could play and an hour later I was exhausted. Although I could not speak their language, there was still a special bonding and love, a respect and sharing that transcended the need for words. Laughing can be so freeing and so uniting at the same time.

Toward the end of my walk the following day, I saw a boy and girl down on all fours looking keenly at the ground next to a beautiful flowering violet tree. I stopped to see what was so captivating. In halting English, their mother told me that for nearly thirty minutes the two children had been engrossed in watching the movement of some ants as they made their journey from the tree to some bread crumbs a few feet away. At that moment I got down on my hands and knees and for several precious minutes I joined the children in their adventure, letting myself get totally involved with them and the ants. It was delightful.

It's fun to be around people who can let their inner child come out to play. These are usually happy, fully functioning people who have not forgotten that it is possible to be happy and responsible at the same time; who aren't afraid of what others think; who can occasionally become totally immersed in fantasy, just as they did when they were children.

Take advantage of the many opportunities you have to let your inner child out for a great adventure. I sometimes get my friends involved. For example, I love to rent videos such as *E.T.* or *Winnie the Pooh* and invite over a few close friends to watch these movies with me—but I make two requests. The first, to come dressed as a little child, and the second, to bring a favorite toy. My very special teddy bear, Golden, and I greet the guests. Ah! To let your inner child out to play is such a glorious gift—free and available to all.

Reflect a moment on your own experiences being around children. What are the children like? How do you feel when you are with them? What qualities do they express to you? Before you read on, write down what comes to mind when you think about children.

Study your list for a moment. How many of these qualities are part of your personality? Which ones would you like to develop or reawaken?

When I wrote my list that evening after my neighborhood party, here is what I came up with: Children are cheerful, alert, eager, trusting, persevering, and open. They are also energetic, caring, sensitive, friendly, and inquisitive. They are enthusiastic, playful, expressive, spontaneous, and natural. They laugh a lot and love to act silly and crazy. They are also incredibly lovable and innocently loving. From my perspective, these natural childlike qualities are the true essence of living fully.

As children grow older they are strongly influenced by the mores and behavioral patterns of their role models and their society. It is a shame to see that the models of adulthood in families, in schools, on television, and throughout society are often negative. This is what the children absorb. Yet those young people who grow up relatively unencumbered by negative cultural models are able to handle people and situations with a sense of involvement, enthusiasm, and spontaneity.

LET YOUR INNER CHILD REAR ITS BEAUTIFUL HEAD

A child lies dormant in every one of us, waiting to be recognized and accepted. It is natural for people to be happy, healthy, creatively alive, and childlike.

We are as young as we think, and the fountain of youth lies within each of us. We simply have to let ourselves shine each and every day as children do.

Some of you may be thinking that there's no way you can act like a child. You have a job with many responsibilities, bills to pay, and many problems and frustrations to deal with. But understand that children have problems and frustrations, too. They have tests in school, difficulties with friends, and problems with parents, and yet they seem to bring a different attitude to life's situations. They handle things as they come up without taking life so seriously. Young people can often show great wisdom. I'm not suggesting giving up adulthood. Rather, I suggest we integrate the child and the adult within us. That's the key to celebrating life.

One way of achieving this blend is to spend time around children. Watch them from afar. Play with them. Get involved. Throw yourself into their activities. Pretend you are a child again. Now if you don't have any children of your own, find a way to be with children at least once a month. You might do volunteer work with Big Sisters or Big Brothers, the Boy or Girl Scouts, the local park, or the pediatric ward of a nearby hospital.

I know it will be valuable and worthwhile for you. Children have a way of revealing much to us about ourselves if we allow ourselves to be open to them. They are like mirrors, showing us many valuable lessons about living.

BE ALL THAT YOU CAN BE

What a beautiful gift we can give to each other. Children know this well. Being all that you can be means being authentic, sensitive, vulnerable, and willing to express your feelings. When we're being who we are, we don't wear masks, we have no pretenses, we are ingenuous. Children exhibit these qualities when they meet a new friend. Even though they might start out with some shyness, when it feels right (and for children it almost always quickly becomes right), they relate as though they were long-time friends.

At my party, three of the children were new to the neighborhood and didn't know anyone. Yet within the first few minutes they were all getting along as though they were best buddies.

Compare this approach with your own feelings and behavior when you meet someone new. How do you respond? How long is your initial period of shyness? Are you likely to feel reserved or suspicious? If you are, perhaps these feelings are related to how you feel about yourself. The ability to trust lies in your mind and is expressed through your attitude. What you believe to be true about yourself and about your world will be duplicated in all your life experiences. Our thoughts have a great influence upon our circumstances. In his wonderful book, *Love*, Leo Buscaglia says, "Love is like a mirror. When you love another you become his mirror and he becomes yours...and reflecting each other's love you see infinity." *You are always in a relationship with yourself, especially in the presence of another*. Acknowledge and be thankful to others for serving as your mirror.

The next time you meet a new person, be aware of your reactions. Notice if you are being cool, standoffish, keeping the person at arm's length with small talk. See if you are wondering what this person is after. Are you feeling a little uncomfortable, uncertain about where this new encounter is headed? Take your cue from kids, who can have a great time together even if they know they may never see each other again. They are not averse to gaining something for fear of losing it. Set right out to find this new person's funny bone, or find some other way to put him or her at ease. When you show that you trust and respect someone, the barriers immediately begin to drop. If you let your childlike trust take over and feel positive about being able to handle anything that comes along, your very attitude of certainty will see you through.

This week go out and meet someone new. Introduce yourself to people, even if it feels funny at first. This will help shake off your inhibitions about talking to strangers. Trust new friends and yourself to make the best of the situation. Find out what it is you have in common. The more you do this, the more you'll discover, as I have, that what we have in common with each other far outweighs the differences, and further, that it's the differences that make friendships stimulating and exciting.

The child in you knows how to deal with everyone and every situation with perfect aplomb. So allow your inner child to show you how to be a friend and how to make new friends.

It is also important to find ways to let your family and friends know you care. You don't have to wait for birthdays and anniversaries. Make every day Valentine's Day. If you have a difficult time expressing your feelings verbally, send a card or note, offer a hug, or send flowers. My mom and I speak often by telephone. When we finish talking we always end by telling each other, "I love you." That means so much to me. Remember too that just because a message might not be received or acknowledged the way you would wish, it's still worth sending. Live today as though it were your last day. Be that friend or loved one you would appreciate having.

GIVE FANTASY ITS WINGS AND FLY

Fantasy, or creative daydreaming, is a healthy experience for both children and adults. Remember how when you were a child your bedroom took on many worlds of its own? Sometimes it was a fortress, other times it was another planet. Remember when you dressed up or when you pretended you were a grocer, doctor, pilot, athlete, or ballet dancer? For both children and adults, creative dreaming provides a practical escape from the pressures of everyday living. It eliminates boredom and enhances creativity. Dreaming creates your reality; in fact, your present realities started with thoughts, dreams, and visualizations. So many of us spend our waking hours thinking about all the negative elements around us or about how others should change to meet our expectations. Dreams and goals give our thoughts positive direction and purpose. When we know what we want and where we are headed, we don't spend our time thinking about what we don't want or don't have. What we think about consistently, we draw into our lives.

This was never more apparent or real to me than it was several years ago on a ski trip when I took to Sun Valley, Idaho with the UCLA Ski Club. Part of the package involved a flight to a city in Idaho where we would later catch a bus for the long ride to Sun Valley. I bought my ticket early and looked forward to the trip for weeks. On the day of departure, my mom dropped me off at the airport. I checked in got my seat assignment, and then boarded the plane. I was puzzled at not seeing any of my friends, who were part of this trip, on the flight, and figured they must be sitting toward the back. After the plane landed I became concerned when I couldn't find any of my friends at the baggage claim area. Bewildered and confused, I headed for the outdoor curb where, according to my ski information packet, the buses would be waiting—no friends or buses anywhere! I called the bus company to find out why the buses were late. The person on the other end of the line was somewhat amused as they informed me: "The buses will be there tomorrow." Tomorrow! In light of the fact that I am an organized, efficient, and accountable person, you can imagine my astonishment. How was it that I marked the day on my calendar, talked with my friends about the upcoming ski trip without discovering the erroneous date, and encountered no problems at the airport when the ticket I offered was dated for the following day?

As is my style, I decided to make the best of it. I made reservations at a nearby hotel with a sauna, gym, and salad bar. After the taxi dropped me off, I called my mom back home and we had a good laugh about my oversight. I then bundled up in my sweats and ski hat and went out for a jog in the freshly fallen snow.

After a while, I came across an inviting health food store. It had a small restaurant and I decided to get some soup. As I waited for the waitress to take my order, I became aware of an elderly man sitting a few tables away. He was staring at me with a weird expression on his face, making me feel very uncomfortable. Then rather quickly, his stare turned from inquisitiveness to a look of shock. I noticed his wife asking him if he was okay. Pointing to me, he continued to stare and his wife turned in my direction.

Apprehensively, the man came to my table. With a noticeable difficulty in forming his words, he asked, "Are you Susan Smith Jones?" I couldn't believe that someone had recognized me under my three layers of clothing and hat. When I answered, he and his wife gasped.

It turned out that one week before, this man had sat in the very same health food store reading an article I had written about creative visualization and the importance of positive daydreaming. I wrote about how if you believed enough, through visualization and creative thoughts you can create any reality you choose. After reading this article, which included a photograph of me, the man said to his wife how much he would like to meet and talk with me. His wife skeptically suggested that he visualize meeting me, which is exactly what he had been doing the week before we met. Most of his daydreams focused on sitting with me and asking me all of his personal health questions.

Neither of them will ever question the validity and power of creative visualization, nor will I. This was not mere coincidence. We talked for a few hours, shared many stories, and I answered countless health questions. The man was contemplating bypass surgery at his doctor's recommendation. I clearly detailed for him the wellness lifestyle program described in this book and my tape albums. I wrote out the diet recommended in chapter two, and suggested he start it immediately. I also encouraged him to begin a walking program, and meditation, stretching, and positive visualizations about his health. As a result of my suggestions and embracing a new health program, his surgery was canceled. His doctor was astonished at the reversal of his coronary heart disease.

From this circumstance and countless others, I've come to realize that there is an unfathomable, yet recognizable, divine order to this universe. It's ever-present and always working in alignment with what we need for our highest good and spiritual unfoldment and growth. I've learned not to analyze or question it anymore. I continue to live in awe at the magnificent adventure life continually is. It was Helen Keller who wrote: "Life is either a daring adventure or nothing. To keep our faces toward change and behave like free spirits in the presence of fate is strength undefeatable." I'm convinced that it's extremely important to always imagine and think about what you want in life, while at the same time letting go of thoughts of what you don't want. Let your imagination work for you and not against you. Make friends with your thoughts. I write about visualization in great detail in the next chapter.

Children have the ability not to place limits on their thinking and dreaming. Anything and everything is possible for those who believe, and children understand this better than anyone. They possess limitless dreams and goals, and express their aspirations easily. I am saddened when I hear parents telling their children that it is silly to make up fantasies about pretend-friends or animals or trips out of the universe. Encourage your children to fantasize and encourage them to share their dreams with you.

To get back in touch with your fantasy life, you might try finding some children with whom to laugh and play, and encourage everyone to share his or her wildest dreams. You will discover how creatively spontaneous children can be, and it will rub off on you.

What are some of your dreams and fantasies? Have you ever wanted to go sailing or windsurfing? Or how about river rafting or body surfing? Maybe you've wanted to take a cooking class, wanted to paint, visit Nepal, learn karate, bake bread, climb Mount Whitney, or spend the night in the mountains. Whatever it is, make a list. It doesn't matter how crazy or silly these things may seem. You don't need to justify to anyone why you want to do these things. Just that you want to do something is reason enough to do it.

Now look over your list. Some things you wrote down will be difficult to do right away. But I'm sure that you listed at least one thing that you can do immediately. Do it today. Keep your list so that you can add to it as well as cross off things as you've accomplished them or changed your mind.

Acting out my fantasies, even in the face of fear, has added enchantment and excitement to my life. Some of the things I've tried that were on my list include skydiving, hang gliding, motorcross, painting, Tai Chi, photography, and camping alone in the mountains. I even tried bungee jumping. Was I scared? You bet! After the jump, I felt like I could do anything I wanted; nothing could stand in my way. The other bonus was that when I jumped, I got a free chiropractic adjustment at the same time. What a thrill! Still left on my list is to design and build my dream home, play baseball with the Dodgers and basketball with the Lakers, take singing lessons, and go horseback riding with Robert Redford. In fact, there are still several items left on my list yet to accomplish but I can assure you before too long, I'll be able to cross them off as completed.

LIVING IN THE PRESENT

Living in the moment is different from living for the moment. Children allow themselves to get totally involved and focused on whatever they are doing right now. Granted, their attention span is not long, but they are still able to focus on whatever is taking place in their lives at the moment. When they eat, they just eat; when they play, they just play; when they talk, they just talk. They throw themselves wholeheartedly into their activity.

I look back on my early childhood and recall that I had no sense of time. My family took frequent long trips in the car. Usually within ten minutes of leaving home I would ask, "Are we there yet?" followed by "When are we going to be there?" This was repeated every ten minutes or so. Two hours away didn't mean anything to me. My only sense of time was now.

I am not recommending we forget the future. I believe in planning ahead, preparing for the future, and fostering dreams. But that has its time and place. Most of the time, be here now. Be open to the touch, feelings, sights of what is around you and in you right now. Appreciate life with all of your senses.

Have you ever noticed that children are willing to try anything at a moment's notice? Even though they might have experienced that same thing before, they will express wide-eyed excitement and wonderment. This is because children don't use a yardstick to measure activities or compare the present with the past. They know they've played the game before, or had someone read the same story just last night, yet it's still as fresh and wonderful as it was the first time.

Often when I'm conducting a workshop, I ask the participants to go outside for ten to fifteen minutes and saunter the grounds, alone, in silence. I have them practice being totally absorbed in what they can see, smell, taste, feel, and hear. To be with nature, letting its beauty into your awareness, is wonderful. What I have discovered in taking this kind of walk (and I do this at least once a week) is that I feel a subtle, gentle communion with nature. The flowers, trees, birds, even the insects seem to be in harmony with me.

When was the last time you walked past a school playground when the children were playing? Notice how totally involved and absorbed the children are when they are playing. They seem oblivious to future problems and appear to have let go of annoyances of the past. They let their spontaneity run free. One moment they are totally involved with other children and participating in a certain game. Then minutes later, they will change games and yet again be totally involved in another.

How spontaneous are you? If you are like many people, your schedule is tightly planned. It's appropriate to have goals, to make plans, to be disciplined with your time. But if you are too rigid, if your schedule is too strict, it will be hard for your inner child to come out and enjoy life. Plato's words, "Life must be lived as play," are important to keep in mind.

Set aside a specific time each day free from any scheduled activity. Then when the time rolls around, see what you feel like doing. How about daydreaming, writing a letter, going to the park, or taking a ride on your bike? Just ride and see where you end up. See what moves you at the moment. As you tune in more to your inner child, it will show you more and more how you can thoroughly enjoy each day and how being more spontaneous will add a new dimension to your life.

If your present is obscured by "if only," or "just wait until tomorrow," try the following exercise. Write down some of your self-limiting thoughts, beliefs, and habits. Take your time. Look deeply within. Include as many as you can think of. Then put your list in a brown paper bag. Close the top securely. Then, as you breathe deeply and slowly, put the bag in a fireplace or big bowl and set it on fire. Watch all of your excess baggage dissolve before your eyes. Just let it go. And as it's dissolving, affirm something such as "I choose to embrace and celebrate life moment to moment."

DON'T BE AFRAID TO MAKE MISTAKES OR FAIL

Failure is only a word and has no power other than what you give it. Children haven't yet learned the adult meaning of the word failure and thus have the desire to take risks most of the time. They intuitively know that to risk is to learn and grow.

Have you ever watched a child learning to ride a bike? A child will try again and again, falling, getting up, and starting over, no matter how many times it takes, because he or she is not trying to prove anything to anyone else. A child isn't afraid of failing repeatedly in order to accomplish a goal. What is failure anyway? Just a delay in results and a way of seeing which choices worked for you and which didn't.

At my party for the children, we played a game that involved laying a large sheet of plastic on the grass. Then we turned on the hose and ran water over the plastic sheet. We ran and slid over it, twisting, spinning, and getting entangled with each other. It was great fun and even though it was easy to slip and fall, as we all did, no one was concerned with how foolish he or she looked. We were all having a wonderful time enjoying the moment. Be more concerned with your own integrity and experience of living than what others might think.

ACCEPT THE WORLD AS IT IS

Children don't resist life. They are incredibly accepting and have the unique ability to take things as they come, and make the most of them.

In adulthood we face many conditions that we wish were different— all the way from world hunger, environmental pollution, crime and drug problems, to rising prices and our fitness routine or diet. Many times, no matter what we do, things don't seem to change fast enough. The key is to get involved, while trying to keep a clear perspective of the situation.

Take the weather. It's clearly a natural phenomenon that we cannot control. Let's say it's early morning and you've just woken up to discover that it snowed heavily last night. Your driveway is full of snow and the roads are a mess. You begin bemoaning your fate, dreading the drive to work. Even if you choose to stay home, you are already convinced that the day is wasted. On the other hand, your children haven't been this excited in days. Either they will get to walk through the snow on the way to school, or if they stay home, they'll be able to play all day in this winter wonderland. What heaven!

Last week a friend of mine had plans to play tennis. Instead, Mother Nature decided to bless us with some much-needed rain. My friend's tennis plans were ruined and instead of finding a way to celebrate the wetness, he sulked around his house all day, angry at the weather. What a waste of precious, sacred time!

It's all just a matter of attitude. Make whatever is going on in your life at the moment okay. Accept what is and what can't be changed, and make the best of it. Be in touch with your emotions, express yourself, complete your emotions, and then let them go. Babies do this so marvelously. Think back to the last time you saw a baby really upset. (For some of you, this might be within the past hour.) A baby will cry his or her heart out and purely express his or her upset. When a baby is crying, I doubt that the baby is wondering if he or she should be crying and probably doesn't feel guilty or embarrassed for crying. The baby purely cries, then lets it go. Similarly, when a baby is angry, he or she will let you know and will also quickly let it go without holding on to it or holding resentment. Babies express themselves fully, then move on. What delightful teachers and what a perfect demonstration of the positive use of energy they are!

It occurs to me that all the magical qualities expressed by children and babies I'm discussing in this chapter are also shared by animals. Perhaps that's why I've always been a great lover of animals, especially dogs, cats, and horses.

The more I pay attention to how children and animals experience and embrace life, and the more I release my fears about being rejected and feeling uncertain, the better life becomes for me and for those people around me, because I become softer and kinder.

I have come to realize that, at times, there's a controlling self within me that can be demanding and a perfectionist and judgmental. Life flows far better for me and for those around me when I am able to replace that person with a more caring, gentle me. When I can forgive and forget, when I can say and feel that whatever happens is acceptable, when I can take people in my arms and embrace them and be embraced and discover that we are each special, unique, and wondrous, then life becomes a great river that will flow no matter what I do. I can flow with it and live in peace or I can slip back into old patterns and live in despair, fighting against the current. The river does not care. It only makes a difference to me and to those around me. The choice is mine. The struggle to be a different person, to respond differently to life and to the people I know, is not a change I made once and no longer worry about. It is an ongoing struggle to be more soft and flexible, to give myself permission to enjoy who I am and what I do, to allow myself to laugh, tease, and relax in undemanding ways that really feel good. When I am successful in allowing those things to happen, my life is better for me and far better for the people around me.

LAUGH AND BE A LITTLE SILLY

When was the last time you really laughed? If you can't remember, you had better read this carefully, because your life might depend on it. Laughter is the lubricant of life. It's the elixir that enables you to experience the fullness and joy of life.

Along with laughter comes smiling. Smile more. It's great for firming your facial muscles; it makes you feel better; it makes people wonder what you've been up to; it's a small curve that sets many things straight; a smile confuses an approaching frown; and it's the shortest distance between two people.

Concomitant with laughter is not taking yourself or life too seriously. Being able to laugh at yourself and the incongruities of everyday situations is the best way to quell stress and to enjoy life. Laugh! Laugh! And do it often every day.

This reminds me of when I took my car to a local automatic car wash. I came back outside after paying and noticed that my car was parked separately from all the others. A few other car owners and most of the car wash employees were standing around my car, some looking shocked, some gesturing wildly, and some laughing. At first I thought they were admiring my good-looking automobile. (I have a large 4-wheel drive recreation vehicle.) As I got closer I saw what all the excitement was about—I had forgotten to close the sun roof and there was a lake inside my car! It was then I noticed a huge sign on the wall that read: "Close all windows and sun roofs." I hesitantly opened the car door and out rushed the water. Suddenly it struck me how funny this all was and I began laughing so hard my stomach hurt and tears rolled down my face. As I sit here relating my story, my car is almost dry. It would have done me no good to get upset, and besides, now I'm driving a car with the cleanest interior for miles around. I have often wondered what happen if I left the sun roof open in a car wash and now I know.

Children are special in this way. The intuitively realize that happiness is a choice—an attitude they create. That's why children often act silly and crazy, making and telling jokes. They also know how to cultivate a sense of humor, which is one of the most important components of wellness.

In Victor E. Frankl's book *Man's Search for Meaning*, he tells the story of his experiences in the Nazi concentration camps. In this poignant account he discusses the importance of humor to well-being and to staying alive. "Humor was another of the soul's weapons in the fight for self-preservation. It is well known that humor, more than anything else in the human make-up, can afford an aloofness and ability to rise above any situation, even if only for a few seconds."

So let your inner child come out and play and orchestrate your day. When you do, you find it natural and easy to look for the good in every person and in every situation, no matter what the appearances. Keep laughing your way through life. Learn to laugh, especially at yourself! Give yourself permission to have fun and be a little giddy. In other words, lighten up. When you do this, the world will seem brighter and more beautiful. Children have so much to teach us in this area.

Every once in a while, a few friends and I go on an adventure I created called a Surprise Hike. Our group starts out from some point and goes for a hike in the local Santa Monica mountains. Every time we get to a fork in the path, one hiker gets to choose where to go next—straight, right turn, left turn, or maybe about-face. We never know where the journey will take us. It's all a surprise. Then the person who chose the direction for that portion must also decide on a surprise adventure on that path, which can be just about anything. Some of the things I've suggested are petting a lizard, talking to a rabbit, singing with the birds, dancing, kissing a tree or plant, imitating a deer, or picking up a pebble that speaks to you. Crazy, you say? Perhaps.

Each day, be a little crazy. Write a silly note and hide it in one of the shoes or pockets of a family member so he or she will find it later. Throw snowballs, fly a kite, hug a tree, skip pebbles over the water, kiss a flower, talk to the animals, or bring home a birthday cake (carrot, of course) even though it's nobody's birthday. Let go of wondering what other people will think of you. It doesn't matter. What matters is that you enjoy being with you and that you have lots of fun in your own company. When you do, other people will too.

Other special times for me occur four times a year, during the change of seasons. These four high-energy days I celebrate by doing things such as lighting candles and buying flowers, both reflecting the season's colors. I dance and sing for the sun and moon. I make special gifts and offer these to Mother Nature. (I also celebrate the full and new moons.) Sure, I've had more than a few people tell me that I'm definitely crazy. I take their remark as a compliment and celebrate it. It gives me a great leeway for oddball behavior.

LOVE UNCONDITIONALLY

The ability to love unconditionally is the most precious quality within us. All life is positively affected by love. Love is an unlimited source of energy and serves as the basic foundation of all life, of all joy. Along with love come the gifts of kindness, tenderness, forgiveness, and service. The great Chinese philosopher Lao Tzu once said, "Kindness in words creates confidence, kindness in thinking creates profoundness, and kindness in giving creates love."

A child's love is the perfect example of these God-given qualities. Have you noticed that children quickly forget their anger and forgive others when they've been hurt? Children accept you totally for your good points and for your not-so-good points too. They don't care about differences in people—about different races, religions, or backgrounds. They just love. In exchange, they are lovable, for that's exactly what they attract to themselves. The more we love, the more we are loved, and the lovelier we are. We attract to ourselves the equivalent of that which we believe and express. Children are prepared to accept people as people, and even if offended or hurt, children will come back to forgive and love over and over again.

Part of loving another unconditionally is serving that person with your true attention and real feelings, and listening to his or her feelings. What a beautiful gift this is—to listen to the other person's hurt, anger, and upset without getting defensive. Be receptive, not reactive. That's the key.

Children have helped me see more clearly that relationships work best when we offer forgiveness to everyone. It is often difficult for us to see the projection process within ourselves, and it's even more difficult to stop our projections. But when we practice forgiveness, all our relationships begin to change.

Because of a child's loving and forgiving nature, he or she tends to be naturally grateful for life's treasures. A few weeks ago I finished a tour of schools of all levels, where I presented lectures and workshops. In one particular school, I focused on healthy self-esteem and I worked with children ages four to eight. I asked them what made them feel grateful. Here are some of the responses I received. "I'm grateful to be breathing, because my breath gives me life." (She was five years old.) "I'm grateful for my birthdays, because that's a day I give my parents presents for bringing me into the world." (He was eight years old.) "I'm grateful for my cat. When she purrs I know she's happy, and that makes me happy." (She was six years old.) "I'm grateful for my new bike, because I love to feel the wind on my face and hair when I ride. I also like to share my bike with my best friend, because she doesn't have a bike yet." (She was seven years old.)

DECIDE TO FORGIVE
The quality of unconditional love was made clearer to me the day of my neighborhood party. Just before it was over, I saw two small girls hugging and kissing each other. Just five minutes earlier they had been angry at each other because one of the girls had taken the last piece of carrot cake. Without any interference by me or the other children, I watched the two girls handle their problem. One girl decided to share the piece of cake, and the other girl thanked her with a big hug and kiss. I was very touched by the girls' generosity. Later I called my friend with whom I had the disagreement, to say that I was sorry for the misunderstanding and also to say "I love you." It was easy and natural, and I felt grateful to those two little girls for showing me how to express my love more freely and unconditionally.

I believe with all my heart that in a world where so much conflict exists between people of different races, religions, and backgrounds, the greatest bridge to understanding and peace is laughter and love. It's through compassion, forgiveness, laughter, and love that we can create a world where everyone wins, where everyone lives in peace and harmony. Never underestimate the power of love; it is the solution to any problem.

Children know this better than most of us. Watch them. Learn from them.

Let's all begin today to live more joyfully, to play at the game of life. Let the child within you blossom. Permit yourself to experience life to its fullest—to celebrate you and life.

Learn from children that the elixir for perpetual youth lies within every one of us. Each day is a brand new rainbow full of love, joy, wonder, and celebration.

CHAPTER ELEVEN

Living Your Highest Vision: Turning Dreams Into Reality

The way for you to be happy and successful, to get more of the things you really want in life, is to get the combinations to the locks. Instead of spinning the dials of life hoping for a lucky break, as if you were playing a slot machine, you must instead study and emulate those who have already done what you want to do and achieved the results you want to achieve.
—BRIAN TRACY

Positive thinking became almost synonymous with success in the 1970s. In its early use in organizations such as Dale Carnegie's success courses, positive thinking meant using willpower and conscious, positive thoughts to achieve goals. Napoleon Hill's maxim of success, "What you can conceive and believe, you can achieve," is a popular positive thinking slogan. Never underestimate the divine potential of positive thinking. If it's rightly employed, this power of the mind is a catalyst that makes possible a wondrous transformation in our lives. It was Ralph Waldo Emerson who said: "The good mind chooses what is positive, what is advancing—embraces the affirmative."

Positive thinking is the belief in our own self-worth and in the value of everyone else and every circumstance. That positive belief leads to self-confidence, respect for others, and a lifestyle based on strong values. Sometimes you slip into the habit of negative thinking because you feel discouraged, depressed, lonely, isolated, or stressed. You want results fast and easy. But life isn't like that. Life is meant to be a challenge. When our minds are full of fear, doubt, and clutter, good ideas can't get through. You get your best ideas and make your best decisions when you're relaxed, open to impressions and responsive to them. Find a way to link the present situation with wonderful opportunities to learn and grow. You can't just sit at a desk and think positively about something and expect it to happen. You have to make it happen—or at least help make it happen. Keeping alive a goal or dream, or even hope, requires action.

For me, the best action I can take is to look for the hand of God in every situation—finding in happy experiences glimpses of His infinite kindness, and in painful ones His guidance and blessings to help me win

Living Your Highest Vision

new victories over my limitations. I try to behold the Divine in everyone and everything.

TAKE CHARGE OF YOUR MIND AND LIFE

If I had my way, I would require that all students each year of their education to take a class I'd call 'mind power.' This would be the science of mind and to cover a variety of topics, including mind strength and clarity—how to be alert yet relaxed. A special section would be devoted to awareness, or mindfulness, and how it affects all areas of our lives. Finally, students would be shown how to choose effective, positive thoughts—to be in control of thinking at all times, instead of allowing thoughts to be in control.

Control of the mind is essential if we are going to be happy and healthy. Train the mind always to be loving and kind and to see the best in others and in everything. When the road of life is steep, keep your mind even.

Making your dreams a reality doesn't happen by luck. Success is not an accident. You can choose to be active and create what you want, or simply respond to whatever happens around you, hoping for the best. Successful people are very deliberate about making the choice to be in charge of their lives. They don't get up in the morning and hope that they'll have a good day. High-achieving people take full control of their lives and if they don't find the circumstances they want, they make them.

Successful people make a choice to begin working on some dream. Nothing will ever happen without your having the courage to begin. This means taking risks, being vulnerable, making mistakes, and even failing. But life can't be lived on the sidelines if you want to be successful. The fun is challenging yourself to something you've always wanted to do.

Our lives reflect our thoughts, dreams, expectations, beliefs, hopes, feelings of self-worth and desires. Knowing this, you can consciously modify your inner states to create and live your highest potential and vision. You are not the victim of circumstance: you are the architect of your life. Your conscious thoughts create an unconscious image of your life, yourself, and your feelings. Your unconscious image reproduces itself perfectly in your circumstances.

Each of us is given free will and we can create our own happiness and our own heaven or hell. You can do it by choosing your thoughts. Choose confident living and positive thoughts and you will produce a heaven of happiness. Complications, conditions, or people do not upset you, but the way you think about them causes your upset. Freedom is not possible until you discipline and retrain your mind. Your beliefs and thoughts create your reality. Right this moment, you can choose to see things differently, to live life from love, peace, and joy instead of from fear.

MY OCEAN SWIM

A few years ago I had a glorious experience that showed me the tremendous power of thought. It was a splendid morning and I was accustomed to going to the beach for an invigorating swim a few times each week. It was very early, just before sunrise. After some stretching exercises and a short run, I was ready for my swim. Because it was the end of summer, the water was still comfortably warm. But this morning there was something in the air that I couldn't quite put my finger on. I felt it deep inside me—a joyful anticipation, a faint knowing that today would be different, that this day would be one I would celebrate the rest of my life. I went out into the ocean, rode a few waves, and then swam past the swells.

I was aware of the peacefulness of the water. Glassy, sparkling, and clear, it rejuvenated my body and soul with each stroke. A few minutes later some old friends joined me, a group of pelicans who seem to enjoy escorting me. They were gliding flawlessly a few feet above my head when suddenly they flew away. Surprised, I waved good-bye as I turned over to begin the backstroke. It was then that I saw something that made my heart plummet.

A large, dark, frightening fin was heading straight for me. Shark! I quickly looked toward the beach. No one was there. I had always taken for granted that I would stay calm in a life-threatening situation. But not this time! As the fin continued in my direction, I simply froze and treaded water. I was so terrified, I couldn't even cry or swim away. And then it happened, a sight that will forever warm my heart and soul. The fin danced out of the water. It was a dolphin followed by a school of about two dozen more!

Less than two weeks previously, I had watched a Jacques Cousteau documentary on dolphins. During my meditation that evening, I visualized myself swimming and playing with a school of dolphins. I accepted and affirmed that that was my desire and reality. I then thanked God for this wonderful experience.

There in the ocean that morning the dolphins stayed with me for the next half hour, swimming, jumping out of the water, and jumping over me. I swam underwater with them, listening to their beautiful sounds, touching their skin, feeling a connection and an exchange of love. For what seemed like hours, nothing else existed except my world of dolphins. I was oblivious to any thought of the past or future. Being right in the moment, I rejoiced in the joy of discovery.

Then, as quickly as they had arrived, they swam off, and I was left alone and immensely grateful. I swam back to the shore, where there was now a group of people who had gathered and watched my dance with the dolphins. I answered many questions and tried to share what the experience had been like for me. I found it was very hard to put my feelings into words. Experiences that speak directly to your heart are often difficult to express clearly.

The others left and I just sat there, enveloped in wonder at this truly remarkable experience. All I could do was cry—what had happened touched me so deeply, so lovingly. The experience was a beautiful lesson in living in the present and appreciating each moment. Because of that experience and so many others, I will never doubt the power of belief and thought to create any reality we choose.

THE PRINCIPLE OF CHOOSING

Let's look at an all-too-common example of how the principal of choice works: weight control. Let's assume that you've always had difficulty controlling your weight. You've tried all kinds of diets and they've never worked, so you have negative feelings about diets. You've tried to limit the amount of food you eat without much success, so you don't have much faith in your self-control. You get on the scale every morning and the numbers reinforce your image of yourself as overweight. It really is a vicious cycle. In order to better understand why you keep repeating the same patterns, let's look at the way your mind works.

Brain researchers see the mind as composed of three primary parts: the conscious, subconscious, and superconscious minds. As the window to the world, your conscious mind runs your daily waking activities, such as making decisions, relating to others, and so on. Your subconscious mind, however, carries memories of all your experiences. It is the storage center for all the information your conscious mind sends it, based on your daily experiences. Your subconscious mind is a computer that is fed the data of your every thought, feeling and experience. The superconscious mind is your connection to the Divine. I'll address that topic in Chapter Fourteen on meditation.

Relating this to the example of weight control, if you get up every morning and worry about what clothes will fit, if you dread getting on your scale, if you dislike being seen in public, if you think about going on a diet but doubt that it will work (they don't—see chapter three on healthy weight), you are programming your subconscious computer in a negative way. Your subconscious mind creates reality according to its programming. If you think of yourself as fat, as having little self-control, as being unable to change, you will see those beliefs reflected in your life—you won't lose a pound.

The same is true for every other area of your life. Your subconscious beliefs and thoughts about yourself, your relationships with others, your money, your material possessions, your job, and so on, will be faithfully re-created in your life. Now you may be thinking: "That isn't true for me; I know that I really want to lose weight and tone up my body (or make more money or have a really good relationship), but I'm not experiencing that in my life." The answer is that there is a vast difference between wanting something on a conscious level and wanting it on a subconscious level.

The conscious mind and subconscious mind are often in conflict. Consciously you may want something, yet subconsciously you create mediocrity or failure. That's why positive thinking as commonly perceived doesn't work. It doesn't do much good to force yourself to think positive thoughts if your subconscious still harbors many negative beliefs. What you need to do is to reprogram your subconscious mind to break the vicious cycle of negative beliefs creating your negative reality. In addition, you must make some behavior changes on a conscious level that will contribute to new beliefs.

The birth of excellence begins with our awareness that our beliefs are a choice. You can choose beliefs that limit you, or you can choose beliefs that support you. The key, says Anthony Robbins in his motivating book *Unlimited Power*, is to choose beliefs that are conducive to success and to discard the ones that hold you back. It is our belief that determines how much of our potential we'll be able to tap, he says. Beliefs can turn on or shut off the flow of ideas. Virgil, the greatest poet of ancient Rome, said, "They can because they think they can."

WHAT YOU THINK ABOUT YOU BRING ABOUT

The law of correspondence says, "As within, so without." It says that your outer world tends to be a reflection of your inner (subconscious) world—like a mirror. What you see in the world around you will be consistent over time with the world inside you.

The law of concentration says that "Whatever you dwell upon grows in your reality." Studies reveal that successful, happy people think about successful, happy things most of the time. By the same token, unsuccessful, unhappy people constantly dwell upon people they dislike, the situations they are angry about and the events that they don't wish to occur in their lives. And whatever we think about most of the time, we bring about in our lives. Those two laws in combination

Living Your Highest Vision

explain much of success and most of failure.

So the starting point in making your dreams a reality is to discipline yourself to think and talk about only those things you want, and to refuse to think and talk about anything other than what you want. These can be tangible as well as intangible things. Besides thinking and talking about the new job or house you desire, talk and think about healthy things such as being grateful instead of unappreciative. Be loving instead of angry. Push all negativity, fears, doubts, and self-sabotaging, limiting thoughts and visions aside. You'll discover that all manner of remarkable things happen in your life that bring you closer to your goals when you take your thoughts off your problems and focus instead on your goals. Don't accept anything less than what you want and focus on that which has your heart.

It's equally important to capture the feeling of the goal fulfilled, of whatever it is you desire, whether it's being prosperous, fit and healthy, being in a loving, supportive relationship or being very successful at work. Then you'll start acting that way and finally become it. The key to the process is to *capture the feeling*, because when you do that you've captured the ability to internalize it. Then it's only a matter of time. Feeling refers to the intensity or amount of emotion you bring to your mental pictures. Emotion is central to all accomplishments. There is a formula: T X F = R. Thought times feeling equals realization. This means that the thought or picture multiplied by the feeling or emotion that accompanies it equals the speed at which it occurs in your reality.

If you see your world only according to what surrounds you right now, you are judging by appearances and limiting what you are going to have. Instead of thinking, "I'll believe it when I see it," think "I'll see it when I believe it."

TRUST IN GOD AND BE PATIENT

Trust in God, the divinity within, regardless of appearances. The very best help for everything in life comes through trusting God and letting God take over, by letting God reveal the highest and best way to us and through us. Trust in Divine order to unfold great and wonderful works in your life.

When you plant seedlings, you know that there is a timing and order before a single flower or fruit appears. Careful cultivation may encourage the buds, but the seedlings follow God's orderly design of growth. The divine plan for you is orderly, too. Favorable conditions for your physical, mental, and emotional needs promote good results, but your spiritual evolution provides complete fulfillment.

Following nature's clues, realize that neither love, friendship, nor worthwhile accomplishment can be forced. So simply be the best kind of friend or co-worker possible and enjoy watching God's order produce wonderful results. Such results may not happen according to your own or another's plans, but they will happen when you live a life surrendered to God. They may be even better than expected.

I believe that trials do not come to destroy you, but to help you appreciate God better. They are the effects of conscious or unconscious action in the past, somewhere, sometime. To overcome your trials you must resurrect your consciousness from the environment of spiritual ignorance. I affirm often: "Heavenly Father, I know that You are coming to my aid, and that I will see Your gift in this challenge bursting forth. My power to overcome is greater than all my trials, because I am Your child. Thank You Father for guiding me and blessing me."

It's from the invisible that the visible is made. William James wrote, "Belief creates the actual fact." So believe, feel, and give thanks in advance (which shows faith in the process) that your goal is now your current reality.

THE POWER OF FEELINGS

You must say what it is you desire. Be specific. You must put in mind that which you choose to bring into your life. You must direct the power within to create what you want. The creative principle works according to the seeds that you plant. Therefore it's imperative that you plant the seeds that you desire to grow. When you plant seeds that you don't want to grow, it's out of a lack of understanding. If you plant love, you get back love. If you plant scarcity, disease, and disaster, you get back scarcity, disease, and disaster. Say what you want, be specific, and act as if what you want were already true.

It's important to understand that belief can be embodied in subconsciousness through the path of emotions. If an idea excites your interest, your interest will stimulate your emotions, particularly feelings of love, and when the feeling reaches the stage of passion it will then be recorded as a belief in the subconscious mind.

Let's take a closer look at the role of feelings in being the person you want to become. Your feelings are the power that creates. Just to simply visualize something without deep, passionate feelings will do little good. From the extensive research I have done in the field of human potential and manifestation, I have come to appreciate the role of feelings. I like to describe feelings as an electromagnetic force field that is so strong it sends up a vibration that pulls like vibrations to itself. It is a magnet for similar energy.

Human behavior specialists know that success begets success and failure begets failure. It is a proven fact that when one makes money, other money comes more easily. A millionaire would tell you that after she or he made one million, the second, third or fourth million came more easily and with little additional work. The more money you have, the more money is attracted to you. It works on a law similar to that of magnetism. After interviewing many highly intelligent, successful people with diverse backgrounds and vast experience, the conclusion I came to was that what you think about and how you feel about things are the determining factors in the way your life works out.

Any feelings we want we can have by simply feeling them. It's this powerful force of feeling that acts as a generator to bring into creation that which we desire. Negative feelings bring negative results. Positive feelings bring positive results.

As I lecture around the country and the world, I often hear statements such as: "I continually affirm, visualize, meditate, and believe in my highest good, but I rarely see results." Most of the time it's because the receiving channels have not been opened. This can be done by practicing forgiveness toward ourselves and others, and by releasing all fear, anger, guilt and any blockages to the presence of love inside you.

POSITIVE ACTIONS BRING POSITIVE RESULTS

Here are some of the external, conscious changes you can make.

If you feel that your beliefs about money are creating negative results in your life, examine the behaviors that support those negative beliefs. Maybe you are frugal in your grocery shopping: you always buy the cheapest of every brand and skip the luxuries. Although frugality might be wise in light of your current financial situation, you should be aware that it also tends to reinforce your belief that you have very little money. One way to attack this belief would be to substitute a new behavior for an old one. In other words, the next time you're in a grocery store, allow yourself to indulge in a little luxury. While you're doing it, imagine that this is your present reality and feel it.

If your problem is loneliness, make it a point to smile at one stranger every day, just as if you had plenty of friends and an abundance of love to share.

If you are overweight, buy yourself something appealing that you would normally have denied yourself because of your present weight.

It's important to remember that living your vision and creating what your heart desires is related to how you feel about yourself. If you feel that you are important enough to ask and divine enough to receive, receiving will be your reward. If on the other hand you feel unworthy, it will be almost impossible for abundance to flow into your life. "Think of how a tree unfolds to all of its magnificent potential, always reaching for the sunshine and growing and flourishing," writes Wayne Dyer in *You'll See It When You Believe It*. "Would you ever suggest to a tree, 'You should be ashamed of yourself for having that disgusting moss on your bark, and for letting your limbs grow crooked'? Of course not. A tree allows the life force to work through it. You have the power within your thoughts to be as natural as the tree." He reminds us that all we need to do is be ourselves.

The more time you spend focusing on your goals and imagining yourself as already having achieved a goal, the more likely and quickly you will be able to achieve it.

WHAT YOU GIVE AWAY, YOU GET BACK MULTIPLIED

Here's another important aspect of changing your subconscious image—the law of circulation which states that what you give away, you get back multiplied. You must first give away the very thing you desire. If you desire increased prosperity in your life, share what you do have with others. Don't hoard it, because that would be a manifestation of a fear that there might not be enough.

When you have decided what you want, it's important to give a tithe. Tithe gifts can be in monetary form or a giving of yourself in time and/or deposits of love. Tithing traditionally meant to give a tenth of your income to your church. But tithing doesn't necessarily have to go to a church. I tithe money to those individuals or organizations who feed my soul and nourish my spirituality and who are making a positive difference on this planet. I also give money and time to those individuals less fortunate than I. It is futile to say, "Yes, when I get this money I will give a tenth of it as a tithe." You must start helping those in need before that. If you do that, you will be living the spirit of "give that you may receive."

One day after writing my prosperity affirmations and goals on cards, I went to the grocery store. While waiting in the checkout line, I suddenly called out to the harried mother in front of me, "I'll pay for those." Needless to say, she was astonished. Quite honestly, so was I. The words seemed to have just popped out of my mouth. After some hesitancy and some excellent persuasion on my part, she let me pay her bill. The pleasure I received made me feel rich inside. Later that same day I ran into a person whom I had counseled several months before. At that time she had been unable to pay and so I wrote it off as an experience. But that day she wrote me a check.

To act 'as if' takes courage and trust. It's hard to start giving when you don't think you have enough. Go out into the world as if you had the courage and you'll find that the courage you wanted is already there. Do the thing and the power is yours. But it begins with a risk. If you don't risk, you don't receive. That's how you generate power.

Your subconscious mind is extraordinarily powerful, but it is a servant, not a master. It coordinates every aspect of your thoughts, feelings, behaviors, words, actions, and emotions to fit a pattern consistent with your dominant mental pictures. It guides you to engage in the behaviors that move you ever closer to achieving the goals you visualize and feel most of the time. If you visualize something that you fear, your subconscious mind will accept that as a command as well. It will then use its marvelous powers to bring your fears, instead of your dreams and aspirations, into reality.

Many people feel that their deepest beliefs and feelings are forever a mystery to them. They feel they don't understand the real reasons behind their actions, and as a result they feel powerless to change their actions. You have the power and ability to recognize and change the beliefs you have about yourself. Although your beliefs may seem mysterious and complicated on a conscious level, on a subconscious level they are usually simple. Your beliefs about yourself are based entirely on your past experiences. All of your experiences program your subconscious, and the result is the person you are today.

That is not to say that all you will ever be is the sum of your experiences. However, unless you take conscious control and choose the kind of programming you are feeding into your subconscious computer, you are destined to repeat your past. Have you ever noticed that your life experiences are all very similar—it's just the people who keep changing?

CHOOSE YOUR THOUGHTS AND WORDS WISELY

Two other effective ways to reprogram your subconscious mind are creative visualizations and affirmations. The idea is to alter your state of consciousness so you can temporarily set aside the conscious mind and focus your concentration specifically on your subconscious. Suggestions given to your subconscious while in an altered state of consciousness, whether they are images or affirmations, will be at least twenty times as effective as suggestions given in a normal state of consciousness, according to brain researchers. One of the best ways to alter or slow down your state of consciousness or brain wave activity is through relaxed deep breathing.

Brian Tracy, friend and human potential expert, host of Nightingale-Conant's Insight Tape program and author of the book, *Maximum Achievement*, is world renowned for his work on the powers of the mind and visualization. He emphasizes the importance of vividness in mental pictures. The more vividly you can see something that you want in your mind's eye, he says, the more rapidly it will materialize in your reality. Most people have only a vague, fuzzy picture of what they want. They say they want to be rich or healthy or happy. But when you ask them exactly what that means to them, they don't really know.

Vividness requires clarity of detail in your mental pictures. The more time you spend examining pictures of your desired goals, drawing your own pictures of them, or writing out clear descriptions of what your goals and dreams would look like when they came true, the more rapidly the pictures are accepted by your subconscious as a command. Your subconscious mind immediately goes to work to coordinate all of your other resources, internal and external, to bring those desires into your life. The clearer and more vivid your goal is in your mind's eye, the more rapidly it materializes in the world around you.

Be precise. Be absolutely definite. Know what you want, visualize what you want, and say what you want. It will not do to say you want a lot of money or that you want a new car or a house. You must state exactly what it is that you want and hold that picture firmly before you.

If you want money, state definitely how much you want. It must be a definite sum. If you are wise, you will not bother so much about money. Strive to gain virtues which will be of use to you when you leave this life. No one has ever taken a single coin into the next world. The more money you have, the more you leave for other people. The more you strive for money, the more you make it difficult for yourself to aspire to and attain spiritual values.

The more good you do for others, the more good you take with you. We can never have too much spirituality. We can never have too much purity of thought. We can never help others too much, for in helping others, we help ourselves. So if prosperity is your goal, make part of your visualization definite plans for how you will help others when you create this prosperity.

Prosperity comes in many shapes and forms, but all are alike in one way—each is a gift from God. A new car, an unexpected check, a smile from a friend or stranger, a breathtaking sunset—these things are among God's wondrous bounty that you can experience every day. When you pray, give thanks to God for answering your prayers. From this day forward, show your appreciation for any future good you will experience by declaring, "Thank You, God, for all the prosperity blessings I have received and will receive." Welcome prosperity graciously and enthusiastically. Bask in the warmth of God's generosity and give thanks for your blessings every day. Thank You, God! My needs are met! I even printed the words 'Thank You, God' on my checks, recognizing that God is my source.

Write down your major goals in the present tense on 3 x 5 cards and review them on a regular basis. As you read a goal on a card—for example, "I earn $250,000 per year"— close your eyes for a few seconds and imagine what it would be like if you were earning that kind of money. Visualize your ideal lifestyle. Get the feeling of success and achievement that goes with that greater income. Then open your eyes, smile, and go about your business, knowing in your mind's eye that you have already succeeded in achieving your goal.

Feed your mind a clear mental picture of your desired goals for the coming day, the coming week, and the coming months just before going to sleep at night. I do this every night for about ten minutes. As you drop off to sleep, your brain wave activity naturally slows down (as it naturally speeds up upon awakening), at which time your subconscious mind is the most receptive to the input of new commands. Since your mental pictures are a command, take those last few minutes before you fall off to sleep to daydream and fantasize about exactly the person you want to be and the life you want to have. Your subconscious mind will then take the picture down into its subconscious laboratory and work on it all night long. What often happens is that you wake up in the morning and have ideas and insights to help make those mental pictures a part of your life.

A few years ago one of my goals and dreams was to have a home-away-from-home, somewhere out in nature where I could go to write and have some quiet and solitude. While I wasn't sure where I wanted this home to be, I was very clear on some of my specific requirements. I wanted the home to be away from a large city and crowds of people, surrounded by trees and nature's sounds. The home itself needed to have lots of wood and windows, a spectacular view, and lend itself to my healthy lifestyle—sun, fresh air, organic garden, and great for working out. So for a few months I visualized this home. I wrote my vision down on three-by-five index cards and gave thanks that it was already a reality.

About six months later, I was invited to give a seven-day workshop in Coos Bay, located on Oregon's southern coast. I had been there before, giving several Sunday services at the Unity-by-the-Bay church and thought it was a beautiful area, but never considered buying a home there. One evening I had a break during my workshop and was invited to visit my dear friends, Wally and Gloria, where they lived on top of a forested hill overlooking Coos Bay. During our conversation in their home, they mentioned that the house next door was for sale. I acknowledged their comment and didn't give it any more thought until later. In the middle of the night I was hit by a cosmic two-by-four and immediately realized I was supposed to buy that house next door to my friends. My realization seemed absurd because I hadn't even looked at the inside of the house. I just knew the house was supposed to be mine and would be the perfect place for personal retreats and to write.

The next morning I called my friends. Upon hearing my decision they were delighted, even though they thought I was a little crazy. I called the realtor, Arch Wilkie, and learned that the house was in escrow and about to close. He would be happy to show me other homes, but this one was no longer available. I told him, "You don't seem to understand. That's my home and I'm not interested in looking at any others." I left Arch my telephone number and asked him to call when it was available. As it turned out, it did become available. I gave an offer and it became my retreat home, God's and mine. It didn't come without roadblocks—the path of least resistance isn't always the best. The whole process of creating a home presented me with one challenge after another and also taught me numerous lessons, like the importance of belief and faith; not judging by appearances; if it's to be, it's up to me; being thankful for everything seen and unseen; and beholding the Divine in everyone and everything. By the way, my home in Coos Bay is on top of a hill, surrounded by trees, overlooking the bay, has lots of light, and is filled with angels. I never thought Coos Bay as a place for my home-away-from-home. Now that I have it, I realize it's the perfect place for me and was made possible because of my partnership with God.

TAKE A WORD INVENTORY

Be aware of everything you say during the day. Take an inventory of what you actually say. Speak only those words that are positive, loving and uplifting. The words you think and speak have a tremendous influence on your life.

We literally live the words that have become a permanent part of our thinking and speaking patterns. If we say positive, joyful, spiritual, life-enhancing words, we begin to live happier, more joy-filled lives. Just as we need to be careful about the food we put into our bodies, we need to be every bit as careful about our words and thoughts, for they are food for our bodies and souls.

I have found that from time to time I get into bad habits with my words. Not too long ago, I was driving with my close friend, Reverend John Strickland. The day was hot and the traffic was heavy. A rude, reckless driver cut me off. I said in a loud voice, "I hate it when someone does that to me!" John looked very startled to hear that come out of me. He said, "Don't use the 'H' word. That's a terrible thing to put into your consciousness. You should say instead, 'I prefer drivers not to cut me off in traffic,' and then silently bless the driver."

I was in no mood to listen to a lecture. I felt like saying to him, "I hate it when somebody lectures me!" But I didn't do that because he was absolutely correct. I have fairly frequently thought about that and other careless statements. Have you ever said, "That burns me up," "They're driving me crazy," or "This is back-breaking work?" These seemingly harmless expressions program garbage into your subconscious mind. The subconscious does not know that you don't really mean it. It plays those ideas out into your life and experience, as if you really mean it.

What can you do to help yourself become aware of self-sabotaging words? I asked a couple of close friends with whom I spend time to call my attention to every word or expression I say which is not positive. I've learned to pay attention to what I say (most of the time) and to interrupt negative expressions. I usually say or think to myself "cancel" or "erase" and then change the words. I have also imagined in my mind's eye a large screen in which I write any negative expressions I've used and then draw an X through them. I've done this on paper, too, and then burned it. Use any method that is effective for you.

It is important to find positive ways to say exactly what you mean. For instance, replace "I'm sorry" with "I apologize." After all, that is what you mean. Change "I'm afraid you have the wrong number" with "You have the wrong number." As you find more ways to speak more accurately, you stop feeding your subconscious mind with misinformation about yourself.

Your words communicate more than you intend them to reveal, for they spring from your deepest thoughts. They tell others how you feel about yourself and the world around you. You are as good as your word. In my opinion, when it comes to keeping your word, there is no such thing as a small situation. Perhaps it would be no big deal for you to say you're going to call someone and then not do it; but it can be very important to the other person. It's very important to me that my friends and business associates be accountable and that their words count. When I learn that someone doesn't follow through on what they say they're going to do, and it's apparent that it's a pattern, I choose not to spend time with that person. I'm inspired by people who make their word count.

To me, a verbal agreement is as important as a written one. In fact, I have verbal agreements, as opposed to written ones, with most of the companies for whom I do consulting. People know my word is good and they can count on me.

Every time my friend, Lynn Carroll, makes a promise, no matter how small or seemingly insignificant, she keeps her word. If she makes plans with someone and then is offered the opportunity to do something more exciting or interesting, she never hesitates, saying: "Thank you, I'd love to do it, but I already have a commitment." Lynn's behavior invariably brings two reactions, both positive. The first friend is pleased because she and Lynn stick to their plan, and the second friend is also impressed. Lynn is not only well liked, she is also very successful. Lynn is as good as her word, friends say of her. To me, there can be no higher praise than that. Make your word count. It's a gift you give to your family, friends, business associates, community, and the world.

Fill your consciousness with positive things. There was a study conducted at Sussex University in which thirty subjects were shown a television news broadcast in which the topics were either positive, negative, or neutral. Not surprisingly, it was shown that negative news broadcasts put the subjects in a bad mood and made most of them edgy. We always have a choice about what we watch and give attention.

When you choose to be filled with a love of life and of God, you communicate joy through your words and actions. Because you know that God is so much a part of you and all that you do, you just naturally express love. Your words reach out to touch and uplift everyone around you. No matter what the subject is, the inner reality of God's presence stays the same. God's love and peace affect you in a deeply personal way, which is revealed through your words and actions. In Proverbs 15:1 we read, "A soft answer turns away wrath, but a harsh word stirs up anger."

YOUR HEART'S HIGHEST VISION

What's life without dreams? Do some people say you are a dreamer, hinting that you are something less than you should be? They don't know that you are using the tools of imagination and faith and painting a scene that is a real possibility for you. You recognize your dream as it takes shape, alert to the good that is unfolding right before you. Be a dreamer—a dreamer of what God has created for you to have and explore and share in this wondrous world. Never let anyone, including yourself, convince you that your dreams can't come true, not when you know they come from the divine good awaiting your acceptance. You dream the dreams that are inspired by Spirit and follow them in ways that bless you and all those whose lives you touch.

Visualization is a powerful tool that can carry you towards achieving your dreams and goals. Your job is to use the power of visualization consciously and continuously to create the kind of future you want for yourself.

What are your dreams? What is your vision? What do you expect to achieve in life? An important part of the process is expectation. Always expect to achieve your highest good, the best life has to offer, and live so that the best may become a part of your experience. Never allow anyone or anything to cause you to doubt your power and ability to live your vision—to manifest your goals and dreams.

There's an unfathomable, yet recognizable, divine order to this universe. It's ever-present and always working in alignment with what we need for our highest good and spiritual unfolding and growth. I've learned not to analyze or question it anymore. It asks only for our trust, faith, and courage.

PATIENT PERSISTENCE IN THE GOOD

I continue to live in awe of the magnificent adventure life continually is. I'm convinced that it's extremely important to always imagine and think about your heart's desires, while at the same time letting go of thoughts of what you don't want. In other words, let your imagination work for you and not against you. Make friends with your thoughts. Know that you are exactly where you need to be in life and, at any moment, you can choose to experience something else simply by taking responsibility and consciously choosing to think differently. This reminds me of the fantastic words by writer Nikos Kazantzakis: "You have your paintbrush and colors. Paint paradise, and in you go."

There is power in what you think and say. In order to change, you must start with your images, thoughts, and words. They will then get stored in your subconscious as reality. Then you will start acting on that new reality. I use visualization for everything from creating or healing relationships, to increasing my prosperity and fitness level, to finding parking spots, to tapping into higher levels of creativity and peacefulness.

When we see evidence of adverse conditions in the world or our personal lives, we may find it difficult to believe that God's power is at work. Yet even in the midst of circumstances that we cannot personally understand, we can affirm that God's love is healing, strengthening, and preparing the way for good. Regardless of appearances, we can always trust God to bring order to chaos and peace where there seems to be disharmony. We accept our own part in the overall scheme by holding firmly to the truth about ourselves and others. Instead of focusing our attention on negative conditions, we let our thoughts be loving and reflective of our true nature. The good thoughts we sow will help us remain patient as we wait for God's good to unfold.

These days most of my visualizations and affirmations have to do with being in perfect harmony with the superconscious mind—the Divine within—and staying open to this guidance. I want to be an open vessel through which God's will is manifest in my life. My human mind is not usually aware of what God's will for me is, but the divinity within me is. Every day, through prayer and meditation, I consciously surrender all to God, holding nothing back, and I ask for awareness, strength, and courage to act on the guidance I receive. In adopting this way of thinking, I have seen more changes and far greater fulfillment in my life than I could have imagined possible.

The indwelling Spirit makes all things new. This Divine power completely regenerates, renews, restores and rebuilds your life and world according to divine reality. I realize that Spirit can do for me only what it can do through me. "When you unlock the human door you are caught up in the life of the universe where your speech is thunder, your thought is law, and your words are universally intelligible," said Ralph Waldo Emerson. In quiet and stillness, that which is for your highest good is waiting for you to claim it. You will never have to search for it.

IN ALL THINGS BE GRATEFUL

I once read a story of a small boy about ten years old who came into a restaurant and sat at the counter. The waitress came over and put a glass of water in front of him. "How much is an ice cream sundae?" he asked.

"Fifty cents," replied the waitress.

The little fellow pulled his hand out of his pocket and studied a number of coins clutched in it. "How much is a dish of plain ice cream?" he asked. There were many people waiting at the counter and the waitress was slightly impatient.

"Thirty-five cents," she said brusquely.

Again he counted the coins. "I'll have the plain ice cream," he said.

The waitress took his money, brought the ice cream, put it in front of him and walked away. When she came back a few minutes later, the boy was gone. She stared at the empty dish and then swallowed hard at what she saw: placed beside the empty dish were two nickels and five pennies, fifteen cents—her tip. That was some time ago, but she still keeps those seven coins as a gentle reminder that little people are just as important as big ones, especially to themselves.

It's so easy to be grateful when all is going our way. But what about when life challenges us? I recall Helen Keller's remark: "I thank God for my handicap, for through that, I have found myself, my work, and my God."

We don't have to have problems to grow. We can grow in spiritual maturity as we turn to God. But it seems to me that only a faith and belief in God and His goodness can give us the understanding and strength to be grateful in the midst of challenge, and the courage to live more from our ever-present inner guidance.

Let go and let God's spirit of love and light direct you. It's in surrender that we find everything we are seeking. Begin each day with an expectant attitude. Look for the special blessing each person and situation has for you. Be open to new good and give thanks that God is always with us on each new adventure.

First thing in the morning and anytime during the day, pause and invite God's spirit of love and light to guide you along your way. At home, in your car, at work, let go of anxious thoughts and let God's spirit of light and love fill your heart and mind. Moment by moment, realize the presence of peace and harmony within you. As you let go of worry and fear, invite God's spirit to fill your mind. Become one with God. You are a beacon of love and light shining forth into the world.

Richard Bach, author of *Jonathan Livingston Seagull* and *Illusions*, wrote "You are never given a wish, without also being given the power to make it true."

When you know your heart's desire, and turn everything over to God, the perfect plan is set in motion as you let God direct you in all matters. You must take action and have complete trust in that action, knowing that God's love is directing you. The more we trust God, the more our minds and hearts and lives will be filled with Divine power, love, and success. When you understand this concept and integrate this knowledge into your life, you will be able to turn your dreams into reality and create a healthier, happier life than you ever imagined possible.

CHAPTER TWELVE

Serenity and Solitude:
Essential Ingredients for Quality of Life

Seek time to be alone; and in the cave of inner silence, you shall find the wellspring of wisdom.
—PARAMAHANSA YOGANANDA

One of the true masters of the art of serenity was the great inventor Thomas Alva Edison. When his factory burned down, he did not bemoan his fate. The newspaper reporters who went to interview him immediately following the disaster found him calmly at work on plans for a new building.

Another master of this art was Ralph Waldo Emerson. As his library of precious books was on fire, writer Louisa May Alcott tried to console him. The great philosopher said to her, "Yes, yes, Louisa, they're all gone, but let's enjoy the blaze now."

Men such as Edison and Emerson mastered the art of serenity. According to Webster's dictionary, serenity has to do with the quality or state of being serene—calm, tranquil, peaceful, quiet, noiseless. But to master this art of serenity, we need also to master another art, that of being alone.

SOLITUDE AND SILENCE

Everyone needs time for solitude and silence. During those precious times can be found the peace of your own company. While few of us would choose lifelong solitude, all of us can benefit from some time to ourselves. We may differ from our friends, colleagues, and partners in the amount, frequency, and urgency of our need, as well as in the way we spend our personal time. We may have trouble carving out periods of privacy, or even feel guilty claiming them, but when we're deprived for too long, we experience distress and lack of balance.

In *Man's Eternal Quest*, Paramahansa Yogananda writes, "Be alone within. Don't lead the aimless life that so many persons follow. Meditate and read good books more...Once in a while it is all right to go to the movies and have a little social life, but mostly remain apart and live within yourself...Enjoy solitude; but when you want to mix with others, do so with all your love and friendship, so that those persons cannot forget you, but remember always that they met someone who inspired them and turned their minds toward God."

It's hard to practice solitude and silence when we are constantly bombarded with a barrage of noises that seem to be part of living in our technological society. When we think we've carved out some quiet time, we become more sensitive to subtle sounds such as the refrigerator motor, air conditioner, heater, distant traffic, or the dripping faucet.

It's not easy to find absolute silence in the outer world, but you can find silence inwardly. Within each of us there is a peaceful silence waiting to be embraced. This silence is the harbor of the heart and when you rediscover it, your life will never be the same. From Psalms 62:1 in the Bible we read, "For God alone my soul waits in silence," and Yogananda said, "Calmness is the living breath of God's immortality in you." He also said the following, which I have posted on my bathroom mirror: "Always remember that seclusion is the price of greatness. In this tremendously busy life, unless you are more by yourself, you can never succeed. Never, never, never. Walk in silence. Go quietly; develop spiritually. We should not allow noise and sensory activities to ruin the antennae of our attention, because we are listening for the footsteps of God to come into our temples."

Mystics, saints, and spiritual leaders of the past and present have all advocated periods of silence for spiritual growth as a practical way to find balance and to be made whole again.

Concomitant with silence is spending time in solitude. Ah, solitude! Even the word evokes peace within me, perhaps because it's such an important and vital part of my life. Henry David Thoreau wrote in his journal, "It is a great relief when for a few moments in the day we can retire to our chamber to be completely true to ourselves. It leavens the rest of our hours."

How do you feel about being alone? There is, indeed, a difference between aloneness and loneliness, the two sides of solitude. Loneliness expresses the pain of being alone; solitude expresses the joy of being alone.

Sometimes finding time to be alone is a difficult thing. One of my friends has three children and rarely has time to herself. She is very busy working and raising the children. She often finds herself rushing between the children's dance lessons, doctor appointments, grocery shopping, and different household errands. When she told me how she spent her days, I became exhausted just listening. I suggested she give herself permission to call some time her own. Now, after she drops off a child at dance lessons, she either pulls out a favorite book and reads in her car or she spends the time in meditation. There are no phones, no people, no distractions.

She has an hour of quiet and solitude to do or think as she pleases.

When I'm conducting a workshop I often ask the participants to go outside for fifteen minutes and stroll the grounds alone in silence. I have them experience and practice being totally involved and absorbed in what they see, smell, feel, touch, or hear. I want them to let nature's beauty into their awareness. No matter what part of the world we are in, I always have participants come to me afterwards and say that this was their first experience of being truly alone and finding peace in their own company.

What I have discovered in taking this kind of walk is that I feel a subtle, gentle communion with nature. I build a garden of the soul. As mentioned in a previous chapter, the flowers, trees, birds, clouds, and even insects seem to be in communication with me. It rejuvenates my entire being and allows me to be more fully aware of my environment, sensitive to nature and connected to feeling my oneness with all life.

I devote a few hours a week to private counseling. With many clients, the session may first begin with an invigorating hike in the beautiful Santa Monica Mountains. I find this to be a wonderful way to let go and surrender to the spirit of life. Listening to the silence and sounds of nature is a great way to feel serene and in touch with your feelings, hence making it easier to express yourself. By the time our session is over, we both feel rejuvenated physically, mentally, and spiritually.

Several years ago, I spent time in a monastery in which disciplined silence was required twenty-four hours a day. At first it was difficult. There was so much I was feeling, experiencing, and seeing that I wanted to share with the others. Then, slowly and subtly, I discovered that the silence was overwhelmingly blissful. It was almost as though a gentle wave of peace rolled over me. There was nothing but silence—all around me, through me, and everywhere expanding and reaching out to touch all creation. Things that touch the heart are often difficult to put into words, and this was one of those experiences. I just knew that I loved the silence, reveled in it, and wanted to have it with me always.

Since that time at the monastery, I carry this silence with me. Even in conversation, I am aware of this quietness beneath the sounds of people's voices. Although I sometimes lose awareness of it, I can recall it and let it once again be a source of great peace and joy, like the awareness of a close and loving friend.

Since my experience at the monastery, I now find time for regular periods of solitude and silence. I recognize that I choose more solitude than most. Not only do I meditate at least twice a day, but I also take off several hours once a week, one weekend a month, and a few days with each change of season to simply be alone and embrace silence. In fact, as

I write this chapter I'm celebrating a new glorious season and am spending a few days in Coos Bay, Oregon away from most of the activity of my usual world. This regular supplement of solitude and silence greatly enhances all areas of my life. It nourishes my soul.

Constant activity and noise enervate the body and leave us feeling drained mentally, emotionally and physically. Quality time alone is renewing. I enjoy exercising alone at dawn. I feel great not only because I am alone, but also because I'm working out and find pleasure in my own company. There's also serenity in being self-sufficient—feeling complete, whole, and satisfied with myself and what I'm doing—whether I'm working or enjoying a respite of relaxation and solitude.

"Silence will help you see clearly exactly what is out of balance in your life," says Barbara De Angelis, Ph.D. in her wonderful book, *Real Moments*. "It creates an opening through which you can receive truth, perspective, strength, healing, revelation."

When was the last time you were alone—I mean really alone—and in silence without radio, video, or tapes, listening to the silence of your heart, being at peace with your own company?

Here are some simple ways De Angelis suggests to create and experience more silence in your life:

CARVING OUT TIME TO BE ALONE

- Drive with your radio turned off. Cars are great moving awareness centers. I consider them 'sacred spaces.'
- Don't turn on your TV if you're not really watching. Background noise keeps your mind restless and suggestible to unwanted influences.
- Keep your telephone from becoming a disruptive force. Turn the ringer off and the volume down on your answering machine a few days each week. Sometimes I gather my messages at the end of the day and return the calls in one sitting.
- Exercise without your personal stereo. If outdoors, listen to nature. It can be more meditative. Move to the rhythm of your thoughts.
- Sit in silence by firelight or candlelight. "Watch the flames. Listen to logs crackle, or watch the wax drip down the side of the candle," says De Angelis. "Imagine the light illuminating all of the dark or hidden places inside of you. Enjoy the simplicity of the moment."

There's an old saying that God gave us two ears and one mouth so we may hear more and talk less. How well we use our ears plays an important part in determining what we learn as we go through life. The more time I spend in silence, the more I appreciate the power of brevity and silence when conversing with others.

Silence is golden. It can persuade, dissuade, heal, inspire, command, console, win elections, promote good health, and bring about greater happiness and harmony in your life. Even when you are with other people, silence can help you communicate ideas, feelings, beauty, strength, or understanding without uttering a sound.

Understanding and accepting another's need for private time is more difficult for those who don't want to be by themselves. Some of us are apt to feel rejected when our company is turned down in favor of the other person's being alone. It is not a rejection, although it may be misunderstood that way.

Often the issue is finding time. You must choose to make the time. Make privacy a priority in your life. Privacy is a universal need. There will always be others who want some of your time. In order to get quiet time to yourself, reserve a regular period in your daily schedule when your family and friends know that, barring emergencies, you expect to be left alone. It helps to explain your needs clearly and specifically to others.

Find a way to fit this privacy into your life. For some, solitary exercise may be all that is needed to maintain that balance throughout the day.

Others spend several minutes alone one or more times a day in some type of meditation. This spiritual exercise allows life's experiences to touch us more gently. Still others embark on longer silent retreats to go more deeply into their own consciousness and clear all channels. Whether for short or extended periods of time, retreating from the outside world will enhance and enrich all areas of your life.

I believe that all the other good things we endeavor to provide for ourselves—sound nutrition, daily exercise, vitamin supplements, material wealth—will be of limited value unless we learn to live in harmony with ourselves, which means knowing ourselves and finding peace in our own company. Peace is a natural consequence of time spent alone. In time spent alone we realize we are never really alone and that we can live more fully by focusing on inner guidance. Too often we look outside ourselves for our worth and forget that nothing will ever be enough until we are enough. When we recognize that we are already enough, everything else will be enough. It all starts on the inside.

As we open our hearts to silence, we access the most powerful healer of all—the healing power of love, of God. In silence, deep within our hearts, each of us knows the truth.

SIMPLIFY, SIMPLIFY!

A natural outgrowth of the practice of solitude is the desire to slow down and forego the hurry habit. There's an American sickness I've seen growing over the past years: the hurry sickness, the busyness sickness. We see it everywhere—instant breakfasts, fast foods, in-and-out cleaners, one-minute managers, and twelve-minute fitness programs. I wouldn't be surprised to see a new book about one-minute sex!

To let go of the busyness of life requires simplifying our lives. Simplify! What a wonderful word and a powerful process it represents. I have discovered great joy in simplifying all areas of my life. This includes my thoughts, what I say, how I choose to spend my time, how I arrange my closets, cupboards, and garage—everything.

To simplify is so freeing and feels so good. For example, look at the foods you eat in one meal. It's hard to appreciate any one of them fully when so many are mixed together. Similarly, you can have a fantastic collection of art objects in your home, but if you have too many and it's cluttered, appreciating each piece is difficult.

In his delightful little book, *How You Can Talk With God*, Yogananda said, "Why do you consider nonessentials so important? Most people concentrate on breakfast, lunch, and dinner, work, social activities, and so on. Make your life more simple and put your whole mind on the Lord."

When your life gets too complicated and out of balance, you become less sensitive to your own needs and the needs of your family and friends around you. When you consciously choose to simplify, your life slows down and you are better able to live in the present moment with a wise awareness of your own inner guidance and divinity. Often we live so harriedly and hurriedly that we don't pay attention to what's really important. Our lives are cluttered with things we don't need.

What can you do to simplify your life right now, today? One surprisingly effective place to start is by cleaning out and simplifying one of your closets, some cupboards, or your garage. Keep that up for fifteen minutes each day until you have finished with your entire home. As a result of this disciplined exercise, you will find yourself easily and naturally beginning to simplify other areas of your life—how you spend your time, what you think, and what you say. This technique is not only freeing and refreshing, it also supports you in feeling more serene and peaceful, and in seeing your life from a higher perspective. The technique works because outside and inside always reflect each other; change one and you influence the other.

LIVING FULLY AND LIVING SIMPLY GO HAND-IN-HAND

In his book, *Voluntary Simplicity*, Stanford Research Institute social scientist Duana Elgin claims there is a trend toward simplicity. He states, "To live with simplicity is to unburden our lives—to live a more direct, unpretentious, and unencumbered relationship with all aspects of our lives; consuming, working, learning, relating, and so on. Simplicity of living means meeting life face to face, confronting life clearly without unnecessary distractions, without trying to soften the enormity of our existence or masking the deeper manifestations of life with pretensions, distractions, and unnecessary accumulation. It means being direct and honest in relationships of all kinds. It means taking life as it is—straight and unadulterated."

Letting go of clutter, living honestly, simply and freely, without pretensions, encumbrances, and superfluity is what living fully and joyfully is all about. Perhaps we can head in that direction by having fewer desires and being more selfless. The venerable Lao-Tzu said: "Manifest plainness, embrace simplicity, reduce selfishness, have few desires."

At one time in my life, I found great pleasure in collecting material things. My income was generous and I would delight in buying lots of clothes, appliances, electronics, gadgets, and cars, until I got to the point that I was seeking fulfillment from what I collected rather than from the divinity within. In pursuit of many material goals, I began to lose sight of my spiritual goals, through which all fulfillment, happiness, and peace come. I was looking outward to my collection of stuff rather than within, to my true nature, for my value and worth as a human being.

Fortunately, I discovered that what the world holds for me is not as important as what I bring to the world. When I realized that, it became clear to me that I wanted to live more simply in every aspect of my life. I have found that I can live well and still live simply. I still buy clothes and other items these days, but more often I'm giving things away and finding ways to make my life more simple, less complicated.

How can you simplify your life in order to fulfill your purpose more easily and live more fully? We can assist each other on our journey through this miracle called life, but no one can live your life for you. In the end, it comes down to choice. Once you become aware that you are choosing everything, you can take over your own life and live it the way your Higher Self knows how to live it. You can choose to let go of clutter and complexity in favor of serenity, peace and happiness—a more spiritual life.

TO FIND HAPPINESS, SERVE

When your life is less cluttered, you have more time to focus on what's really important, like being of service and letting God's will navigate your thoughts, words and actions. Albert Schweitzer said, "I don't know what your destiny will be, but one thing I do know: the only ones among you who will be really happy are those who have sought and found how to serve." I believe that service is the key to a happy life, to a spiritualized life—and it is also the key to spiritualizing business.

Whether or not we belong to a church or service organization, or have a job that provides meaningful service opportunities, not a day goes by that we can't at least serve another human being by making deposits of unconditional love. It's not the deed that is essential; the important thing is the loving serviceful attitude—success and saintliness are more a product of inner consciousness and attitude than efficiently improving the world's outer condition.

Yogananda said: "Instead of making money and greater profits your goal in business, make service your goal, and you will see the entire plan of your life change. Business for private profiteering is wrong." That doesn't mean that we shouldn't make a legitimate profit. It just means that service, not money, should be our goal; then profit follows automatically. Profit is the natural result of service. As the best entrepreneurs know, values can be profitable.

There is intrinsic security that comes from service, from helping other people in a meaningful way. One important source is your work, when you see yourself in a contributing and creative mode, really making a difference. Another source is anonymous service—where no one knows it, no one necessarily ever will, and that's not your concern, but rather your concern is blessing the lives of other people.

Yogananda suggests that each day we find ways to do some good. Perhaps give to a worthy cause or help some individual. Sometimes all a person needs is some understanding, attention or compassion. See God in everyone, no matter how erring the person may be. When you mentally put yourself in the position of others, it is easier to understand them, to act with kindness, and to help. "The one thing that will help to eliminate world suffering—more than money, houses, or any other material aid—is to meditate and transmit to others the divine consciousness of God that we feel. Everyday radiate His consciousness to others," explains Yogananda.

Someone once said, "Service is the rent we pay for the privilege of living on this earth." And there are so many ways to serve.

CHAPTER THIRTEEN

Acts of Kindness: The Joy Factor

Of course I love everyone I meet. How could I fail to? Within everyone is the spark of God. I am not concerned with racial or ethnic background or the color of one's skin; all people look to me like shining lights!
—PEACE PILGRIM

I could hear the frustration in her voice the moment I picked up the telephone. My friend Rose called me because she was on the verge of quitting her job, even though she loved her work. She needed some guidance.

Rose is a very talented window dresser for a popular store on Rodeo Drive in Beverly Hills. She loves what she does, but she had been having a very difficult time with her boss. During our telephone conversation, she described how she was convinced that she was unjustly criticized by her supervisor and felt that some of her best work was rejected and unappreciated. She also felt he was deliberately rude and unfair to her.

Because I believe that we always attract to ourselves the equivalent of what we think, feel, believe, and put our faith in, I lovingly suggested to my friend that maybe she, rather than her boss, was the one in need of a new attitude. I asked her how she felt about him.

Rose confessed to me that her mind was filled with criticism and unkindness toward this man and that she rarely felt positive in his presence because of the way he treated her. She even revealed to me that every morning as she walked to work, she visualized the entire scenario of how she knew she would be treated by him that day. Rose confirmed my observation about the law of correspondence. I explained that he was merely bearing witness to her conception of him.

When Rose realized what she had been doing, she agreed to change her attitude and only think of him in a loving, kind way. I recommended that before drifting off to sleep at night, she visualize her boss congratulating her on her fine designs and creativity and that she, in turn, see herself thanking him for his praise and kindness.

To her delight, after only seven days of practicing her visualizations, the behavior of her employer miraculously reversed itself. Rose proved the power of imagination and kindness. Rose's persistent desire to replace love and tenderheartedness for unkindness influenced his behavior and determined his attitude toward her. It is always the same—as within, so without.

Humans are powerful spiritual beings meant to create good on the earth. This good isn't usually accomplished in bold actions, but in singular acts of love and kindness between people. It's the little things that count, because they are more spontaneous and show who you truly are. The amount of love and good feelings you have at the end of your life is equal to the love and good feelings you put out during your life. It's that simple. "What a splendid way to move through the world," writes Jack Kornfield in *A Path with Heart*, "to bring our blessings to all that we touch. To honor, to bless, to welcome with the heart is never done in grand or monumental ways but in this moment, in the most immediate and intimate way."

THE RELIGION OF KINDNESS

The Dalai Lama said, "My religion is very simple—my religion is kindness." Gentleness and kindness go hand in hand. Gentle means kindly, mild, amiable, not violent or severe. Gentle also implies compassionate, considerate, tolerant, calm, mild-tempered, courteous, and peaceful. But I think the best synonym for gentle is tenderhearted. I love being around people who are tenderhearted. What about you? Think about those people you love to be around the most, with whom you feel the most enthusiastic and positive and can be yourself. You'll probably say they're loving, supportive, kind, and maybe even tenderhearted.

To be treated with tenderheartedness and kindness, we must first offer that quality to the other person. Respond to others exactly as you would want to be treated. No one likes to be belittled, ignored, or unappreciated. Everyone likes kindness, patience, and respect. In Ephesians 4:32 we read, "Be kind to one another, tenderhearted, forgiving one another, as God in Christ forgave you."

"Random acts of kindness" is a slogan that's been catching on around the country. Acts of kindness are those lovely things we do for no reason except that for a moment, the best of our humanity and heart comes forward. Every day we are presented with hundreds of opportunities to practice kindness towards our fellow humans. These gestures aren't expected or anticipated. Don't ever underestimate the power of kindness. In the process we are transformed. We become, in a sense, an angel for a moment and touch the Divine when we give to another pure love and joy without expecting something in return. We become twice blessed, for in blessing another we bless ourselves. In showing love and kindness to another, we also increase our self-esteem. Acts of kindness connect our heart with the heart of another person and create pathways through which our love can flow.

Sometimes these acts of kindness are made anonymously and sometimes not. But in the process, we can't help but be changed ourselves. In giving of our highest selves, purely out of love, our body, our heart and our environment change, and for an instant we realize that loving and being loved is the one true human vocation. We feel connected to the love in ourselves and the love in others.

I'll never forget the morning of January 17, 1994. It was 4:31 AM and I was meditating on the floor in front of my altar. My first reaction was that God was speaking to me! A couple of seconds later, I knew it was the biggest earthquake I had ever felt. I will never forget the terrifying sensation of holding on to the corner of my bed and listening to everything in the house crashing. It felt and sounded like the end of the world had arrived. I felt certain that I was going to die. Most everyone who went through this experience felt like the epicenter was under their own home, and that it was more like four minutes than forty seconds. For those moments and for the hours that followed, I was living totally in the present moment.

But what's important here is the response from the community. Adversity always brings gifts and powerful lessons. Families, friends, and even strangers reached out to one another with true compassion and kindness. Sharing the same experience brought people together on common (if shaky) ground, opened our hearts, and woke up our spirits. Southern California was invigorated with a newfound compassion and kindness.

It permeated everywhere and lifted the hearts of all. In the days following the earthquake the crime rate was at the lowest in years. We were forced to slow down and to see more clearly what's truly important and essential in life: not the things you possess or the work that you do, but the people in your life, the heart-to-heart connection you have with others and the love you give.

Antoine De Saint-Exupéry wrote in *The Little Prince* that what's truly essential is invisible to the eye—it can only be seen and felt with the heart. "When strangers start acting like neighbors, communities are reinvigorated," says Ralph Nader. Acts of kindness send out a positive ripple into the world and help bring us back to the feeling that people are basically good and kind. The love you have to give never runs out, for the more you give, the more you have to give.

Sometimes we get so caught up in our responsibilities and commitments to family, friends, work, and doing what's expected of us that there's little left to give to others, let alone ourselves. That's when we need to step outside the ordinary and enter into the realm of the extraordinary and magnificent. With willingness and a little effort, you can create miracles in your life and the lives of others. You can become an angel, transforming the lives of others simply by giving with love.

For random acts of kindness to flourish we need to begin in perhaps the most difficult place of all, our own hearts, with simple acts of kindness toward ourselves. It is essential that we refuel our own spirits so that we will want to be compassionate to others. Then we can truly give to others from a heart overflowing with loving kindness. "Let us not be satisfied with just giving money," says Mother Teresa. "Money is not enough, money can be got, but they need your hearts to love them. So, spread your love everywhere you go."

KINDNESS AT THE AIRPORT

Not long ago I was moved by a gesture of love at the airport. I was leaving Portland, Oregon to fly to Los Angeles. Because of stormy weather, most flights were delayed and some were canceled. The airport was crowded yet my flight on Alaska Airlines was scheduled to leave on time. As they announced the final boarding, I noticed a harried man run up to the counter with his briefcase in one hand and ticket in another. He was told by the ticket agent that his reservation had been cleared and his seat given away. She told him that she would do everything she could to get him a seat on a later flight.

Well, he went ballistic. Everyone in the terminal could hear his frustration. He had an important meeting in Los Angeles that he couldn't miss. I felt for him because I've been in similar situations where I couldn't afford to miss a flight. In his tirade he yelled out that he wanted to see a supervisor.

All of a sudden a woman who looked to be in her seventies walked up to this man and said that she wasn't in a hurry and would be happy to give him her seat. As you can imagine, this man stopped right in his tracks. It almost looked like he was going to cry. He apologized to her, to the ticket agent, and to everyone around for his behavior and thanked the woman for being an angel in his life. He boarded the flight smiling, relieved, and much wiser. What a blessing for the lovely woman, too. The man wasn't aware of this, but the airline got the woman on another flight just three hours later, and also gave her a free round-trip ticket to any destination served by the company. So she was truly twice blessed.

LET YOUR HEART-LIGHT SHINE

Reaching out with a kind act or word of praise or appreciation can be so simple. Yet sometimes we assume that others have it together and don't need our kindness. Wouldn't it be better to move beyond our assumptions and to offer the kind of thoughtfulness we would appreciate receiving—a compliment, a smile, a hug, a pat on the shoulder, a note of thanks, or just a question that shows concern? If your kind gesture goes unnoticed or is refused it doesn't matter, because in giving to another, you give to yourself.

Take smiling. Everyone can do it. If you're not used to smiling, practice in the mirror by pulling up on the corners of your mouth! It's so simple and yet so effective. Learn to smile sincerely, from your heart. Did you know that it takes more muscular effort to frown than it does to smile?

Smile at family and friends, at strangers, everyone you meet or pass during the day today. Do you realize how many lives you can touch simply by smiling? You smile at one person and he or she catches the good feeling and smiles at another person, and so on until your smile has indirectly affected the lives of several thousand people in one day.

Or how about writing a note of thanks or appreciation? You don't need a special occasion to send a card or note to someone. You think you're too busy to send a card or note? It doesn't take much time. I love to write letters and am very faithful, as most of my close friends will attest. Sometimes I'll go to a card store and purchase several dozen cards to have on hand. Isn't it fun to receive a card from a friend for no reason at all? It may even be quicker than the telephone.

Last week a friend and I were having dinner at a local restaurant. It was early evening and the restaurant wasn't very busy, and my friend and I had the opportunity to visit with our waitress. We found out that she was a single mom in her early twenties with two children and was putting herself through college and working two jobs just to make ends meet. In spite of all her challenges, she was cheerful and a joy to be around. When we got our bill, my friend and I decided to do something special. Even though the bill was under $30, we left a $100 tip. What a great feeling!

Sometimes the kindest gestures may go unnoticed. When I walk down the street, I love to put coins in parking meters if I find some that have expired. The drivers of the cars may never know, but it makes me feel good. Some times I send a note anonymously with a kind word or a few dollars when I know the recipient is in need. It takes so little to do so much.

Sometimes gestures are very much noticed. Not long ago when I was in Coos Bay, Oregon, my wonderful friend Helen Guppy accompanied me to a radio station where I was scheduled to do an interview from 11 PM to midnight. When the interview was over, the radio station closed and everyone left. Helen and I walked to my car only to discover that it wouldn't start. I lifted the hood to see if anything looked out of the ordinary. Helen reminded me that we were not in the best area of town and blocks from a telephone. It was cold and beginning to rain. I told Helen that we needed to imagine and affirm that an angel would help us out of this dilemma.

As we were getting back into the car to see if an angel would start the engine, a cab drove by. The driver stopped and asked if we needed nay help. Helen whispered to me to have faith, even though he didn't look like the angel she imagined. I agreed. The cab driver looked under the hood and immediately checked the battery. It was out of water. He had a jug of water in his cab and filled the reservoirs. He also told us an interesting story. He had just dropped off a passenger several blocks away and was heading home since his shift was over. Something inside him guided him to take a totally different route that evening, one he had never taken before. He thought it was odd but did it anyway. That's when he saw Helen and me looking under the hood and wondered if we needed help. We told him that he was our imagined angel. He smiled. The cab driver followed us back to my home to make sure the car didn't stall, then said good-bye.

That's not the end of the story. The next day I found a book on angels left "anonymously" on my doorstep. But Helen and I both knew who left it.

William Penn described well the act of kindness when he wrote, "If there is any kindness I can show, or any good thing I can do to any fellow being, let me do it now, and not deter or neglect it, as I shall not pass this way again."

REACH OUT AND TOUCH SOMEONE

Each of us can make a difference in the world. By our intentions and through our attitudes we can choose to see heaven or hell. Alan Cohen writes in his delightful book, *Joy Is My Compass*, that "the difference between a saint and a sourpuss is that the sourpuss sees his daily interactions as a nuisance, while the saint finds a continuous stream of opportunities to celebrate. One finds intruders, the other angels. At any given moment we have the power to choose what we will be and what we will see. Each of us has the capacity to find holiness or attack all about us." Make a difference in your world by giving deposits of love and kindness every chance you get. You never know how profound your gesture can be in someone else's life.

A few years ago a friend and I went to see a play in Los Angeles. After it was over, we decided to get something to eat at a coffee shop down the street. It was late and few people were in the restaurant. After awhile I noticed a ragged woman who obviously didn't feel good about herself. The waitress told us that this woman came in every Saturday evening at the same time. As I was talking with my friend, I couldn't help but notice the woman's appearance. In her mid-fifties, she had dirty clothes and matted, greasy hair, and carried a backpack as her purse. I could sense her sadness and loneliness. I was keenly aware of my desire to reach out to her, but I didn't really know what to do.

My friend had to leave, but I decided to stay. I went over to the woman's table, touched her hand, and asked her to keep me company while I finished my meal. At that point she started to cry, and I thought to myself, "Susan, you certainly misread your inner signals this time." As I sat down to try and mend the situation, this woman, Gloria, told me I was the first person to approach her with genuine warmth and caring in years!

Gloria and I talked for an hour and she invited me to her apartment a couple blocks away. In her cramped and disheveled one-room apartment I listened through the night to her life story.

I found out that Gloria hadn't worked for months and that she had no family and rarely had visitors. As she spoke of her love for children, I remembered a telephone call I had received two weeks before. A friend who owns a day care center had called, asking me if I could recommend someone for an opening as a teacher's aide. I will never forget the sparkle in Gloria's eyes as I told her the details of this possible job.

It was now eight o'clock in the morning. I suggested she take a shower and then we could return to the coffee shop for breakfast. We also called the day care center owner. The position was still open and I arranged for Gloria to have an interview later that day.

In the meantime, I helped Gloria curl her hair, showed her how to apply some makeup, and helped her to pick out a clean dress to wear for the interview. It was wonderful to see her transform before my eyes. Gloria got the job and began work the next week. After several weeks, I paid a surprise visit to Gloria at the center. I could hardly believe my eyes. She looked ten years younger and was aglow with enthusiasm. The children all loved her and so did the center's owner. She invited me to her apartment for dinner that evening. I didn't recognize her home either. She had cleaned and painted every inch and even had a couple of plants on her dresser. I was so touched. Gloria was radiantly alive and happy, as she was meant to be.

From this experience I truly learned the value of reaching out to someone even though you have no guarantee of the outcome. I believe that's what living is all about—person to person, heart to heart. Life is not a spectator sport. Participate in the adventure of life. You cannot induce permanent change in someone by doing for them what they can and should do for themselves, but you can be a catalyst for change. With love in your heart and a willingness to risk and be vulnerable, all will be right.

It takes a strong person to be gentle and kind. "Tenderness and kindness are not signs of weakness and despair," writes Kahlil Gibran, "but manifestations of strength and resolution." When we relax and get centered in the divine flow, we can feel God's gentle presence within us and express that gentle kindness toward ourselves and others.

There have been many teachers in my life who have taught me about kindness and have shown me by example that angels walk among us. My mom, June B. Smith, is one such person. She lives her life doing kindnesses for others and has been my greatest inspiration. I'm always telling Mom that when I grow up, I want to be just like her.

Another angel is my dear friend Helen Guppy. Although her wings are invisible, they are quite obvious to me. Her greatest joy comes from helping others, whether she knows them or not. Her life is about blessing the lives of others and, in return, she is filled with joy and happiness. Along with my mother, Helen has taught me the true meaning of unconditional love and kindness.

THE HEALTH BENEFITS OF SMALL PLEASURES

To be gentle and kind to others, we must first be gentle and kind with ourselves. There's no need to be hard on yourself, to beat yourself up when you make a mistake, choose incorrectly, or repeat the past. Be kind and understanding of yourself. Be especially kind to yourself if you behave in a way that you dislike. Always talk kindly to yourself, and be patient when you find it difficult to be a 'holy' person. Forgive yourself, and then when you do not act as you want, use your actions as a reminder of where you are and where you are not. Be your own best friend.

A study has uncovered a surprising benefit to working small joys into your day-to-day schedule. It can help give your immune system a boost. Researchers in the Department of Psychiatry at State University of New York at Stony Brook asked one hundred volunteers to fill out an evaluation of daily ups and downs. They compared this information with antibody activity in the participants' saliva, which indicates immune system fluctuations. They found that the stress of a negative event weakens the immune system on the day it occurs, but a positive event can strengthen the immune system for two days or more.

"In other words, positive daily events help immune function more than upsetting events hurt it," says Arthur Stone, Ph.D., the psychologist who conducted the study. Among the everyday events that boosted subjects' immune systems: pursuing leisure activities (such as jogging) and spending time on a favorite hobby or special interest. Take time to be kind to yourself with life-affirming pleasures and activities.

THE HEALTH BENEFITS OF LOVE AND KINDNESS

Just as God forgives us, we must continually forgive ourselves. Forgiveness is an act of self-love, rather than some altruistic saintly behavior. In working with countless people over the years, I have come to the conclusion that an absence of forgiveness is tantamount to staying imprisoned in an unawakened life. Forgiveness is as important to learn and practice as are all of the other principles in this book.

The more you extend kindness to yourself, the more it will become your automatic response toward others. Fill yourself with love even toward those who would do you harm—which is what all spiritual leaders of all times have said—and see if you still feel anger and revenge. One of my favorite Bible verses is John 13:34, "Love one another." This is a crucial part of learning to forgive. True forgiveness begins with love. When we learn to love others as God loves us—unconditionally, and without thought for what has happened in the past—we will not have any trouble forgiving them. We will be led out of the darkness of doubt and confusion and into the light of understanding. We will release the painful experiences of the past and invite more positive ones into our lives.

Love and kindness are intimately related with health. This is not simply a sentimental exaggeration. One survey of 10,000 men with heart disease found a fifty percent reduction in frequency of chest pain (angina) in men who perceived their wives as supportive and loving.

Tender loving care is a valuable element in healing. In the insightful book, *Healing Words: The Power of Prayer and the Practice of Medicine*, by Dr. Larry Dossey, I read about a fascinating study by David McClelland, Ph.D., of Harvard Medical School. He demonstrated the power of love to make the body healthier through what he calls the "Mother Teresa effect." He showed a group of Harvard students a documentary of Mother Teresa ministering lovingly to the sick and measured the levels of immunoglobulin A (IgA) in their saliva before and after seeing the film (IgA is an antibody active against viral infections such as colds). IgA levels rose significantly in the students, even in many of those who considered Mother Teresa too religious or a fake. In order to achieve this effect in another way, McClelland later asked his graduate students simply to think about two things: past moments when they felt deeply loved and cared for by someone else, and a time when they loved another person. In both cases there was an increase in IgA levels in the students.

THE HEALTH BENEFITS OF FRIENDSHIP

I highly value and feel a great sense of gratitude for the love and support I receive from my friends, and for the opportunity to care deeply for others. The only way to have a friend is to be one. Friends help sustain us when we're down, comfort us when we're sad, and offer counsel when we're confused. Friends are truly the best kind of wealth we can have—a wealth not calculated in numbers, but in the priceless value of a true friend. Show love and appreciation for your friends. Practice forgiveness and seeing your friends as beloved children of God. Never take your friends for granted. Friendship is as sacred a commitment as any other; our friends are sent by God, for us to help them and for them to help us.

Often in today's society we put our selfish interests first, before loyalty or integrity or commitment to higher values. Since what emanates from us will come back to us at some point, this is ultimately not a winning attitude. We must do what is right for the sake of doing what is right. To have a true friend you must be a true friend. The love shared between two people is the most precious gift we have. I love what Sir Hugh Walpole said: "The most wonderful of all things in life, I believe, is the discovery of another human being with whom one's relationship has a glowing depth, beauty, and joy as the years increase. This inner progression of love between two human beings is a most marvelous thing, it cannot be found by looking for it or by passionately wishing for it. It is a sort of divine accident."

I am reminded of my beautiful friend, Molly. Well into her seventies when I met her, she knew how to celebrate life and the importance of being kind and loving to everyone. That was evident in her many friendships. The times we spent visiting together will always be special to me. A vibrant, alive, positive woman, Molly spent her days swimming, walking, doing yoga, or volunteering at the UCLA hospital.

Molly was diagnosed with terminal cancer. The shocking news darkened her sunny disposition for the first three days, then she adjusted to it and decided to make the most of whatever time she had left. She continued her routine and seemed as radiantly alive and cheerful as ever.

The last month of her life was spent in the hospital. I was away on a lengthy speaking tour and when I returned I immediately visited Molly in the hospital. I wasn't prepared for what I saw. During my absence she had lost nearly half her body weight, all her teeth, most of her color but, astonishingly, not her cheerful attitude. Although she was physically unrecognizable, her spirit shone through when she said, "Sunny, I know I've looked better. Let's see if you can perform your magic and fix me up." I brushed her hair, washed her face, and applied a drop of her favorite perfume. Although she could barely move, and she had a difficult time speaking, she still told me a couple of jokes. She also spoke with great appreciation about the flowers in her room and the birds singing to her from the tree outside her window.

She then asked me to lie down next to her, because she needed to talk and she didn't think she had much time. That final hour she spoke to me about the light and colors she saw and about the peace and joy she felt. She was ready to go to the other side and was actually eager to make her transition. Just before she died she said to me, "Life is meant to be joyful. Don't ever get too serious about life. Laugh every day and live each day as though it were your last. Continue to find ways to give love to others like you have always done with me. Follow your heart and let the beauty of life into your spirit." And then she passed on.

Molly reminded me that we must embrace all of life and live every day as though we were born anew. Erich Fromm said, "Living is the process of continuous rebirth. The tragedy in the life of most of us is that we die before we are fully born." My experiences with Molly also make me think of something Elisabeth Kubler-Ross said in her book, *Death: The Final Stage of Growth*. "What is important is to realize that whether we understand fully who we are or what will happen when we die, it's our purpose to grow as human beings, to look within ourselves, to find and build upon that source of peace and understanding and strength that is our individual self. And then to reach out to others with love and acceptance and patient guidance in the hope of what we may become together."

Through love and forgiveness, we can live from the heart and in the heart of God. My unshakable belief in the ever-present goodness and availability of God underlies everything in my life. I've come to know that, with God as my source of inspiration, I have a well that will never run dry. Each day is a fresh new possibility to be kind to ourselves and others. And when we live in the heart of God we can let our kindness shine in everything we think, say, and do.

SHOWING KINDNESS DAY TO DAY

Every day you have countless opportunities to practice kindness towards yourself and others. Here are some ideas to add to your list.

- Go to your local shelter and adopt a pet.
- Offer a ride to a friend who can't get around.
- Volunteer time at your local library.
- Pick up some trash as you walk down the sidewalk.
- Ask your friends and co-workers to tell you their stories of random acts of kindness. Have a party for telling such stories. Emphasis on the pleasure of giving with no strings attached inspires us to do more.
- Give another person your parking spot.
- Let another driver get in front of you if they want. Wave and smile at them, too.
- Surprise a forgotten friend or relative with a phone call.
- Give a present to an underprivileged boy or girl, or to someone for no reason at all.
- Take the clothes you haven't worn in a year to a homeless shelter. Organize neighbors on your block to do the same.
- Wave hello to pedestrians when you're in your car, even if you don't know them. It will lift their spirits as well as yours.
- Let the person behind you in line at the grocery or hardware store go in front of you.
- Pay for the groceries of the person in front of you. If they are hesitant, just tell them it will make you feel terrific.
- When you're in line for a movie, anonymously pay for the ticket of someone behind you in line. Then watch their face as they receive the news.
- Order a mail-order gift anonymously for a friend or someone you know who needs to be cheered up.
- Slip a $20 bill into the pocket or purse of a needy friend or stranger.
- If you drive on a toll bridge, pay for the next few cars after yours.
- Laugh out loud and smile often. Even when you're not in the mood to smile, do it. It will lift your spirits. Don't take your life so seriously. Play the game of life and show kindness.
- If you know someone who's having a difficult day, do something special and wonderful for that friend without telling them you did it.

- Tell your family and friends often how much you appreciate them and how blessed you are to have their presence in your life.
- Tell your boss or employees the same things. Everyone wants and needs to feel appreciated.
- Get your children to go through their toys and select some to give to those less fortunate. Let the children go with you to take the toys someplace they are needed and will be appreciated.
- Plant a tree or flowers in your neighbor's yard where it's needed —with their permission, of course.
- Take some beautiful plants to your local nursing home, fire station, hospital, police station, or doctor's office.
- Make sandwiches, drive by a city park, and give them out to the homeless people.
- Leave a flower anonymously on someone's windshield.
- Look in the mirror every day and tell yourself how beautiful and wonderful you are.
- Compliment others throughout the day.
- If you see someone who appears stressed or unhappy, visualize them surrounded by light and love.
- Be loving and kind to yourself every day, knowing you are a child of God and deserve to live a joy-filled wonderful life.

CHAPTER FOURTEEN

Meditation and Prayer:
The Key to Transforming Your Life

What joy awaits discovery in the silence behind the portals of your mind no human tongue can tell. But you must convince yourself; you must meditate and create that environment.
—PARAMAHANSA YOGANANDA

Meditation is an ancient art going back long before recorded history. Stone seals have been found in the Indus Valley of India dating back to at least 5,000 BC showing people seated in various yoga postures. For all these millennia, meditation has survived as a vital science of living.

Only during the past three decades has scientific study focused on the clinical effects of meditation on health. Meditation is so thoroughly effective in reducing stress and tension that in 1984, the National Institutes of Health recommended meditation over prescription drugs as the first treatment for mild hypertension.

The first research on the physiology of meditation was conducted by Dr. R. Keith Wallace at UCLA. Studying Transcendental Meditation, Wallace found that during meditation the body gains a state of profound rest and the brain and mind become more alert, indicating a state of "restful alertness." Studies show that after meditation, reactions are faster, creativity greater, and comprehension broader.

HEALTH BENEFITS OF MEDITATION

Dr. Herbert Benson, of the Mind-Body Institute at Harvard University, determined that meditation practice can bring about a healthy state of relaxation by causing a generalized reduction in multiple physiological and biochemical stress indicators, such as decreased heart rate, decreased respiration rate, decreased plasma cortisol (a stress hormone), decreased pulse rate, increased alpha (a brain wave associated with relaxation), and increased oxygen consumption.

Scientists are finding that meditation also helps keep us wrinkle-free and healthy. One study showed that people who had been meditating for more than five years were biologically twelve to fifteen years younger than non-meditators. A comparison of hospital records of 2,000 meditators and 2,000 non-meditators revealed that the meditators required only half as much medical care. They have eighty-seven percent less heart disease, fifty-five percent fewer tumors and eighty-seven percent fewer nervous disorders.

The late Dr. Hans Selye, a pioneering Canadian stress researcher, described two types of stress—negative stress and positive stress. The difference between the two depends upon whether or not you feel in control of the stress. By becoming more aware of your reactions to stress, meditation can assist in providing an increased internal sense of control.

Another medical expert who advocates meditation is Dr. Dean Ornish, a well-known physician from California and author of many books, including *Love and Intimacy: The Scientific Basis for the Healing Power of Intimacy*. In his groundbreaking book, *Dr. Dean Ornish's Program for Reversing Heart Disease*, there are easy-to-follow instructions for a calming routine that includes meditation, yoga, and progressive relaxation.

Dr. Jon Kabat-Zinn at the University of Massachusetts Medical School, author of *Wherever You Go There You Are*, founded the Stress Reduction Clinic in 1979 to help people suffering from chronic pain and chronic diseases such as cancer, heart disease, and AIDS, as well as stress-related disorders such as abdominal pain, chronic diarrhea, and ulcers. According to Dr. Kabat-Zinn, these conditions are often the most difficult to treat, and the patients have frequently tried other, more conventional forms of medicine without complete success.

Dr. Kabat-Zinn designed a stress-reduction program to test the value of using mindfulness meditation to help patients develop effective coping strategies for stress, and to see whether meditation would have any effect on their chronic medical condition. Kabat-Zinn's stress-reduction program patients also make a commitment to practice on their own each day. As it turned out, the majority of people improved in a number of different ways.

- Virtually all patients, whatever their diagnoses, show dramatic reduction in physical symptoms over the eight-week period.
- Psychological problems—anxiety, depression, hostility—also drop over the eight weeks. Follow-up studies four years after completion of the course show that both physical and psychological improvements are consistent over time.
- Symptom reductions are greater than with other techniques, such as drug intervention, indicating that results don't come

Meditation and Prayer

from a placebo effect. Somehow the patient's inner
for healing are being tapped.
* Patients' self-perceptions change. They view the
healthier and better able to handle stressful situatic
suffering destructive effects. They feel more in con
lives, view life as a challenge rather than a series of obstacles,
and feel they are living more fully.

In general, Kabat-Zinn concludes that meditation is effective in: decreasing pain; reducing secretion of stress hormones, including adrenaline and noradrenaline; decreasing the amount of excess stomach acid in people with gastrointestinal problems; lowering blood pressure; and increasing relaxation.

MEDITATION AND THE BREATH

Although meditation can take many forms, most techniques can be grouped into two basic approaches: concentrative meditation and mindfulness meditation. Both gradually train you to focus your attention and strengthen your concentration with the result of eventually quieting the mind.

Concentrative meditation focuses the attention on the breath, an image, or a sound (mantra), in order to still the mind and allow a greater awareness and clarity to emerge. To sit quietly and focus on your breath is the simplest form of concentrative meditation. This form of meditation can be compared to the zoom lens of a camera that narrows its focus to a selected field.

Concentration is the ability to tell yourself to pay attention to something and then do exactly that! Our minds tend to drift. We have continuous mental conversations. Most people talk to themselves nearly every minute of the day. Through meditation we control, limit, and finally eliminate this internal chit-chat. An effective way to control and master your mind is through breath awareness.

The connection between the breath and one's state of mind is a basic principle of yoga and meditation. Think back to a time when you were frightened, agitated, distracted, or anxious. Whether or not you noticed it, your breath was probably shallow, rapid, and uneven. On the other hand, when the mind is calm, focused, and composed, the breath will tend to be slow, deep, and regular. It also works in reverse. By consciously taking slow, deep, and regular breaths, the mind will become calm. Focusing the mind on the continuous rhythm of inhalation and exhalation provides a natural object of meditation.

Breath control is the tool that allows you to alter your existing mental state. Inhale slowly and rhythmically through your nose, breathing quietly and deliberately. The incoming breath fills (in sequence) the abdomen, the ribcage, and the upper chest. After you draw a full, comfortable breath, hold it for a count of one to three, then release it slowly at the same rate and rhythm as you drew it in. The exhalation procedure is the exact opposite of inhalation. First expel the air from your upper chest, next the ribcage, and finally the abdomen. Allow the abdomen to power the breathing process. Try to breathe silently.

Breathe with concentration for a few minutes. Do it now. Settle into your posture and relax (don't slump). Sit on a bench, in a chair or cross-legged on a cushion, folded towels or pillow. (I sit on a quarter-moon-shaped pillow.) The crossed-leg position (with elevated buttocks) is great for smooth breathing and proper posture. Place your hands in either of the two following positions. The Zen mudra position is right hand palm up on lap, left hand on top of right hand, also palm up, the balls of the thumbs touching lightly. Another hand position is to place left hand on left thigh, right hand on right thigh, both palms up, gently touching your thumb to your index finger. By monitoring the breathing, maintaining proper posture, and using one of the hand positions, you stay alert and focused. You are meditating. Notice as you do this that your mind becomes more tranquil and aware.

I use a meditation technique called Kriya Yoga which I learned in the inspiring Self-Realization Fellowship Lessons of Paramahansa Yogananda (see Resource Directory). This is a very effective way to increase our inner receptivity to God's guidance.

MINDFULNESS MEDITATION

The other type of meditation is mindfulness meditation. According to Dr. Joan Borysenko, "Mindfulness meditation involves opening the attention to become aware of the continuously passing parade of sensations and feelings, images, thoughts, sounds, smells, and so forth without becoming involved in thinking about them." The meditator sits quietly and simply witnesses whatever goes through the mind, not reacting or becoming emotionally involved with thoughts, memories, worries, or images. This helps the meditator gain a more calm, clear, and nonreactive state of mind. Mindfulness meditation can be likened to a wide-angle lens—a broad, sweeping awareness that takes in the entire field of perception.

Mindfulness is an ancient Buddhist practice which has profound relevance for today, says Dr. Kabat-Zinn. Mindfulness has nothing to do with becoming a Buddhist, he explains, but is a way of "waking up and living in harmony with oneself and with the world." Mindfulness is paying complete attention to whatever we're doing, allowing the "mind to be full" of the experience. The opposite of mindfulness is mindlessness, to do things without thinking, without much feeling, automatically, and unconsciously like a robot. In mindfulness, we examine who we are, question our view of the world and our place in it, and cultivate some appreciation for the fullness of each moment we are alive. Most of all, it has to do with being in touch with yourself and your world.

We are often more asleep than awake to the unique beauty and possibilities of each present moment as it unfolds. We're usually absorbed in anticipating the future—planning strategies to ward off things we don't want to happen and to force outcomes that we do want—or in remembering who did what to whom and why. Most of us spend very little time aware of the present moment. Such mental manipulation leaves one enormously agitated.

While it is the tendency of our mind to go on automatic pilot, our mind also holds the deep innate capacity to help us awaken to our present, mindful moments and use them to advantage. Those moments are really the only moments we have to live, to grow, to feel, to love, to learn, to give shape to things and to heal. The essence of mindfulness is paying full attention. We come out of automatic pilot and observe more deeply. This allows us to feel more connected to what's going on around us and to develop a greater understanding of the order of things. Just as a garden requires attending if we hope to cultivate flowers and not weeds, mindfulness also requires regular cultivation. The beauty of it is that we carry this garden with us, wherever we go, wherever we are, whenever we remember. It is outside of time as well as in it. Kabat-Zinn calls mind cultivation "wakefulness meditation."

The meditative disciplines, whether concentrative or mindfulness, reintroduce calmness and stability into our lives.

WHERE TO MEDITATE

You don't have to travel to the Holy Land or the Himalayas to find sacred space. Dr. Ornish began reserving a space at home for his meditations when he was an undergraduate in college. "I was living in a one-bedroom apartment, and I didn't have a room I could use for that purpose," he says. "I didn't even have a corner of a room. But I had two closets. One I used for clothing; the other was for meditation," which he

he floor. He suggests dedicating some space exclusively
ditation. Doing so enhances your meditation, and makes
your home more sacred.
edicate a personal sacred space. Ornish suggests, "you
ture of a religious or holy person, or someone whose
sense of calmness or peace and love, or just set up a
candle—whatever has the meaning for you of being sacred or inspiring."

A sacred place is where you find tranquillity, where you will relish moments of rich solitude. "In your sacred space, things are working in terms of your dynamic," explains Joseph Campbell, "and not anybody else's. Your sacred space is where you can find yourself again and again."

For some uplifting and practical reading on effective prayer and meditation, I recommend the following books: *Healing Words: The Power of Prayer and the Practice of Medicine* by Larry Dossey, MD; *Handle with Prayer* by Alan Cohen; *Enter the Quiet Heart* by Sri Daya Mata; and *In the Sanctuary of the Soul, How You Can Talk with God, Journey to Self-Realization*, and *Autobiography of a Yogi*—all by Paramahansa Yogananda.

HOW TO BEGIN

First, decide where you are going to meditate. For more than twenty years I have devoted a corner of my bedroom as my place of meditation. Create some type of altar with inspiring books, pictures, or objects like statues, candles, or flowers. Keep it simple and clean. On my altar (which is really a wicker basket) I have placed a natural cloth covering and have some items which inspire me including pictures of Jesus and Paramahansa Yogananda, the Bible, a candle, and some fresh flowers. I usually sit on a pillow designed for meditation on the floor.

Carve out a regular time to meditate every day. Make it a top priority in your life. Firmly resolve that you will meditate on a regular schedule. As Roy E. Davis in his wonderful book, *A Master Guide to Meditation & Spiritual Growth*, suggests, "Consider your meditation session as your daily appointment with the Infinite, and keep that appointment without fail." I devote the early morning before sunrise to meditation and well as the early evening. This disciplined practice helps me to start and end the day on a positive, uplifting note. Whenever you choose to meditate, pick a quiet time of day, if you can. Ear plugs are sometimes helpful.

If you aren't comfortable sitting on the floor, find a chair where you can sit with your spine straight—posture is important. Avoid sitting with your back supported by the chair's back. Tilt the chair forward slightly so the seat is parallel to the ground. Sitting with your back and neck straight will make the energy flow more easily through your spine. Find a fairly comfortable position to sit in. Lying down is not recommended because it encourages falling asleep.

As in physical activity, it is better to start small and develop a regular practice than sit in meditation for hours a day and give up in frustration. I recommend starting with ten to fifteen minutes once a day. In the beginning it is most important to establish a regular time for meditation and to stick with it. Later you may want to sit more frequently or for greater lengths of time.

Regardless of the technique you use, you'll find the mind wanders and the body experiences unusual sensations. Most traditions suggest you should avoid trying to stop thinking or being distracted. When you realize you are distracted, gently bring your mind back to the object of concentration. Each time the mind wanders and is brought back, your ability to concentrate has been strengthened. Your mind is being trained to respond to you rather than you responding to the whims of the mind.

Let's say that you have chosen to focus on your breath as you slowly and deeply inhale and exhale. As soon as you're aware that you're not focusing on your breath, gently but strongly refocus on it. By this process of focusing and refocusing on one point, eventually your internal noise is lessened, your head is quieter, and your energy higher.

Deeper levels of meditation begin after the initial noise and distracting thoughts have been cleared away. Usually, periods of quiet—when it's easy to focus—alternate with periods of random thinking. As you continue to meditate, times of easier focus, greater clarity, and inner quiet lengthen. These times of quiet joyfulness are the first goal of meditation. There is no limit to the depth, energy, and peacefulness that can be achieved in meditation.

Meditation should be continued until a quiet mental state is reached. Don't stop in the middle of a lot of thoughts when it's difficult to concentrate. Stop when you are quiet. These periods of noise and quiet will alternate as your meditation breaks through layers of thought and tension. Stop whenever a more stable place is reached. You don't have to reach samadhi (bliss) to have a great meditation.

Start your meditations with your energy as high as possible. It's nice to have showered first. Feel awake. The higher your energy is and the more awake and alert you feel, the easier it will be to focus and meditate. It's also best to meditate on an empty stomach or at least before eating a heavy meal.

Don't be too rigid in your practice. On occasion, find other special places to meditate. I often become immersed in meditation in nature—at the beach, in the mountains, out in the desert, or in the local park. I enjoy the sounds of nature when I meditate outdoors. Being out in nature helps you to see things more clearly and become one with your surroundings.

NATURE MEDITATION

In Joseph Cornell's book, *Listening to Nature*, I learned about a nature meditation he refers to as "stillness meditation." Here's the technique, which I usually do while out in nature. It helps to quiet restless thoughts and sometimes brings wonderful calmness.

FIRST, RELAX THE BODY: Do this by inhaling and tensing all over: feet, legs, back, arms, neck, face—as much as you possibly can. Then throw the breath out and relax completely. Repeat this several times.

TO PRACTICE THE TECHNIQUE ITSELF: Observe the natural flow of your breath. Do not control the breath in any way! Simply follow it with your attention. Each time you inhale, think 'still.' Each time you exhale, think 'ness.' Repeating 'still...ness' with each complete breath helps focus the mind and prevents your attention from wandering from the present moment.

DURING THE PAUSES BETWEEN INHALATION AND EXHALATION: Stay in the present moment, calmly observing whatever is in front of you. If thoughts of the past or future disturb your mind, just calmly and patiently bring your attention back to what is before you, and to repeating 'still...ness' with your breathing.

Stillness meditation, explains Cornell, "will help you to become absorbed in natural settings for longer and longer periods. Use it when you want to feel this calmness, indoors or outdoors, with eyes open or closed."

WHITE LIGHT MEDITATION

The following meditation is one that can be done anywhere and is easy for beginners as well as advanced students of meditation.

- Sit in a straight backed chair with spine erect and feet flat on the floor. (You can also sit cross-legged.) Fold your hands together in your lap, or hold them in prayer position. Eyes may be opened or closed.

- Feel yourself relaxing as you take several long, slow deep breaths. Imagine a beautiful white light completely surrounding you. This is your protection as you open sensitive energy

Meditation and Prayer 215

centers. You can do this with any of your meditations.
- For about ten minutes, gently concentrate on a single idea, picture or word. Select something that is meaningful, uplifting, and spiritual to you. You could even focus on some peaceful music.
- If your mind wanders from your object of focus, gently bring it back to your awareness.
- After ten minutes, separate your hands and turn them palms up in your lap. Close your eyes if opened.
- Relax your hold on the object of concentration and shift your mind into neutral. Remain passive, yet alert, for ten more minutes. Gently observe any thoughts and images as they may float by. Just be still, detached, and be with whatever you are experiencing.
- Open your eyes after ten minutes, close your palms and again imagine that you are surrounded completely by a white light. This is your continued protection as you go about your daily activities with peace and joyfulness.

This twenty-minute meditation recharges your energy field and nourishes creativity and tranquillity. At other times during the day, allow a sense of light and love to flow from within your being, and let it fill your entire body. It's very easy to do, and puts you into a meditative state.

For a variety of other meditations you can use, refer to my book *How to Meditate*. If you prefer my guided relaxation meditations, I have included six different ones as part of my seven-tape audiocassette album *Celebrate Life!*, which incorporates music and nature sounds. I also have a longer guided meditation on my audiocassette *How to Achieve Any Goal: The Magic of Creative Visualization*. (Refer to the Resource Directory for more information on these tapes or to order).

SPIRITUAL BLESSINGS FROM MEDITATION

The longer an individual practices meditation, the greater the likelihood that his or her goals and efforts will shift toward personal and spiritual growth. As I travel around the country giving talks and meeting people, it delights me to learn how many people are taking responsibility for their health and lives and embracing a holistic program including meditation. It's not uncommon for me to hear: "I began meditating to decrease my stress and to feel a sense of control in my life. But as my practice deepens, not only do I feel more relaxed, I also am developing a more open heart—more sensitivity, greater compassion, and less negative judgment toward others."

Many individuals who initially learn meditation for its self-regulatory aspects find that as their practice deepens they are drawn more and more into the realm of the spiritual. Meditation is all about breaking through the everyday world of tension and thoughts to create greater inner peace, calm, insight, and enlightenment. It will change your life because it changes you. Find the method or methods which suit you best.

The goal is to truly integrate spirituality into every area of our lives. It takes discipline, courage, and a warrior's strength. It's not for the faint of heart or the weak-minded. Jack Kornfield writes: "To open deeply, as genuine spiritual life requires, we need tremendous courage and strength, a kind of warrior spirit. But the place for this warrior strength is in the heart. We need energy, commitment, and courage not to run from our life nor to cover it over with any philosophy—material or spiritual. We need a warrior's heart that lets us face our lives directly, our pains and limitations, our joys and possibilities. This courage allows us to include every aspect of life in our spiritual practice: our bodies, our families, our society, politics, the earth's ecology, art, education. Only then can spirituality be truly integrated into our lives."

In her work with many cancer and AIDS patients, Dr. Borysenko has observed that many people are most interested in meditation as a way of becoming more attuned to the spiritual dimension of life. She reports that many die 'healed,' in a state of compassionate self-awareness and self-acceptance.

Quiet your mind in meditation to experience the perfect rhythm of the universe. When you go within and allow yourself the freedom to be at peace without judgment, simply meditating and experiencing the oneness of it all, you soon start to find that energy which is blissful and enlightening. If practiced enough, that quiet mind state will convince you of the oneness and perfection of it all.

We are all one in spirit with God and with each other. Although we may look different on the outside, we are still one with God, one with each other, and share the same innate spirituality. It's easy to forget this truth in today's tumultuous world. When we watch the news or read the newspaper, it's easy to forget that we're all children of God. By meditating and following God's guidance, we naturally live together in peace and harmony. If we are faced with or witnessing intolerance from others, meditation can give the strength to bless the situation and acknowledge that there is a divine power in charge. Although others may seem worlds apart from us, the peace gained in meditation reminds us that we all look at the same sky, bask in the glow of the same sun, and are blessed by the same all-knowing, innate power that is God. Meditation helps keep our heart connected to God and our eyes focused on our vision. Obstacles are what you see when you take your eyes off the vision and separate yourself from God.

THE DIVINE SURRENDER

During my meditation period, I often incorporate prayer, visualization, and affirmations. Most often my prayer involves surrender to the Divine. A prayer of surrender can be one of the most powerful and blessed aspects of meditation.

What is it that we surrender? Our negative feelings, negative thoughts, fears, resentments, addictions, and resistance. Resistance to change is nothing more than hardening of the attitudes. Many people are addicted to stress-producing stimuli. We become needy, neurotic people when we look to the world for what the world cannot give us. When we have lost our peace, we look for it everywhere. In fact, we seek desperately. Until we remember that our own capacity to love and be connected to God is what we truly seek, we are doomed to endless compulsion to look for happiness where there is none and for satisfaction where there is only more longing. Life's difficult situations force us to be more conscious of our dependence on God and the need to deepen our connection with Him—to perfect our faith and trust and love.

Surrender means to trust in the forces and principles that are always at work in the universe. With surrender, an inner knowingness and contentment overtakes us. With surrender we trust the perfection and beauty of it all, and at the same time know the paradox that all of the suffering that seems to go on all over our planet is a part of that perfection, as is our own strong desire to help end it. The best way to surrender is to make a personal commitment to forgive every single person that we have ever had any conflict with.

The inevitable result of surrender is to draw closer to God. When we surrender to the Divine our compulsive negative thoughts, fears, addictions, and resistance, our lives will be transformed. No part of our lives is unimportant to God. Whatever our need—whether it deals with health, finances, or human relations—nothing is beyond God's presence and power. There is nothing we cannot turn over to God.

To surrender all to God—letting go and letting God—brings out the gifts of love and peace that are within us. Strength and understanding may not come all at once, but as we prove our desire is real, as we are willing to follow and trust, God shows the way. In everything, trust God. That's true surrender.

Yogananda taught me a prayer of surrender: "Lord, no matter what I'm going through, I love You. I am your child; You are with me always." In that prayer of perfect surrender, we feel our life to be in God's divine embrace, and know that everything is well. Or "God I trust in Thee. Show me the way."

Take time to become quiet, to listen within, and to place all in the hands of the One who created and loves you. God knows what is best for you and sees the good that you may not see. God will help you and show you the way. Be open to the lessons you need to learn. Life is a persistent teacher. It keeps repeating lessons until we learn them. Trust that everything that's happening can be for your highest good. As you remember to trust God in everything, give thanks for the special relationship you have with the One presence and power.

Surrender brings with it gratitude. Gratitude, an overflowing feeling of thanksgiving, is the instant response of the soul touched by the awareness of the Divine. Sri Daya Mata, president of the Self-Realization Fellowship says that with even a momentary awakening to God's presence, such joyous freedom bathes our consciousness—a blessed release from all the tensions and fears and anxieties that weigh us down in this world—that in wordless praise our whole being pours forth a ceaseless "Thank you! Thank you! Thank you!"

THE POWER OF AFFIRMATION

Too often we fail to see God's beauty and goodness right around us. We can overcome this careless forgetfulness by training the mind through repetition of a simple thought-affirmation: "Lord, Thou art in me. I am in Thee."

I usually repeat spiritual affirmations like this one loudly at first, then softly, then in a whisper. I repeat them mentally, again and again, until they become automatic. At that point it has reached my subconscious mind which will keep it going on its own. And if I keep affirming with even deeper concentration, it reaches the superconscious mind—"the magic storehouse of miraculous powers," as Yogananda said.

Affirmations can—and should—be used for spiritual success. One very simple affirmation I repeat often is: "I am a child of God." When we repeat that to ourselves often enough and with deep enough concentration, it reaches the superconscious mind and we realize, through direct experience: "I am a child of God!" Then everything in our lives is transformed—our attitudes, our abilities, the way we go about our daily lives.

Let the mind dwell on these positive affirmations when it is not otherwise occupied. With continuous repetition, feel the truth of what you are affirming. By repetition, the reality of His sustaining presence becomes ingrained in our consciousness. A profound certainty grows within us that in every way we are being provided for. Gratitude and joyous praise then flow naturally. Begin now to celebrate this inner thanksgiving, whether you're meditating or not.

I sometimes end my meditations with what I call a 'meditation prayer.' I also say these before I fall asleep so that the positive, uplifting thoughts can be carried into my subconscious and superconscious mind during the night. Write some of your own and keep them with you to read whenever you have extra time. I keep different ones in my purse, briefcase, and car. These can be recited out loud or silently, but make sure you say them with feeling. Here are two of my favorites.

POSITIVE MEDITATION PRAYER

Every day, each and every moment is a new opportunity to begin again, to celebrate the gift of life. There is no past or future. There is only now, a blessed moment filled with unlimited opportunities for good. I live every moment to the fullest by releasing memories that are no longer useful, by letting go of things that can limit me, and by opening my mind and heart to experiences that will uplift me and encourage me to stretch and grow. The past has no power to control me. With God, I can live fully and freely in each moment of my life.

Every thought of not being valuable, of being afraid, of uncertainty and doubt, is now cast out of my mind. My memory goes back to God alone, in whom I live, move, and have my being. A complete sense of happiness, peace, certainty, and love floods me with light. I have confidence in myself because I have confidence in God. I am sure of myself because I am sure of God.

The Spirit of Love within me knows the answer to any problem which confronts me. I know that the answer is here and now. It is within my own mind because God is right where I am. I now turn from the problem to the Spirit, accepting the answer. In calm confidence, in perfect trust, in abiding faith, and with complete peace I let go of the problem and receive the answer.

I know exactly what to do in every situation. Every idea necessary to successful living is brought to my attention. The doorway to ever increasing opportunities for self-expression is open before me. I am continuously meeting new and larger experiences. Every day brings some greater good. I prosper in everything I do. Now there is no deferment, no delay, no obstruction or obstacle, nothing to impede the progress of right action, of Divine order in every area of my life.

I identify myself with abundance. I surrender all fear and doubt. I let go of all uncertainty. I know there is no confusion, no lack of confidence. I know that what is mine will claim me, know me, rush to me. The Presence of God, of Love, is with me. The Mind of God is my mind. The thoughts of God are my thoughts.

Today I bestow the essence of love upon everything. Everyone I meet shall be loving to me. My soul meets the Soul of the Universe in everyone. This love is a healing power touching everything into wholeness. I am one with the rhythm of life. There is nothing to be afraid of. There is nothing to be uncertain about. God is over all, in all, and through all. God is right where I am. I am at peace with the world in which I live. I am at home with the divine Spirit in which I am immersed. I am in love with God and with life itself.

Spirit of Love within me, thank you for this precious gift of life. Today, and always, I choose to honor and serve you by loving myself and everyone else unconditionally and by acknowledging your Presence in everything I think, feel, say and do.

AMEN

PEACE MEDITATION PRAYER

Love is here. God is here. Truth is here. Peace, the wonderful peace of God, is right here where I am.

In this beautiful moment of eternity, I turn my attention within. I feel the peace of God that is in me always; the peace that transcends all fear, all concern, all sense of anxiety; the peace that is everlasting. I am a center of perfect peace. Let there be peace on earth and let it begin with me.

Dear Lord, let me be an instrument of peace in my world. Open me to the realization that peace in the world begins with peaceful hearts. I open my heart, my mind, and all that I am to Your peace. In this moment, nothing can disturb the calm peace of my soul.

Every atom, cell, tissue, and fiber of my being is filled to overflowing with the peace of God. I allow that peace of God within me to come forth and bless my family, my loved ones, my friends, and my co-workers. I see and experience the peace of God in my neighborhood, my community, my city, my state, and my country.

I use my God-given power of vision to see and to feel the peace of God flooding the hearts and souls of all the citizens of this country.

I affirm and I speak with power the word of peace. Peace is made manifest in my world. The peace of God moves through the hearts and minds of all people everywhere in all countries, all world leaders and all world citizens. I take this moment, now, to bring that vision closer to reality. I recommit myself to my own inner peace and to peace in the world in a moment of silence.

Let peace radiate in me, O God. Let Your light of peace within me shine forth so brightly that all darkness and doubt are dispelled. For this power, this realization of peace in my heart and in my world, I am eternally grateful. I give thanks for this precious gift of life.

AMEN

PRACTICING THE PRESENCE

Just imagine your days filled with nothing less than peace, contentment, and happiness. These things are natural when you are constantly aware of and give thanks for God's love and presence in your life. Our only problem is that we're disconnected from the power of our soul.

To see God's presence everywhere, we must see through all forms of illusion or maya (an Eastern term for the illusion of the material world). We must ask God to help us see more clearly by seeing with God's eyes. Ask God to open your heart, quiet your mind, and experience a richer, happier, transformed life. God is your source of instant, constant peace.

I don't quite understand why we feel more peaceful when we turn our attention to God, but that doesn't matter. I don't know all about electricity, but I can still flip a switch and get light. I know from experience that when I tap into the peace of God within, I get tranquillity. When I face the challenge of giving a lecture, making a presentation, writing an article or book, or when anything seems to be testing me, I remind myself to flip that switch. We can all learn to be peace-filled people, for no matter what is going on around us, God is there.

Make meditation and prayer a top priority in your life. In time, and with disciplined practice, your life will become a moving meditation and prayer devoted to God. Meditation and prayer are the medium of miracles. When you meditate and pray, you can't not change. By living a meditative, prayerful life, the joy you receive from sharing with God can be continuous.

Some of the prayers I say to God each day include:

God, may my mind be filled with thoughts of You.
Make me an instrument of peace and harmlessness, through the grace of God.
God, give me a new heart to see everyone in my life as an innocent child of God.
I am the peace of God.
God, guide my thoughts, feelings, words, and actions to reflect your love and light.
God, show me how I can best serve You today.
I behold the Divine in everyone and everything.

Be willing to live a God-surrendered life and to love more. It's in the willingness that lives are changed. The more you can love everything and everyone, and possess an attitude of gratitude, the healthier and happier you will be.

CHAPTER FIFTEEN

Self-Mastery: The Power to Be Your Best

We become experts at preparing to live, but have a difficult time fully enjoying the process of being alive, right now.
—BARBARA DE ANGELIS, PH.D.

No man is free who is not master of himself.
—EPICTETUS

Just for a moment, close your eyes, breathe slowly and deeply a few times, and imagine yourself as a master of the universe. As a master you have the ability to create anything you want, even something that has never existed before. Be outrageous in your thinking and envision what you most want now.

You have this power within you—it is the birthright and potential of every human being. The only real limitation to all possibility is your thought, belief, and imagination. Once you have a clear vision of what you want, focusing on the result and not just the means, then the natural play of universal forces will lead you to the accomplishment of that goal. Og Mandino said, "Use wisely your power of choice." Henry Ford encouraged us to believe in ourselves when he wrote, "Whether you think you can or not, you are right."

When you compromise your dreams and values and instead live a life that's expected of you rather than what your heart asks of you, you give your power away. In her perceptive book, *Anatomy of the Spirit*, Carolyn Myss, Ph.D. offers that when you compromise your dreams and values to live a life that is expected of you rather than what your heart asks of you, you give the power away and disconnect from your soul. It takes courage to embrace the unfamiliar and allow miracles to occur. It takes boldness to go after our dreams even though we're navigating uncharted territory. Don't give up. "It takes a lot of courage to release the familiar and seemingly secure, to embrace the new," says my friend, author and motivational speaker Alan Cohen. "But there is no real security in what is no longer meaningful. There is more security in the adventurous and exciting, for in movement there is life, and in change there is power."

You and only you have the ability to create miracles in your mind and life. The choice is always with you. It has nothing to do with luck and everything to do with believing in yourself as a part of the divine force that suffuses everything in the universe. The great rule is this: if you can conceive it in your mind, then it can be brought into the physical world.

Living in such a fast-paced world constantly conspires against inner peace. The intense pace and stress of our daily lives can very easily put our peace, happiness, and health, not to mention our spiritual lives, at risk. It's easy to get caught up in the whirl of today's hectic lifestyle—especially if we've forgotten the truth of our potential. This leaves us less time for self-fulfillment. Deteriorating standards and values lead to low self-esteem and rob many of us of our dignity.

If we feel an inner emptiness, we may be tempted by the easy solution, since life is hard and learning to live fully takes more time. But the fact is we can slow things down. We can face our own challenges, however large or small, with aplomb and equanimity, on terms that are our own, our heart's guidance. We can choose to experience aliveness and become masters of our lives.

In the 1960s, Abraham Maslow wrote his famous *Toward a Psychology of Being*, which helped turn around the emphasis of psychology. Psychology was my undergraduate major at UCLA and I was drawn to Maslow's work. He chose to study high-functioning people—those living their highest potential—rather than people with problems as was usually the case in psychology. Maslow developed a 'psychology of being,' not of striving but arriving; not of trying to get someplace, but living fully. He found a common denominator among all his high-functioning subjects. They all had a vision, were committed to it, were self-motivated, and believed they had the power to master life. Do you believe you have the power to master life?

IF IT'S TO BE, IT'S UP TO ME

Self-mastery begins by taking inventory of your life. According to Socrates, "The unexamined life is not worth living." Mastery involves taking responsibility for our lives and what we've created rather than blaming other people and circumstances for our lot in life. Blame is a convenient excuse for why our life is not exactly what we would like it to be. Mastery also involves being self-disciplined, being courageous, moving through fear, and recognizing our inherent divine power—using it to bring our vision to life.

Millions of masters-in-the-making like you are awakening to the concepts of self-responsibility and choice. Its proof is in the success of teachers such as Dr. Deepak Chopra, Marianne Williamson, Dr. Wayne

Dyer, Dr. Bernie Siegel, Oprah Winfrey, Carolyn Myss, Ph.D., Dean Ornish, MD, Paramahansa Yogananda, and many others who help people bring spirituality and wholeness into everyday life. Once introduced to these empowering ideas, people are giving up being victims in favor of being masters. Self-mastery is true heroism in action.

When you have the tendency to blame another person or circumstances for how you feel or for what you are experiencing, stop, check yourself and remember: what you feel is up to you. Your feelings are governed by your mind. You can't think one thing and feel something else. Feelings and experiences always correspond to thoughts. The habit of blaming others or circumstances has to stop if you are to become master of your life and live your highest potential. The circumstances and conditions are only tests.

Instead of whining "why?" and pointing the finger of blame, masters say: "This is the situation. I take responsibility for it. I realize I created this emotional stuff. I know I have the power to make new choices about how I view any event and my reactions to it. I am powerful enough to uncreate this situation and re-create something healthy and joyful. I now choose to see everything through the eyes of love."

Love empowers you to higher levels. Nothing will transform and enrich your life more quickly than the consistent experience of love. Let others know that you love them. Tell them and show them, often. Don't wait until it's too late, for you don't know if they will still be here tomorrow. My spiritual teacher, Paramahansa Yogananda, used to say that if we want to live our highest potential, all we have to do is teach the mind how to think differently—how to be gentle, calm, loving and centered on God. Seeing through the eyes of love is the same as seeing through the eyes of God. When you know that you are a spiritual being in a physical body, and you live from that awareness moment-to-moment, your life will be transformed. It's simply an internal shift—an eighteen-inch journey from your mind to your heart. You will find yourself more certain, fulfilled, successful, content, and peaceful than ever before. You will be living in a state of grace.

Anyone who goes about his or her own life with a sense of serenity, contentment, and grace has no need to manipulate others. A well-adjusted person who's master of his or her life doesn't try to control others or circumstances. It is rare for a person who is reasonably satisfied with his or her life to try to run someone else's. Such a person continues to grow through a living process of discovery and renewal.

As paradoxical as it sounds, this is the mind-set for self-mastery: to surrender, trust, turn away from habits of accumulation, outer achievement and quick fixes, and to allow yourself to be purposeful through inward guidance.

The more you live from inner guidance—that peaceful, loving center within you—the more you'll find that everything you need to meet your wants and desires will be provided. The essence is knowing that you are already complete, already whole, and that nothing external to yourself in the physical world can make you any more complete.

YOUR REALITY REFLECTS YOUR THOUGHTS AND INTENTIONS

You create your thoughts, your thoughts create your intentions, and your intentions create your reality. Intention is directional energy. With understanding and skill, intentional living is one of the most useful ways to achieve happiness, health, and wholeness and to banish obstacles to spiritual growth. When life is lived with conscious intention, insights unfold more easily and life is lived more gracefully. What you see around you, whom you associate with, how you function daily, what your relationships are like, how much money you make, how you get along with others, the shape of your physical body, and virtually everything about you, is the result of your intention.

It is usually fairly easy to be happy and peaceful and to feel somewhat saintlike when removed from social circumstances and relationships; but to always be happy, peaceful and soul-centered, regardless of personal and environmental conditions, is evidence of real spiritual growth. Your personal and environmental condition tends to adjust toward harmony as you become more soul-centered.

Your values and higher spiritual Self reflect your intentions. If you view the world as a giving place, you are probably optimistic about other people being kind and considerate and you see goodness in others and in all situations. You experience much gratitude and are teaching others to be loving. You usually find yourself surrounded by others with similar values.

In your relationship with others, what really matters is the heart-to-heart or love connection. At the level of the heart, we are all connected by love. The love that connects us also makes us complete and whole beings within ourselves. In all kinds of relationships, whether with friends, business associates, or lovers, you must not collapse yourself into that union. Maintain your individuality as you unite so the winds of heaven can dance between you always. Let Spirit guide you. The essence of who you are is spirit. Spirit makes us all equally special and precious.

Our main job while here on earth is to take our focus and attention off criticizing and finding fault, and instead find ways to serve others, share the peace and joy of our hearts and let others know we appreciate them. When we continually find fault and criticize another, he or she withers up like a flower without water. Show love, respect, and appreciation to another and they will blossom. Isn't that what we all want—simply to be loved and appreciated? Give this a try: for a day or two, treat others as if the fullness of God resided within them. Imagine that their physical-world attributes are nonexistent.

Being a master of my life means that I put God first before everything. I choose to live in the presence of God (or love) and allow God's thoughts to direct my thoughts, intentions, words, and actions. This requires that I live my highest and best at all times and in all circumstances. I know the loving presence will give me the strength and courage to follow through on my commitments. Being centered on God also means that I give up any dependency on people, circumstances, and material things as my source of happiness and fulfillment. I'm putting God first in my life, trusting that my life's higher purpose is being revealed to me. Knowing my connection to God, I choose to put my faith in God and in my inner guidance.

SUCCESS IS AN INSIDE JOB

For years I've done research on what makes people successful. I recently came across Daniel Isenberg, a business professor at Harvard Business School. He's a very popular teacher there. He said that for years his former students would come back to him and say, "We really like your courses, but now that we're out in the real world, what they teach us in the Harvard Business School doesn't make much sense."

This bothered Isenberg because he wanted to teach his students something useful. So he got the names of the twenty-five most successful executives in the country, and got permission to follow each of them around for a week to try to find out what it was they did that made them successful. Isenberg followed each one for a week, listened to their phone conversations, listened to them talk to their friends and family—and came to the conclusion that what made these people successful had nothing to do with what they teach at the Business School. He discovered two important characteristics shared by all the successful people he observed.

One thing these successful achievers had in common was a commitment to putting their values first. There comes a time in our lives where our goals are in conflict with our values; a time when we want to do something in business, with children or friends, or in a relationship, but we know it's a little unethical or a little judgmental, so we're in conflict between what we want to do at the moment and what we feel or know is right. What these most successful people had in common is loyalty to their values. Without commitment to your values, either you don't achieve your goals, or if you do, they're not really worth achieving after all.

The second thing these highly successful achievers had in common was an incredible faith in their intuition. They all exhibited spiritual sensibility. Some of them were churchgoers, some were not, but they all had a sense of a deeper intelligence in the universe that operated through them. They all made their decisions based on their intuitive feelings about what was going on with their businesses or professional lives. How in tune are you with your intuition—God's whisperings?

THE ROLE OF THE BODY IN SELF-MASTERY

Because we live, move, and have our being in God, being centered on God also means appreciating and respecting our magnificent bodies. Your body is the temple of the living, loving Spirit and therefore deserves reverence. Treat yourself with dignity. Don't wait until you're sick to appreciate the miracle of your body. Honor the love inside you and the love you are. If you want to become healthier and be the best you can be, begin with how you feel about yourself and at the same time recognize your body as God's temple. Heaven on earth is inside each one of us at this moment. "In this life," says Meister Eckhart, "we are to become heaven so that God might find a home here."

We are all composed of a body, mind, and spirit and already have everything we need to be the best we can be, to become masters of our lives simply because we are divine beings. So it starts with taking loving care of yourself. Cherish and respect your body temple unconditionally—no matter what its current shape.

I believe that we need to learn to be a friend to our bodies. Every body needs tender, loving care. Getting mad at our bodies only makes matters worse. Although our bodies are but temporary homes for our spiritual being, we must still take care of them because they are sacred vehicles for this earth journey. So love your body and be committed to being fit for your life journey.

Start today by tuning in more to your body. It is a fantastic feedback machine. If you listen, you will discover that it actually talks to you. When you get a headache, your body is trying to tell you something. Listen to your body's signals. The key is your willingness to listen and act. If you feel a pain, what is your body trying to tell you? It may be telling you that you're eating too much, or eating the wrong kinds of food, or smoking or drinking too much, or not sleeping enough, or not drinking enough water or getting enough exercise. It could be telling you that there's too much emotional congestion in your life.

It's normal to be healthy. It's our divine birthright to be well. We just have to get out of our own way. Listen to your body. Respect and appreciate it. Take loving care of it. Choose your doctor carefully—one who practices a wellness lifestyle and who listens to you. There is a tendency today for doctors to turn to technology and all kinds of elaborate testing first before listening to you or their own intuition. I don't think it's a good trend. Ask both of these questions: what can the doctor do for me? and, how can I help myself?

LOVE IS THE MAIN INGREDIENT TO BEING A MASTER OF YOUR HEALTH

One of the best things you can do is to love yourself unconditionally. Have you remembered to love yourself today? To love and honor your own inner Self and treat yourself with respect and dignity is the simplest way to experience peace and the joy of living.

Love yourself. Remind yourself to do that all day. Put notes up on the refrigerator and mirrors around your home if you need the reminder. Erich Fromm said, "Our highest calling in life is precisely to take loving care of ourselves." When you change your attitude about yourself from negative to positive, everything else in your life will change for the better.

One of the extraordinary secrets of this world is that life flows outward. It originates inside and is projected outward where it is perceived as the external world. We are not affected by other people or by situations and circumstances in the way we normally think we are. We are affected only by what happens inside us. We are affected by our own feelings and our own thoughts. Nothing outside us has the power to affect us.

Most people denigrate and belittle themselves all the time. In this way you create your own problems. If you think that somebody else hurts you or somebody else makes you happy or feel good or bad about yourself, that is delusion. Nobody else is responsible for your pain or pleasure. Nobody else is responsible for your sorrow or joy.

When you get in touch with your innermost Self and you come in contact with that infinite invisible intelligence that is always a part of you and your daily life, then you know what you should think, do and say. Embrace your feelings—all of them. Don't be afraid of the darkness for it is the harbinger of light. "The dark night of the soul," says Joseph

Campbell, "comes just before revelation. When everything is lost and all seems darkest, then comes the new life and all that is needed." Turn everything in your life over to the divinity within you. That divine Self, that light and love within you, exists within everybody, but is being wasted by those who don't take the time to turn within.

Make it a personal policy never to put yourself down. Never debase yourself or think negatively about yourself. Tune in to the inner guidance that is with you twenty-four hours a day. We need to become more dependent on God. The reason we are dependent on external things is that we do not have the knowledge of our own Higher Self, the power within us. To have this knowledge, you have to practice.

DIVINITY IS ANOTHER MAIN INGREDIENT

Start the day with remembrance of God. Live the day in relationship with God. End the day absorbed in awareness of the presence of God. This is not a naive, simplistic approach to living life well. When natural and sustained, it is the culmination of spiritual practice.

A most useful way to begin each day is with prayer and meditation. This not only affirms our understanding that our most important relationship is with the Infinite, it establishes us in the ideal relationship with God—that of knowing that God is our higher True Self and we are in this world to learn to let God's will be done through us.

Make meditation a top priority in your life. The process of meditation is nothing more than quietly going within and discovering that higher component of yourself. Meditation allows you to empty yourself of the endless activity of your mind and to attain a calmness. Regular meditation is a natural process to attain peace of mind, strengthen the body's immune system, slow biologic aging processes, awaken regenerative energies, enliven the nervous system, and nurture enhanced creative abilities. Meditation will enable you to be more peaceful, soul-centered, and God-conscious. With progressive spiritual growth, your understanding of your relationship with the Infinite will improve. You will be more insightful, more intellectually and intuitively capable of discerning the difference between truth and untruth. Ultimately, when you adopt meditation as a way of life, you'll be able to go to that peaceful place anytime and bring that peace and joy to all circumstances in your life.

Listen to the genius of Franz Kafka: "You do not need to leave your room. Remain sitting at your table and listen. Do not even listen, simply wait. Do not even wait, be quiet, still and solitary. The world will freely offer itself to you to be unmasked, it has no choice, it will roll in ecstasy at your feet."

A daily spiritual practice routine is most helpful, but how we live every waking moment is the proof of its value. It is in the arena of everyday circumstances and relationships that we are provided ample opportunity to explore the depth and clarity of our understanding. If you are not living well—freely and productively—you are not growing spiritually. How you experience life is in direct relationship to your inner condition: your psychological health, maturity, your understanding of your purpose for living, and your willingness to do what it takes to live your life successfully.

Avoid becoming addicted to your spiritual practice routines or indulging yourself in inner work to the exclusion of meaningful activities and relationships. Balance your regular sessions of meditation, inner reflection, and prayer with worthwhile involvements in your outer life. In this way you fulfill yourself and your purpose in life.

It doesn't matter what your level of health or spirituality is right now. Regardless of how unspiritual or unhealthy a lifestyle you've chosen, you can at any moment choose differently. You can use your past mistakes or poor choices and learn from them. For some people, it takes being at the bottom before they awaken to the fact that they can choose something else. This is exactly what happened to a friend of mine who I'll call Melissa.

MELISSA TRANSFORMS HER LIFE

Not long ago I was giving two talks in Los Angeles on "SoulCaring: Inspire Yourself to Greatness" and "The Main Ingredients of Health and Happiness: Living a Balanced Life." I shared my thoughts about our power and ability to become masters of our lives and create health, success, peace, and happiness beyond our highest visions when we surrender our lives to God. I said that surrendering is an act of the heart and the equivalent of putting inspiration into your life. When you are inspired, you feel purposeful. When you trust in the invisible intelligence of the universe, you feel empowered and guided. This process is natural, not something that requires mastery of an esoteric curriculum. It can happen in a moment and it often occurs just that quickly. In Zen, this process is called satori, which translates roughly to 'instant awakening.'

After my presentations were over and most people had left, I went into the ladies' room and noticed a woman crying. I remembered her because she sat in the front row and cried through much of my talks. Since I had no plans for dinner, I asked Melissa to join me. Surprised, she gratefully accepted.

Melissa's husband had recently left her for a woman half her age. Her two children had been taken away and given to a relative to care for until Melissa got her life together. She was almost one hundred pounds overweight and had no job, and was depressed, afraid, and considering suicide. That morning when she felt like giving up and was at her lowest, she took a walk and, as providence would have it, saw a flier for my talks that afternoon in the window of a health food store. Something inside her told her she must attend—even though she had never gone to a health or motivational talk before. She arrived about thirty minutes early and I watched her as I set up. I went over and introduced myself and told her I was grateful she took the time to come and hear my presentations. I could sense her sadness and gave her a hug. That was the initial contact until I met her in the ladies' room after the talk.

Melissa believed in the ideas I discussed but didn't know how to implement them in her life. Everything seemed to be going downhill for her and she didn't know how to climb out. She wanted more than anything to turn her life around—find a job, get her children back, and get in shape as she had been a couple of years before.

I told Melissa that if she was willing to make a commitment with every fiber of her being and was willing to do whatever it took to live her highest vision, then I'd be happy to work with her and guide her. She was delighted. For most of that evening, I had her share with me her highest vision and write down answers to questions. If she couldn't fail and if she were living her best self right now, what would that look like? I also gave her all my books and tapes and told her to peruse everything over the next week. Finally, I wrote out a walking program I wanted her to start the very next morning.

Over the following week, I became her daily health and fitness coach. We went over a new nutrition program and cleaned out her refrigerator and cupboards of all junk and unhealthy foods. I took her to a few natural food stores and showed her how to shop for health. I trained her at the gym with aerobics, weight training, and stretching. I also taught her how to meditate and visualize her goals and dreams. She was an inspiration to me—dedicated and committed. Within three weeks, she found a part-time job which eventually led to full-time employment at a florist shop. Melissa missed working in her garden; since her husband had left she was living in a studio apartment. Within four months she had saved enough money to move into a new apartment and, happily, she got her children back.

Today, Melissa is down to her ideal weight, works out, frequents health food stores regularly, manages the florist shop, is engaged to be married, and is feeling empowered and divinely guided. Last month, her ex-husband even wanted to get back together with her—which she knew wouldn't be for her highest good. Melissa has learned firsthand that breakthroughs and miracles occur when she is willing to live her vision and commitment, with her life surrendered to God.

THE POWER OF COMMITMENT

There is power in commitment. When you're committed, you allow nothing to deter you from reaching your goal. If you're committed, you are disciplined even when you are not feeling motivated. Discipline is the ability to carry out a resolution long after the mood has left. There were times when Melissa didn't feel like exercising but she exercised anyway, and there were some slips when she indulged in unhealthy foods such as cheese, ice cream, meat, processed foods, and creamy sauces. Instead of beating herself up with guilt and anger for doing something 'bad,' she came to see that these were choices from which she could learn and perhaps make better ones the next time. She admitted that splurges on unhealthy food made her feel very enervated the next few days and quickly came to realize that the momentary taste pleasure wasn't worth hours and days of feeling sluggish and fatigued.

When you make a commitment, you are willing to put all of your resources on the line and take responsibility for the outcome. Commitment—to a project, a relationship, a health and fitness program—lends stability to the chaotic whirl of everyday life. Daily acts that reaffirm your commitment will increase your feelings of empowerment and self-esteem. The better Melissa felt about herself, the more easily and effortlessly she would make choices that were for her highest good, like going to the gym earlier than usual some mornings because of a busy schedule, or like choosing to eat more fresh raw fruits and vegetables even when she felt like eating something unhealthy.

It's through everyday behavior that we learn what really counts. Commitment must be woven through all of life, our thoughts, our emotions, our words, and our actions. I often hear people say they are committed to being healthy, yet they continually let excuses get in the way. They say they'll have to wait "until next Monday or the day after" to exercise because they're "just too busy now," even though they've made a commitment to exercise each day. Or they won't be able to eat nutritious meals for the next two weeks because of birthdays, anniversaries, travels, or because they are "just too stressed out" to make a major change right now.

Commitment means that you get past your excuses and follow through on what you said you were going to do. Make your word count. How do you ever expect someone to make a commitment to you, or how will they ever expect you to follow through on a commitment to them, unless you first show a commitment to yourself?

If you are committed, you will immediately arrange your personal circumstances so that your lifestyle totally supports your commitment. You will do whatever it takes, whatever you need to do to put your life in order, let go of excess baggage and superfluous non-essentials, and consciously focus on what is important.

Lack of commitment is near epidemic proportions in our society. Just look around. People say they're committed to creating a healthier, more harmonious planet, yet they continue to litter, don't recycle, and drive cars that pollute. They say they're committed to their relationships, yet they lie, are unfaithful, are unwilling to be vulnerable, or walk out at the first sign of difficulty or challenge. People say they're committed to aligning with the spiritual side of their natures, but they make no time for meditation, solitude, or communion with God.

Many people wish they felt more committed and wish they had something really big to commit to. These people don't realize that you can't be committed to anything if you aren't first committed to yourself. By really committing to yourself, by following through on your convictions and decisions and allowing nothing to stand in the way of your becoming master of your life, you will gain tremendous power.

TURNING ADVERSITY TO ADVANTAGE

In my life and the lives of many people I know, the most growth, the greatest lessons, and the most rewarding transformations occur from the greatest adversities and challenges. If we have worked through them, life has a way of making certain past misfortunes pay extra dividends in the future. Or, if we haven't worked through or learned from them, they have a way of reappearing in worse form.

Blaming, complaining, and taking no action will keep you in a rut. You must have the vision to see beyond the appearances of your life. You must choose to look at your life from a higher perspective. Practice seeing all life around you as an aspect of yourself. In this way you shatter the illusion of separation and with it the need to blame and complain.

In quiet and solitude, ask this question: *What is it I need to learn to finish this business so I can move on in my life?* You can choose to turn adversity into opportunity. This transformation begins with taking responsibility for everything you've created in your life. To take responsibility is to accept the consequences of your choices, both good and bad. When you are responsible, you don't transfer blame to other people or circumstances. You must be willing to own everything that happens.

When I began taking responsibility for everything I was or wasn't creating in my life, I was scared. If my life wasn't working, I could blame nobody but myself, and yet, at the same time, I realized that taking responsibility can be very empowering and freeing. This is what living is all about—mastering our lives by becoming all that we were created to be.

Avoid making routine matters and everyday relationships complicated. Your life is your gift to yourself and your thoughtful service to others. Unfailingly and enthusiastically welcome each day with joy and thankfulness because of the limitless opportunities it provides to learn, grow, flourish, and be truly happy and fulfilled. If this approach to each new day has not been your habitual response to life, make it first in order of priorities from now on. Practice the presence of God.

Our challenge is to trust and love ourselves as much as we are loved by God. We live in a friendly universe that is always saying "yes" to us. Our responsibility is to identify and transform those beliefs that have been sabotaging us from accepting and receiving that goodness. When you remove the blockages to God's presence and align with the love that you are, then abundance, prosperity, peace, health, success, and happiness will be yours.

MARATHON MYSTERY

After devoting a whole year to training, I ran my first marathon in Culver City (Los Angeles area) on the first week of December, 1975. When race day arrived, my emotions were mixed. On one hand I was eager and excited to run, although I was not quite sure what to expect since I had never done this before. On the other hand, I was feeling sad because the day of the race was the one-year anniversary of my grandmother Fritzie's death. Fritzie had been instrumental in teaching me about my own spirituality, self-reliance, simplicity, and living fully. As I was driving to Culver City the morning of the race, I felt a tremendous longing to visit with her. I missed her so much. I was actually talking out loud to her in the car, as a way to soothe the ache in my heart. I even said that I was open to her spirit and energy. I asked her to let me know somehow if she could hear me. I asked her to help me through the marathon.

When I arrived at the race site, there were lots of people getting ready. I wished I knew someone so I wouldn't have to run alone. The starting gun went off and so did a few thousand runners. For the first three miles I was alone and felt great—confident, relaxed, and energetic. Around the fourth mile, a man who looked to be in his mid-twenties ran up next to me and we began talking. Before we knew it, we were at mile ten, then fifteen, then twenty. It's amazing the things you'll tell someone you've never met before when you are running together. I think it has something to do with the release of certain chemicals in the body and a change in the electrical activity of the brain during aerobic exercise. We talked about our lives, families, interests, dreams, and goals. I was feeling extremely grateful to him because our conversation made the miles sail by.

Before we knew it, we were at mile twenty-five. At this point in our conversation, we started talking about where we lived. I told him I lived in Brentwood and he told me he lived in Studio City. "That's interesting," I said. "My grandmother used to live in Studio City. What street do you live on?" When he told me the street, I gasped. It was the same street as Fritzie's. At this point we were close to the finish line. I has just enough time to inquire about his exact location. We crossed the finish line as he told me he had moved into an apartment there eleven months earlier, and that the lady who lived there before him had passed away. I could hardly breathe and not because I was tired, but because of what he was telling me. He had moved into Fritzie's old apartment.

Out of all the thousands of people in the race, I ended up running with the person who lived in my grandmother's apartment, and only a few hours after I had asked Fritzie for some sign that she was receiving my communication. Coincidence? I don't think so. Only believe, have faith, and trust your inner guidance.

The key to mastery and living fully lies in turning within and asking God to take charge of every aspect of your life. Look deep within to get in touch with the truth of your being and the unlimited possibility that awaits you. To assist in the process, you may also want to ponder and answer these thoughts and questions, as I had Melissa do at the start of her commitment program.

PERSONAL COMMITMENT STATEMENT

Answer the following:

> What would my life be like if I were now living my highest vision?
> I commit to do the following in support of my vision:
> These are the ways I will now rearrange my lifestyle to totally support my commitments:

> The non-useful behaviors I will discontinue are:
> The new constructive behaviors I will implement are:
> Since I am a spiritual being living in a physical body, I will now nurture my spiritual self by:

Write out the following Personal Commitment Statement at the bottom of your answers and read it out loud (preferably) with feeling, sign your name, and date it. Reread it often. This is your personal commitment. From time to time, as you achieve your goals and live your vision at higher levels, you will want to re-write and refine your Personal Commitment Statement.

> I am passionately, unshakably devoted to my vision of how I want my life to be. I am committed to making my vision a reality for I know I have the power and ability to live my vision. Everything unlike my vision is dissipating, easily and effortlessly. With God as my ever-present help, I agree and affirm that I will do my best to help myself to total wellness and spiritual growth, and share my increasing radiance with my world. What I sincerely desire for myself, I also see and allow for others. Thank you for this precious gift of life. Today, as always, I honor and serve God by loving myself and everyone else unconditionally and by acknowledging God's presence in everything I think, feel, say, and do.

YOU ARE NOT SEPARATE

You can make a profound difference in other people's lives by how you choose to live yours. I'm reminded of the story of a young boy walking down the beach picking up starfish and throwing them back into the sea. A man observed this and finally caught up with the youth. He asked him, "What are you doing this for?"

The boy answered that the stranded starfish would die if left in the morning sun.

"But the beach goes on for miles and there are millions of starfish," countered the man. "How can your effort make any difference?"

The boy looked at the starfish in his hand, threw it to the safety of the waves, and replied, "It made a difference to that one!"

It makes a difference for those around you when you are loving, peaceful, happy, and healthy. It makes a difference every place you go when you are master of your life. You make a difference.

Our bodies are made up of billions of cells. In order to maintain optimum health, each of these cells must operate at peak performance.

When we have sick or weak cells, the healthy or stronger ones must work harder so that our body as a whole will be healthy.

Our planet is like a body, and we are all its individual cells—we are all cells in the body of humanity. Ultimately, we are not separate from others. There is no room for negative thinking, unforgiveness, bitterness towards others, or selfishness. It is your responsibility to this body that we call our planet to be a healthy, happy, peaceful, loving cell that radiates only goodness, positiveness, and joy. In this way, you can help make the world harmonious.

The separation and division that has so long colored our thoughts and beliefs regarding our lives on this planet must now be examined and corrected. To create peace on earth, we must stop dividing the world, the nations, the races, the religions, the sexes, the ages, the families, and the resources, and know that it's time to come together and live in harmony, forgiveness, and love. Awareness of our oneness must precede our thoughts and actions as a part of our belief system. We are all connected to this living, breathing planet. It's our choice. We can choose to make a difference with the way we live our lives.

In his book, *The Hundredth Monkey*, Ken Keyes, Jr., tells of a phenomenon observed by scientists. The eating habits of macaque monkeys were studied on several islands. One monkey discovered that sweet potatoes tasted better when washed before eating them. That monkey taught her mother and friends until one day a certain number (the ninety-ninth?) of the monkeys knew to wash their sweet potatoes. The next day, when the hundredth monkey learned how to wash sweet potatoes, an amazing thing happened: the rest of the colony miraculously knew how to wash their sweet potatoes too! Not only that, but the monkeys on other islands started washing their sweet potatoes as well.

Keyes applies this 'hundredth monkey' phenomenon to humanity. When more of us individually choose to make a difference with our lives—when human beings realize we each make a difference and start acting like it, more and more of us will learn this truth until we reach the 'millionth person' and peace and harmony spreads across the globe.

Where it starts is right here. I believe that we can't change the world, but we can choose to know and change ourselves and, as we do that, the world will be different. It takes all of us together, committing to being healthy, happy, powerful, peaceful, and pure in heart. We must choose to do the things that make a difference—that support wellness, that serve humanity, and that serve all creation.

We're here on earth not to see through one another, but to see one another through. We are here to experience the fullness of life. We are here to become the best we can be. We owe it to ourselves. When we change ourselves, we'll change the world. Says Unity minister and author Eric Butterworth, "It is not so much ours to set the world right, rather it is ours to see it rightly."

Afterword

Choose to live in the full spectrum of wholeness. Suppose you see a rainbow. You notice one or two colors you don't like. Would it still be a rainbow without all the colors blending with one another? All that's taking place in your life is what you've asked for or needed, even if you don't realize it. It's your thoughts and attitudes toward what is happening that make the difference. Let go of judgment. What takes place in the present does not have to be a duplication of your past.

If we could grasp the entire story, we would realize that no problem ever comes to us that does not have a purpose. Everything contributes to our inner growth.

Several years ago I trained as an emergency medical technician. For about a year I volunteered in emergency rooms of local hospitals. One day's experience will be forever vivid in my mind as the saddest and most poignant. It was Christmas Day and for a while the emergency room was quiet. The only cases were one patient with a sprained ankle and another with a severe stomachache. Then all at once three more patients came—three attempted suicides. Two made it through; the third didn't. The thoughts and beliefs of the two survivors were much the same. The woman had experienced several painful relationships which led her to withdraw to protect herself. She was unable to recognize that she had other choices. She was unwilling to risk more pain. The man had lost his job and felt worthless as a human being. He felt that there must be something better somewhere, but not here on Earth. They both dreaded pain and did whatever they could to avoid it. They didn't understand that to live without pain is to be only half-alive. Your life is precious and valuable, pain and all.

Once when Gandhi's train was pulling out of a station, someone ran up to his window and asked to be given some helpful message. To that, Gandhi answered, "My life is my message."

The choices we select in life clearly determine the quality of our lives. With consciousness about who and what we are, and with a commitment to ourselves and to each other, we can make life work for everyone on this planet. We are here to learn about love and to grow from love. This world was made to work. We have everything that it takes for our world to grow harmoniously and fruitfully, to be fulfilling and joyous for every human being and living creature. It is only when we start acting with these truths in mind that we will make the world a better place.

You make a difference in the world. Since your birth you have touched countless lives. If you weren't here the tapestry of life would be incomplete and lacking. Don't give up. It's been my experience that the very moment I feel like giving up, I'm only one step from a breakthrough. If you hang on long enough, circumstances will change. Trust in yourself, your dream, and Spirit. One of my other favorite quotes is by Henry Wadsworth Longfellow who wrote:

Let us, then, be up and doing
With a heart for any fate;
Still achieving, still pursuing,
Learn to labor and to wait.

Follow your heart's desires. Commit to your dreams and regardless of appearances, don't give up. Persevere and you'll find a way to freedom.

You are already free, and more than you could ever imagine. You can simply be happy and whole because that's already your divine nature.

For just a moment, close your eyes and see the planet in your mind's eye, viewing it from outer space as the astronauts have seen it. Notice the land masses and oceans without man-made boundaries or borders. See our earthly home in resplendent hues of green, aqua, blue, and white—magnificence overflowing with natural resources to supply everyone's needs.

Now take a closer look. Focus on the people who inhabit our planet. Look past nationality or race, and recognize that we as the human family are overwhelmingly more alike than different. Notice the shared humanity and spirituality of all human beings and of all creation. Now look closer into the hearts of all beings and see the great depths of compassion and caring, people who love their families and neighbors, people whose goals are peace and harmony for all.

All life is interconnected. We are all one—and as we choose to be healthy and live heart-to-heart, person-to-person, in cooperation, the quality of life on our planet will be transformed. We are all members of a glorious global family. As we let go of the illusion of separation and awaken and commit to being radiantly healthy and fully alive, we will recognize the profound oneness of all life. By acting from this awareness and linking with other members of our family, we will create a living system that sharply accelerates the peaceful transformation of our planet.

Make a conscious choice to give of yourself today and every day. I believe that it first starts in the hearts of each one of us. We have choices to make as to how we want to live and how we want our world to be. Health is a conscious choice. Peace is a conscious choice. Forgiveness is a conscious choice. But it all starts with you—your attitude, your feelings, your thoughts, and your words. Take a good look at your life, and if you want to change it, change your attitude, feelings, thoughts, and words. You make a difference. Choose to take responsibility for your life and your world.

One of the most difficult journeys we ever have to take is the eighteen-inch journey from the head to the heart. As we live from our hearts (from love and surrender) and less from our heads (analyzing, criticizing, controlling, and judging), we will 'lighten up.' It will be easier to look for the good in every person and situation. We'll be able to bring harmony into any situation. When we have peace and love in our hearts, we reflect it into our surroundings and into our world. Lighten up, let your heart light shine and give love and forgiveness to yourself and others.

When we reach out to another and offer unconditional love and forgiveness, joy and peace are the result. We can enrich the quality of life on our planet and together we can create a world where everyone wins. Don't feel that you are powerless or insignificant in affecting a change in what appears to be overwhelming obstacles or major crises on our planet. Everything you do or feel or think or say makes a difference. Every action you take is contributing to the whole. And just perhaps, you will be the one our world has been waiting for.

Embrace life. Live fully. And extend your blessings of love, appreciation, forgiveness, Light and oneness to every person in your world and you will be making a difference.

—SUSAN SMITH JONES

If this book has moved you into action and enriched your life, do yourself and others a favor by giving copies as gifts. As you give, you receive. Remember, we're all here on this earth not to see through one another, but to see one another through and assist others on their journey. Share this book with your relatives and friends. Those wishing to have their own copies may obtain them by calling: (800) 843-5743 (PST).

APPENDIX

Workbook: Self-Discovery Questions and Action Choices

The following questions and ideas are designed to support you in learning more about yourself and in applying the material presented in this book to your life in a direct and personal way. Space is provided to write your responses in the book. Many of you will require more space to write. Please don't hesitate to use extra paper.

This is your personal exploration of your authentic self, to help you to "know thyself." This workbook will assist you in deeper study and self-discovery, and provide future reference. It has been designed to help you make positive changes in your attitude, thoughts, beliefs, actions, and lifestyle. I have grouped the Self-Discovery Questions and Action Choices emphasizing specific themes. Don't skip over this part.

CELEBRATING MYSELF

Self-Discovery Questions

1. What does it mean to me to be healthy?

2. What value have I gotten from being ill in the past (for example, by being sick, would someone pay more attention to me)?

3. In the past, who (or what situations) have I blamed for my failures?

4. People treat me in accordance with how I've taught them to treat me, that is, how I treat myself. What changes can I make in myself and my behavior that will support my newfound magnificence?

5. In the past I may have felt limited in what I could be or do because of what others have said. As I let go of limiting opinions and beliefs and tune in to my own inner signals, what new possibilities become exciting and available to me?

Action Choices

1. Following is a list of at least five things I love about myself:

2. Following is a list of some things I am going to change to improve myself:

3. These are a few things I can do to increase my self-confidence and self-image:

4. Because I must take myself with me everywhere I go, I now choose to start loving myself unconditionally and consistently.

In the following space I describe myself as the radiant being that I am:

5. I now choose to find myself more attractive than ever before. I am wonderful. I now take a few minutes to mentally picture myself as the exquisite person I am, emphasizing my many positive qualities:

EMBRACING MY AUTHENTIC SELF

Self-Discovery Questions

1. Here are some of the many reasons why I deserve to be optimally healthy and fully functioning:

2. What am I feeling angry about? This is how I'll let the anger go:

3. What am I feeling upset about? This will help me let the feeling go.

4. What am I feeling depressed and hopeless about? I'll release it by doing this.

5. What am I feeling happy and joyful about?

6. In the past I have chosen to feel anxious about the following things. I now choose to let this anxiety go.

7. When can I set aside time each day to be by myself and to relax?

8. I can ask the following people to help me to be more positive.

Action Choices

1. Sit quietly with your eyes closed for the next few minutes, envisioning yourself as a peaceful, relaxed, confident, and happy person. Describe how that looked and felt:

2. Every night before you go to sleep, sit quietly and forgive yourself and others that you feel have hurt you in any way. List those people that need your immediate attention:

3. Think of one person with whom you have not been feeling in harmony. Close your eyes and see both of you sitting facing each other in a circle of white or pink light. Now lovingly share your feelings with that person and resolve any conflict. Finish with seeing your hearts connect and loving each other unconditionally.

4. If you need to forgive a person who has died, sit down and write that individual a letter. Pour out all your feelings and finish it by offering forgiveness and love.

5. If you know someone who's experiencing lots of stress, anxiety, depression, hopelessness, or helplessness, contact that person as soon as possible. Encourage him or her to express feelings to you as you listen without judging, criticizing, or offering advice. Sometimes all we need is someone who cares and will take the time to listen and be our friend. List here who you'll be contacting:

6. From this day forward, I will give _____ hugs a day.

7. I now know that the better I handle stress, the healthier and happier I'll be. Here are some ways I've handled stress in the past. Here are the ways I now choose to deal with stress that support my immune system and well-being:

LIVING MY HIGHEST VISION

Self-Discovery Questions

1. What are my goals in the following areas?

   Relationships

Career

Financial

Fitness

Interests and Hobbies

Health

Spiritual

2. If I knew I couldn't fail, what would I change in my life?

Action Choices

1. Following is my ideal vision of myself, which includes all areas of my life. If I were living my ideal life right now, what would my life be like, what would the world be like, and how would I feel?

2. Am I living this life now? If not, why not? What immediate changes can I make toward this goal?

3. Listed below are the words and phrases that I now choose to eliminate from my vocabulary:

4. My relationships can be more like what I want them to be, not by trying to change anyone else, but by changing my own thoughts and attitudes in the following ways:

NOTES

CHOOSING TO BE HEALTHY

Self-Discovery Questions

1. What foods do I need to eliminate from my diet because they don't support my health?

2. What are ways I have been treating myself without love through my eating behaviors?

3. How can I change the way I prepare food that will support increased well-being?

4. What beliefs do I hold about food that are sabotaging my healthfulness?

Action Choices

1. For twenty-one days I will eliminate the following from my diet and add the following to my diet:

2. This is the book, magazine, or tape I will use to assist me in my health program right now:

These are others I will use in the near future:

3. Listed here are some supplements that I now choose to include in my nutritional program to enhance my health:

4. Following are at least five affirmations that support my being vibrantly healthy:

5. Listed below are the foods I have normally eaten that I know are not healthy and will eliminate on my 21-Day Rejuvenation Program:

6. Each day I choose to spend at least ten minutes visualizing myself as a healthy, radiant being who treats himself or herself respectfully and lovingly. (Describe in a paragraph how this vision appears to you.)

FITNESS FOR LIFE

Self-Discovery Questions

1. What is my resting heart rate and my target exercising heart rate?

2. How do I feel about exercise?

3. What beliefs do I have about my exercise that have been working against me?

4. What excuses seem to frequently come up that interfere with my exercising?

5. Here are my exercise and fitness goals for the following month, three months, six months, and year:

6. The areas of my body that need special attention are:

7. My body is miraculous. Here are a few of the numerous body functions for which I am grateful:

LETTING MY HEART-LIGHT SHINE

Self-Discovery Questions

1. In what areas of my life am I too serious?

2. Would I describe myself as a happy, positive person? Am I the type of person I would like to have for a friend?

3. How do I feel being around children?

4. What qualities do I see in children that I'd like to integrate more fully into my life?

5. In what areas of my life am I too rigid and orderly—too 'adult'?

6. Do I give myself permission to act silly and crazy?

7. How often do I truly embrace the moment? Do I spend my present moments feeling guilty about the past or worrying about the future?

Action Choices

1. If I were to regularly let the child in me out to explore, play and be spontaneous and creative, my life would change in the following ways:

2. In order to get more in touch with my inner child, I am going to spend some time observing children at play as well as participating with them. I can do this in the following ways:

3. Following are fun things to do for those I care about (for example, write a special note, send flowers, or record a song):

4. Here are some things I tried in the past six months that I had never tried before:

5. Here are some new ventures I choose to undertake in the coming six months:

6. Here are some changes I can make to become a little less serious and to lighten up:

7. The following are people I have wanted to meet or get to know better. I'll choose one of them to get together with next week.

8. Following is a description of myself as a happy, positive, magnificent person:

9. Each day I'll set some time aside to envision my ideal life. I will now spend the next few moments imagining one of my goals as already achieved. Here is what I visualized that to be:

EMBRACING THE SACRED WITHIN AND AROUND ME

Self-Discovery Questions

1. What do I want most out of life?

2. What is my personal definition of success?

3. When I feel negative emotions, do I usually blame someone else?

4. When do I feel most happy and at peace?

5. How do I feel about being alone?

6. What are things I do to avoid being alone and having quietude?

7. How old do I feel?

8. What changes can I make in my attitude that will enrich my life?

9. If I knew I had only one year to live, what changes would I make in my life? Why aren't I making those changes now?

10. What does peace mean to me?

Action Choices

1. This is the time during each day that I have set aside just for me:

2. Following are ways I choose to simplify my life:

3. In the past, my negative emotions have sometimes immobilized me. This is ending because I now choose to do the following instead:

4. Following are at least ten things I love about myself and my world:

5. Here is a list of affirmations that support my magnificence:

6. If this were the last year of my life, the following things would be most important to me:

7. These are some changes I can make in my life to experience more peace:

8. Here are some things I am going to do to enrich life on this planet:

APPENDIX

Questions and Answers

The goal is for you to be truly healthy and happy in every dimension of your being, and to be free from any kind of compulsion.
—JOHN ROBBINS

Through the years I've been asked countless questions at lectures and workshops, television and radio interviews, or when consulting and counseling. I've noticed that there are several questions that, although worded a little differently each time, come up most often. You may have similar questions or find these further reflections on attaining health and happiness helpful. My answers are more than a summary of the book's content and go a little deeper for those who are seriously looking to change their lives.

Q: Susan, you are a proponent of slowing down to smell the flowers. Yet it appears that you live an extremely busy, high-pressure life. How do you keep yourself balanced?

A: Although I am busy, I still keep a peaceful mind in everything I'm doing. I truly believe that we have a choice, and I make certain choices. What I do every morning is to arise before dawn to begin my day with meditation. That sets a tone of peace, joy, and enthusiasm for the day. I have learned that my quiet times in the silence with God can be the most revealing and inspiring times of my life. Realizing that God is not remote but an integral part of me, I understand the need to be quiet and listen within. Worries fade away and insignificant matters take their rightful place. A gentle whisper or a certain knowing reveals the truth to me. Silence and meditation are the best way I know to stay balanced. At the very heart of the silence, I realize the presence of God. Wrapped in the safe, protective mantle of God's presence, I feel rested, refreshed, and renewed. God alone is sufficient, for in Him lies all love, all life, all happiness, all joy, all peace—everything that even in your wildest dreams you could not imagine. Cultivate a relationship with Him.

Practice the presence of God every day and never go to bed at night until you have practiced meditation and are filled with that joy. When you feel that eternal peace and balance within, then whoever comes to you shall feel your peace, be uplifted by it, and feel more balanced themselves. Within your being, you carry all the conditions of happiness by meditating and attuning your consciousness to the ever-present joy which is God. Don't allow your happiness to be subject to any outside influence. Whatever your environment is, refuse to allow your inner peace to be touched by it. That's how you stay balanced.

Of course, I also exercise regularly and practice sound nutrition, both of which help keep me in balance. Another choice is how much or how little I attempt to accomplish. You don't have to go faster just because everybody else is. When we push beyond our natural rhythm we grow insensitive to our body's needs and the needs of those around us.

Q: Do you believe in coincidence?

A: It's been said that God orchestrates a coincidence but chooses to remain anonymous. Throughout our lives, coincidences lead us toward the attainment of our life's purpose. By increasing our awareness and remaining connected to our Source, we see that coincidences are happening all around us when we ask the right questions. The answers are easy—it's the questions that are sometimes difficult. We must keep our energy at maximum level to be receptive to the messages that come to us through intuitive thoughts, daydreams, night dreams, and especially from people who show up on our path.

Q: How do you develop intuition?

A: The best way is just to sit still and listen. Turn within and pay attention. Too often we run away from ourselves, filling up our lives with constant activity. We don't take time to be still.

The word intuition means to guide and protect. I believe it's the voice of God within us. Intuition can be nurtured in a variety of ways which I have written about in Chapter Fourteen on meditation. The more you act on your intuitive hunches, the stronger and more readily available they become. As you become more sensitive to your oneness with God and life, you will become more intuitive. Receiving those inner messages clearly comes when you learn to give up the analyzing, reasoning, doubting, and limiting part of your mind.

Q: Do you have a particular meditation and spiritual practice?

A: Yes. My meditation practice is based on Kriya Yoga. For years I have been studying the lessons from Paramahansa Yogananda's Self-Realization Fellowship. Those lessons are invaluable and truly help me look at all the aspects of my life from a new perspective. The essence of the lessons is that we need to live more in the presence of God, and to look inwardly for the answers to life rather than outside of ourselves. I have always had those beliefs on my own, but the lessons were very practical in terms of reminding me that I can live a more spiritual life in a physical world.

Self-Realization means "to know the Self as soul, made in the image of God." Fellowship stands for "fellowship with God, first, and through Him, fellowship with humankind." The Self-Realization Fellowship techniques provide practical step-by-step methods to enable one to recharge the body with cosmic energy; awaken the unlimited power of the mind by concentration; and expand the consciousness by Kriya Yoga meditation to receive the omnipresent love and joy of God. These are definite scientific techniques that have been used for centuries. When Yogananda was alive he always emphasized 'plain living and high thinking.' That's how I choose to live. I want my life to radiate my devotion to God and my loving reverence and concern for all fellow beings, creatures and life itself.

Q: When you say 'God' and 'spiritual,' what do those terms mean to you?

A: My concept of God is the essence of life...love...the universal force that both surrounds us and is within us, and which connects us all to each other. For me spirituality is more than performance of sacraments, prayers and songs. I express my faith by the way I live and by my belief and faith in a Creator—by my reverence for nature and my desire to nurture humankind. Being spiritual also means being honest with myself and practicing self-discipline in every aspect of life. Henry David Thoreau expressed it well when he said, "Our religion is where our love is." I am deeply in love with all people, all creation, and with life itself. Life is sacred and every step we take is on holy ground.

Life teaches us how to live. Honoring the sacredness within and around us heals and enriches life. The life force within us is diminished by judgment far more frequently than by disease. We have a tendency to approve or disapprove of others and ourselves, according to superficial standards and labels of acceptability and achievement, rather than learning to love. Some of the basic tendencies that limit the expression of the healing life force within us are our wrong attitudes about pain and growth, our limiting beliefs and destructive self-definition. We must come back to and embrace our authentic selves—a sometimes difficult thing to do. Actually, we are all more than we know. Wholeness is never lost, it is only forgotten.

Q: Do you feel that today's busy world can put one's spirituality at risk?

A: The intense pace and stress of our daily lives can very easily put our sense of living a spiritual life at risk. It's easy to get caught up in the whirl of today's hectic lifestyle—especially if you've forgotten the truth of your being. We all need a strong foundation of practical spirituality based on the realization that we are co-creators with the ultimate source of power and creativity. With that type of partnership, anything and everything is possible.

Q: What do you mean by 'co-creators,' and how do you see that operating in our practical lives?

A: There is a way to accomplish all of our dreams and live up to our highest visions. We all have access to the universal creative power. We are tied directly to it. Our dreams can always be made a reality by taking them seriously, by continuously focusing on what we want. When we do this, the natural pull of the universe will serve as a co-creative force that leads us to any goal we truly want and feel worthy to receive. We must stop judging from the appearances of so-called 'reality' and have enough faith to choose a loftier perspective on life. Then we can move toward what we want by taking action.

What I see happen with so many people is that they give up easily when their quest is challenged. I have found in my own life that stumbling blocks and challenges are just opportunities to learn and grow. Our only real limits are our own thoughts and self-imposed limitations.

Q: What would you say to the person who is struggling to find purpose in his or her life? How can one come to clarity?

A: I would ask, "What did you want to do as a young child? What would bring you so much joy and enthusiasm you would do it even if you didn't get paid?" Attaining a clear vision of what you want your life to be should be your number one priority. Thoreau said, "The world is but a canvas to your imagination." It all starts with a mental vision of what you want. You are here to experience and celebrate life and to be enlightened, happy, and joyful. This is your true destiny. Take your vision seriously. Why not become the best you can? You owe it to yourself to do that. No one is going to do it for you.

Often we don't begin the one thing we really want to do in life because of fear. The greatest possible growth and personal development is achieved through recognizing and facing our pain and fears. I like what Jack Kornfield says about this in his wonderful book, *A Path With Heart*: "The compartments we create to shield us from what we fear, ignore, and exclude exact their toll later in life. Periods of holiness and spiritual fervor can later alternate with opposite extremes—bingeing on food, sex, and other things—becoming a kind of spiritual bulimia. Spiritual practice will not save us from suffering and confusion, it only allows us to understand that avoidance of pain does not help."

Q: Do you feel that fear can be empowering?

A: Absolutely. We often just live in the 'comfort zone.' But you can learn so much about yourself when you look at what creates fear in your life. Then the challenge is to step out beyond your fear, even though you may not have a clear idea of what you want to do.

What I like to tell people in my workshops is that the time you feel least like starting something is precisely the time to forge ahead. Just the physical act of beginning will create the momentum and energy that will allow you to develop beyond your fear and toward your greatest accomplishments. Every step you take is on sacred ground. Everything about your life is sacred. The path to the sacred is your own body, heart, and mind, the history of your life, and the closest relationships and circumstances of your life. If not here, where else could we bring alive joy, compassion, freedom, and happiness? Don't place any limitations on your dreams or your Creator by doubting that you can accomplish your soul's desire and live a sacred life. Like Jesus, you can call on spiritual power and authority that will allow you to overcome whatever it is you need to overcome, achieve whatever you desire to achieve.

Q: How do you recommend we build our goal-seeking muscles?

A: I recommend you start with very easy-to-achieve goals so you can have success and feel empowered. Visualization is a very important part of the process. You must be able to see yourself achieving your goal. Don't push your goal too far out into the future. One thing that I always do when I am visualizing a goal is to accept it and give thanks that it is already part of my reality. Simply put, 'act as if.' I always end my visualizations with, "This or something better I now accept in my life." I do that because even though I may be clear on what I want, I am always living in the presence of a Higher Power that has a better sense of what is best for my highest good.

Q: What can we learn from your personal success?

A: I remember as a child I wanted to speak to people about being happy and peaceful. When I was about seven or eight, I had dreams of visiting world leaders of different countries and helping them resolve conflict. I always believed in peace, not war. I also knew I wanted to be active and do something involving health and fitness. I got in touch with those early visions and made conscious, faith-filled choices based on them.

Another major key to my success in life is discipline. Discipline is the ability to carry out a resolution or commitment long after the mood has left. Part of discipline is to give enthusiasm to whatever you are doing, have faith in yourself, be tenacious, and have high personal standards and integrity. If you do that, your life will blossom.

Pay attention to your feelings and what your body, mind, and heart are telling you. You are getting messages all the time. Focus directly on what is right in front of you. When any experience in body, heart, or mind keeps repeating, this is a signal asking for deeper and fuller attention.

Another key is regular visualization: seeing in your mind's eye the end result of what you want to achieve and feeling the sensation associated with the wish being fulfilled. I spend time each day visualizing. It really helps to set aside a few minutes each day to focus on one or more goals that you want to bring into your life.

What happens when you live with these attitudes is that you resonate at a higher frequency. Scientific studies have shown that when we are enthusiastic and positive and have faith in ourselves, the frequency of vibration of our molecules is increased at a base cellular level.

Finally, make sure your path has heart. This is essential on any spiritual journey. Be sure that your path is connected with your deepest love. Don Juan, in his teaching to Carlos Castañeda, put it this way: "Look at every path closely and deliberately. Try it as many times as you think necessary. Then ask yourself and yourself alone one question. This question is one that only a very old man asks. My benefactor told me about it once when I was young and my blood was too vigorous for me to understand it. Now I do understand it. I will tell you what it is: Does this path have a heart? If it does, the path is good. If it doesn't, it is of no use."

Q: You are a proponent of ongoing personal change. Would you please explain your change concept?

A: Ben Franklin once said that whatever you do for twenty-one days will become a habit. He is now supported by behavioral scientists. If you meditate or exercise, or perhaps stop smoking or drinking coffee, for twenty-one consecutive days, your body will accept your new behavior as a habit and no longer crave what you gave up. This is a wonderful way for a person to begin to take control of life in a non-threatening manner. Most people can commit to a simple twenty-one days. If you are really committed, then you'll arrange your personal circumstances and lifestyle to support your commitment.

I have done this monthly for over ten years, and I have made twelve beneficial changes every year. I'm not saying this is always easy. Often when you make a commitment to something, things may get worse in your life before they get better. I believe this is so because making a commitment causes everything unlike your goal to surface. Only then can you take responsibility for such things and let them go. Quite often the most rewarding transformations come from our greatest adversities and challenges.

Q: What do you feel are the most basic keys to personal mastery?

A: Seven important things immediately come to mind.

- Have a very clear vision of what you want in your life.
- Be totally committed to that vision.
- Live with faith—believing, even when appearances or experiences may show you something other than your vision.
- Acknowledge that in surrender to the co-creative power within, you will find and create everything you are seeking in your life.
- Maintain an attitude of gratitude. No matter what's going on in my life, I am grateful because I know that I can learn and grow and be a better and stronger person for everything that happens.

- Acknowledge the sacredness of your body and life, and walk a path with heart.
- Always let love be your guide. As Mother Theresa suggested, "Do ordinary things with extraordinary love."

Q: What does 'commitment' mean to you?

A: You've noticed that I am very much into commitment! It's through our everyday behavior that we know what we're really committed to. If we're committed, then everything we think, feel, say, and do is in alignment. Commitment is also an excellent way to free yourself from tension, because then your mind is no longer indecisive.

Lack of commitment seems to be a disease of our generation. Just look around. People say they are committed to a healthier planet, yet they litter, don't recycle and eat lots of animal products—all of which drain our planet's natural resources. People say they're committed to aligning and nurturing the spiritual side of their being, but they make no time in their lives to meditate or commune with their Higher Power. Sometimes a person will get seriously ill or have an accident. That will be their 'wake up call.' It will force them to get in touch with what is really essential in life. But it's easier just to take time each day to turn within and connect with your Higher Self—to pay attention to what is important, then carry that out into the world.

I'm committed to a practical, self-disciplined, day-to-day spirituality as a way of life and always recognizing the sacredness of our lives.

Q: The entire world seems to be in one crisis or another. How do you view our times?

A: I believe that everything is a reflection of our consciousness. If I watch the news and get really upset or angry about what's going on, then what I'm doing is adding to the turmoil already out there. I like to be informed, but I feel that what I can do best is just choose to live my life as peacefully, positively, and lovingly as possible. Everything begins in our own hearts. If we can all live more loving and peaceful lives, then we can add those feelings to the mass consciousness and in some small way make a difference. "As we receive God's love and impart it to others, we are given the power to repair the world," says Marianne Williamson. Attaining and expressing self-realization is what we're all here to do. It's about loving God, knowing our oneness with Him, and then bringing that love, peace, happiness, and realization down into practical application in our daily lives.

What we must sometimes do to survive is not what it takes to truly live. Embracing life deals with the true value of learning to accept life as a whole, and not resist the difficult lessons it may bring us. We all can influence the life force and we all have the ability to heal one another through the power of love. We must recognize and reclaim the capacity we all have to heal each other, the enormous power in the simplest of human relationships: the strength of a touch, the blessing of forgiveness, the grace of someone else taking you just as you are and finding in you an unsuspected goodness.

I believe that healing our world and ourselves begins with regaining our connection with God, and the awe of living in God's world. I'm convinced that the roots of illness and crisis in our individual lives and world are ultimately spiritual—a loss of awareness of the sacred within and around us.

Q: What do you feel are the main ingredients for optimum health?

A: Nutrition and exercise are essential, but I believe there are also other equally important elements, including deep breathing, fresh air, sunshine, pure water, and periodic fasting. Don't forget positive attitude, forgiveness toward yourself and others, and releasing any negative emotions. To this list, I would also add visualization, affirmations, simplifying your life, learning to relax, and becoming more childlike. Then, of course, you want to add meditation, some time for solitude, unconditional love for yourself, living more from inner guidance, and letting go and letting God.

Q: Why do you recommend eliminating dairy products from our diet?

A: Dairy products cause excess mucus, which in turn causes over-acidity. Cow's milk is a high-fat fluid designed to turn a forty-five-pound calf into a 400-pound cow in eighteen months. As my friend Michael Klaper, MD says in his book, *Vegan Nutrition: Pure and Simple*, "It has a 'bovine' mixture of casein protein and saturated fat, and simply is not a natural food for man, woman, or child." Consider the fat content of these popular dairy foods:

Butter = eighty percent
Cream = forty percent

Ice Cream = twenty to forty percent
(luxury ice creams have the highest content)
Cheese = twenty-five to forty percent
Milk Chocolate = twenty-five to forty percent

Animal fat from cow's milk clogs the arteries. Dairy products have been conclusively linked with heart attacks, strokes, and cancer growth (see Chapter Two on nutrition). Dairy products also contain animal proteins, like casein, that can contribute to allergic/inflammatory reaction, such as chronic runny noses, asthmatic bronchitis, and other inflammations of joints, skin, and bowels.

Commercials proclaim that dairy products are good sources of calcium, vital for strong bones, and preventatives against osteoporosis. In actuality, milk, cheese, yogurt, and ice cream are not really wholesome sources of calcium. In addition to significant amounts of saturated fat and allergy-inciting cow protein, these dairy foods contain a large load of phosphate, which can neutralize the benefits of calcium. Studies disclose that dairy products do not prevent osteoporosis. The nations with the highest levels of dairy product consumption are also the nations with the highest rates of osteoporosis. In one study (sponsored by the Dairy Council) women consuming three eight-ounce glasses of cow's milk per day still lost calcium from their bodies and remained in negative calcium balance, even after a year of consuming almost fifteen hundred milligrams of calcium daily! It is not a diet insufficiently high in calcium, but a diet high in protein, laden with poultry, fish, meat, and dairy products that robs the body of calcium. If you are already experiencing osteoporosis or may be at a risk for it, you can slow the rate of calcium loss by adopting a vegan diet; eliminating caffeine, soft drinks, and smoking—all of which leach calcium from the bones; and incorporating weight-bearing exercise (such as lifting weights, climbing stairs or hills, or hiking) outside in the sunshine every day.

In place of milk, my favorite beverage, and the one I recommend in my workshops, is Silk™ by White Wave. This delicious one hundred percent dairy-free soy beverage is perfect poured over cereal and as a non-dairy creamer. Silk is fortified with vitamins A, B_2, D, and calcium, low in fat, and cholesterol free. It's made from whole soybeans that are grown without herbicides or chemical additives. I also use and highly recommend White Wave Rice Silk. It's a cool, rich, great tasting, "full bodied" rice beverage that appeals to adults as well as children. Low fat and one hundred percent lactose and cholesterol free, White Wave Rice Silk is fortified with calcium, vitamins A, B_2,

B_{12}, and D. Silk is also easy to use in cooking and baking, as it maintains the same fresh quality and smooth taste associated with milk products. Both of these products are available in the refrigerated section of your natural foods store. (See Resource Directory for more on White Wave's soy and rice beverages.)

Q: You advocate eating lots of raw food. Why is this beneficial?

A: Healthy raw plant foods are filled with enzymes. Enzymes are involved in every process of the body. Each body cell has an excess of 100,000 enzyme particles necessary for metabolic processes. Enzymes rule and far outweigh the importance of every other nutrient, yet they cannot function properly without the presence of coenzymes: minerals, vitamins, and proteins. For life to continue, you must have a constant enzyme supply, which requires continual replacement of enzymes.

Enzymes are the dynamic factors that break down protein, fat, and carbohydrates into their basic building blocks so that the body can digest and use them. Protein molecules are the carriers of enzymes. They are the life force, the electrical energy factor, the invisible activity that takes place in all aspects of our being alive.

As I mention in Chapter Two and learned from nutritionist Paulette Suzanne (see Resource Directory), there are three basic types of enzymes. Metabolic enzymes are made by the body and are responsible for its biochemical processes, available as needed. Digestive enzymes are made by the body and are active in digestive juices and chemical breakdown of food. Plant enzymes occur naturally in raw, unprocessed food, helping digest food and serving many other purposes.

According to Dr. Edward Howell, who has done more than fifty years of research on enzymes, we are born with only a certain amount of enzymes and the body will not waste its own precious enzymes for digestion unless it is forced. When food is cooked, processed, or heated over 115 degrees F., enzymes are destroyed. Enzyme-deficient food puts a tremendous strain on the body as it tends to deplete the body's enzyme potential and greatly overworks the digestive system to the detriment of the entire body.

Raw, living foods are easily digested, cheaper than packaged food and expensive animal products, easier to prepare and clean up after, help the body achieve ideal weight, do not cause or support degenerative diseases, eliminate body odor, keep you calm and emotionally stable, and boost your immunity. The bonus is that raw foods also taste delicious!

Living foods and living nutrients are found in the supplements Juice Plus+, Green Magma, Sun Chlorella, and Bio-Strath. These supplements bring the needed life force and electrical potential into our cells to detoxify, regenerate, nourish, and actually activate light at the cellular level in enormous quantities, supporting the process of healing and awakening. Nutritionist Paulette Suzanne says, "I have seen tremendous benefits on all levels of life when people choose to activate life and light on cellular levels within themselves. The body begins the healing process by letting go of all it doesn't need any longer (detoxification). Then the cells can be filled with nourishment and high energy vibrations which charge the body and the mind (regeneration). As the body receives more energy and light activation, then acceleration of consciousness, personal growth, and spiritual awakening powerfully uplift the whole person."

Dr. Humbart Santillo, author of *Food Enzymes: The Missing Link to Radiant Health*, pioneered this new whole live food supplement called Juice Plus+. He designed this product by juicing approximately eight pounds of pesticide-free fresh, ripe fruits and vegetables, removing the water and sugars, and cold drying at very cold temperatures to preserve all the enzymes, vitamins, minerals, plant actives, antioxidants, and more. These capsules or tablets contain the nutrition of apple, cranberry, orange, peach, pineapple, date, and prune in the fruit supplement. The vegetable supplement contains the nutrition of broccoli, beet, cabbage, carrot, garlic, kale, parsley, spinach, barley, and oats. This very special selection of fruits and vegetables has been chosen for their powerful nutritional components including cancer-preventive food actives, antioxidants, and living enzymes. In addition, extra food enzymes have been added along with acidophilus and soluble and insoluble fibers, to ensure digestive support.

When you take the Juice Plus+ capsules with your meals, you will not only benefit from all the nutrition of eight pounds of juiced fruits and vegetables, you will also benefit from the live enzymes, which will help your digestion, elimination, immune system, and overall good health. (See Resource Directory for more on Juice Plus+.)

Green Magma is also a superior whole food concentrate. This is evident in the way the Green Foods Corporation organically grows, cultivates, and processes their barley grass, taking the utmost care in transferring live essential nutrients to an easy-to-use, convenient powder form that is easily and quickly assimilated by our system.

There's a way to test if the green powder has not been heated. Try this experiment. Put one teaspoon of Green Magma in a clear glass of hot water. Put one teaspoon of another green product in a clear glass of hot water.

Stir both and let sit for a few minutes. The Green Magma will coagulate at the top, forming a solidified mass. The other product will mix uniformly. Why? Because Green Magma is being heated for the first time, which is stripping the proteins and killing live enzymes within. The other product's content probably has already been heated, or denatured, and then powdered. A similar phenomenon is an egg; egg is a protein that has never been heated. When you boil an egg, it forms a hardened mass. This is because the protein is being heated for the first time as with the Green Magma.

I start each day with Green Magma and Juice Plus+ in a large glass of water or juice (I also add Veggie Magma and Magma Plus powders). I also take Sun Chlorella (see Chapter Five on chlorophyll and greens), Bio-Strath, and Kyolic capsules two times each day, along with Ester-C.

Q: What kitchen appliances do you use and feel are essential in creating a health-friendly kitchen?

A: Besides a set of top quality knives, a salad spinner, a rice/grain cooker, a large chopping board, and juicer (see chapter six on juicing), I recommend a good set of stainless steel cookware and the Vita-Mix Total Nutrition Center. Neova stainless steel cookware is what I've chosen for my kitchen. It is beautiful and durably constructed and carries a lifetime warranty. With Neova cookware, foods won't stick even at medium high heat, which means you can reduce the fat in your diet. The covers fit tightly and the handles remain cool. I can sauté vegetables and tofu and even pop popcorn with without oil, all with great success. Their steamer is excellent, too, and used often in my kitchen. I have Neova's entire set of stainless steel and highly recommend it for every health kitchen.

The Vita-Mix Total Nutrition Center is also indispensable in my kitchen, and I've used it for over twenty years. You can turn fruits and vegetables into whole food juices in less than four minutes, freeze a half gallon of all fruit ice cream in less than sixty seconds, and grind whole wheat into flour for bread or pancake batter in seconds. This marvelous machine performs thirty-five processes in all. It makes being healthy easy and effortless. It also comes with a marvelous recipe book and instruction video. The Vita-Mix TNC delivers to your body the balanced nutrition found only in whole foods, which ultimately can improve the way you look and feel.

Both the Vita-Mix TNC and Neova stainless steel cookware make excellent gifts for weddings, anniversaries, birthdays, and other special occasions. For more information or to order, refer to the Resource Directory.

Q: I carry most of my stress in my back. Sitting at my desk for several hours a day doesn't help. What do you suggest to help take the pressure off of my back?

A: Stress and the negative effects of gravity can certainly create havoc in our bodies and lives. Just sitting and standing all day, and sleeping with our heads propped up on pillows all night, enables gravity to work against us twenty-four hours a day. Just as gravity keeps water from flowing upwards, it also keeps our blood from flowing freely upward and into our heads. Our eyes, ears, gums, scalps, complexions, and brains—all areas above the heart are where blood circulates least—are the first to deteriorate in our heads-up lifestyle.

We must learn to work with the law of gravity instead of allowing gravity to work against us. There are a variety of different yoga positions where the legs are elevated higher than the upper body, achieving this increased circulation to the upper torso. For more than twenty-five years, I have practiced lying on a slant board (BodySlant), which puts the legs higher than the heart and the head lower than the heart. In this position, the pull of gravity on your face, neck, back, internal organs, legs, and feet is naturally and effectively reversed.

In his book, *Look Younger, Live Longer*, Gayelord Hauser states: "In the slant position, the spine straightens out and the back flattens itself. Muscles which are ordinarily tense, are relaxed and at ease. The feet and legs freed from the customary burden and the force of gravity, have a chance to release accumulated congestions in the blood stream and tissues, and thereby reduce the possibility of swollen limbs and strained blood vessels. Sagging abdominal muscles get a lift, and the blood flows more freely to the muscles of the chin, throat, and cheeks, helping to maintain their firmness. The complexion, hair and scalp benefit from increased blood circulation, and the brain is also rested and cleared."

I use and highly recommend the BodySlant (see Resource Directory). Resting in the incline position on the BodySlant is as easy, safe, and comfortable as resting on a bed. I especially love using it after heavy physical and mental activities. The calm, peace, and relaxation it provides is wonderful. And it's the best way I know to *prevent* and alleviate back pain.

Q: There are so many so-called 'energy bars' on the market. Is there one that really tastes good and is healthy, too?

A: Yes. PowerBar Performance provides energy before, during, or after athletic performance. Over the years, athletes 'fueled by PowerBar' have set numerous national and international records. Millions of active people have come to rely on these powerful bars as an excellent source of lasting energy.

The other bars I eat and recommend is the PowerBar Harvest. Made by the same company, this energy bar was created to meet a broader range of everyday energy needs. It provides energy-related vitamins and minerals that life's daily marathons can deplete. Toss one into your child's lunch bag. Try one between meals. Whatever your busy schedule throws at you, be prepared with a PowerBar Harvest bar in your briefcase, purse, or glove compartment. They are moist and crunchy, combining the goodness of whole grains, chunks of real fruit, and natural sweeteners. My favorite flavors are Apple Crisp, Cherry Crunch, and Strawberry.

Q: I've decided to give up meat. What alternatives can you recommend to make sure I get enough protein?

A: Scientific studies reveal that if you eat a variety of plant foods—such as fruits, vegetables, whole grains, legumes, nuts, and seeds—on a daily basis, you don't need to be concerned about getting enough protein. All foods contain some protein, though some more than others. An excellent source of plant protein is soybeans and soy products such as tofu. Studies have found that *tofu* and soy products offer the following health benefits:

- Helps prevent ulcers by neutralizing stomach acid.
- Helps prevent breast and prostate cancer.
- Mimics estrogen's positive effects on the skeletal, reproductive and cardiovascular system while blocking estrogen's carcinogenic effects on breast tissue.
- Decreases LDL cholesterol and helps prevent heart disease.
- A good source of calcium and prevents osteoporosis.
- Low in allergen factors, highly nutritious, rich in vitamins, amino acids, and free of pesticides and other synthetic toxins when grown and processed organically.
- Easy for adults and infants to digest; has no cholesterol, no lactose, and is very rich in essential fatty acids (EFAs).
- Substantially higher as a dietary source of protein and iron than dairy milk.

- Inexpensive, readily available, and virtually tasteless on its own, tofu is easy to add to all of your favorite recipes. Many different soy food products are now available.

In just twenty years, the White Wave Vegetarian Cuisine Company of Boulder, Colorado had grown to become one of the largest soy food manufacturers in the United States and a leader in the vegetarian foods industry. In an interview, president Steve Demos said, "Our mission is to creatively lead the integration of healthy, natural, vegetarian foods into the average American diet. Our interest is in promoting the use of foods we consider the world better off with, rather than without."

One of the company's biggest success stories has been the introduction of its refrigerated soy milk called Silk (also available in chocolate and rice). These good-tasting beverages appeal to vegetarians as well as mainstream consumers who are looking for fresh, non-milk products for breakfast and cooking or baking.

Demos says the company's success has come from providing consumers with affordable, good-tasting, healthy products made from whole soybeans grown without the use of synthetic herbicides, pesticides, or chemical fertilizers. "We have always supported sustainable agriculture," Demos commented. "The future for White Wave and its products is based on our support of folks whom we consider to be the caretakers of whole, healthy foods—the farmers who are carefully, successfully managing sustainable agricultural systems. This is where we started, where we are, and where we are going."

In addition to White Wave's delicious beverages, I also use and recommend all of their other products, including Baked Tofu, Reduced Fat Tofu, Organic Hard-Style Tofu, Tempeh Burgers, Seitan, Dairyless Soy Yogurt, and White Wave Stir Fry. Look for White Wave's top quality products in the refrigerated section of your natural food store.

Q: What type of diet do you eat and recommend for optimum health?

A: For twenty-five years I have embraced a philosophy of living called Natural Hygiene. Harvey and Marilyn Diamond based their bestselling book, *Fit for Life*, on Natural Hygiene. Natural Hygiene teaches that the best way to achieve optimal health is right living—developing self-esteem and a positive attitude towards life; eating fresh, whole, natural foods; exercising regularly; getting plenty of rest, sleep, fresh air, and sunshine; learning to handle stress; and avoiding all negative influences of life.

Sounds like common sense doesn't it? It is. Natural Hygiene recommends a whole-food, plant-based diet of fresh uncooked fruits and vegetables, steamed vegetables, baked potatoes, squashes, raw unsalted nuts, and whole grains, designed to meet individual needs.

Natural Hygiene is unique in its contention that health is normal, as simple as living in harmony with Nature. Health and disease are a continuum—the same physiological laws govern the body in sickness and in health. Healing is a biological process, except in extraordinary circumstances, healing is the result of actions undertaken by the body on its own behalf. Natural Hygiene is for people who are looking for the good life, and not just a pretty good life, a *very* good life. Natural Hygiene offers you the opportunity to live the healthiest, happiest life possible. And you deserve the best!

For more information about Natural Hygiene, refer to the American Natural Hygiene Society in the Resource Directory. I encourage you to become a member. You'll receive a wealth of information that will enrich the quality of your life for a small annual fee. Members receive numerous benefits including a subscription to *Health Science*, the Society's award-winning magazine in which my articles are featured, discounts on seminars and books, and so much more. The Society's book, *The Natural Hygiene Handbook*, eloquently and cogently explains Natural Hygiene. It's also through their magazine that you'll learn about all the health conferences they offer each year. I participate at many of these conferences with lectures and workshops.

Q: Do you recommend dehydrated foods?

A: Dehydration is the oldest form of food preservation and the simplest. From ancient mariners on long voyages to wandering nomads, dried foods were essential. Dates, pears, nectarines, seeds, and herbs, when dried, were lightweight, full of nutrition, and could be preserved for extended periods of time. It was simple because only the sun was needed. But dried foods needed protection from birds, insects, cloudy days, and thieves. And it took time. Today, it's not only simple, but with your own Excalibur dehydrator, it's also easy. The machine does the work.

When purchasing a dehydrator, you want to keep the following six qualities in mind: good electrical design, adjustable thermostat, speed of drying, durability, easy-to-clean, and versatility. It is impossible to design a round unit that meets all of the above criteria: the electrical components will always be below the food being dried and clean-up is almost impossible in a round dehydrator. The dehydrator I recommend is the Excalibur because its design meets and exceeds the six qualities. It has a Parallexx Drying system, removable trays, a rear-mounted heating element to warm the air, an adjustable thermostat to control the temperature, and a fan to push the air horizontally over each tray.

The sky's the limit when you think about what you can dehydrate. Most fruits, vegetables, and herbs can be dried. Many grocery stores carry dried apricots, bananas, pineapple, peaches, pears, prunes, dates, garlic, onion, peppers, spices, and of course grapes (raisins), which are all very expensive. Excalibur owners enjoy an expanded list at a low cost, including such exotic fruits as papaya, mango, and kiwi fruit, and strawberries, tomatoes, and all sorts of vegetables.

I dehydrate many different fruits and vegetables. I even make fruit powders, powdered vegetables, and herb seasonings in my dehydrator. In fact, I dry combinations of different vegetables and herbs such as peppers, garlic, onions, celery, parsley, dill, thyme, basil, and tomato and then blend them together to make my own seasonings. Homemade, dehydrated foods make wonderful gifts for Christmas, birthdays, anniversaries, or for no reason at all. You'll put a smile on the face of a loved one when you give them with a basket of your own homemade dried papaya, mango, pineapple, apricot, strawberries, nectarines, and herb seasonings.

For more information or to order the Excalibur dehydrator, please refer to the Resource Directory.

Q: Both my husband and son have been diagnosed with attention deficit disorder (ADD). Their doctors said that the only thing that will help is to take the drug Ritalin. Are there natural things they can do?

A: Attention deficit disorder is typically a problem of an inability to concentrate on one task for any length of time. This leads to easy distraction, resulting in a tendency towards disruptive behavior and failure to complete assigned tasks. This can occur in individuals of any age. As children with attention deficit disorder get older, their behavior may not be as disruptive. However, they continue to have trouble concentrating for long periods of time and completing tasks in any organized or satisfactory way. As adults, while they may be highly intelligent and even well educated, they often have trouble holding jobs and earning a living. Typically, they move from one occupation to another, trying to find something that can hold their interest. The problem is not lack of interest, it is the inability to concentrate. Make sure your child has been correctly diagnosed. Studies reveal that fifty percent of children are misdiagnosed and don't have attention deficit disorder.

Dr. Ronald G. Cridland, MD, medical director of the Health Promotion Clinic in Rohnert Park, California, has discovered that his patients with ADD who follow the Natural Hygiene approach feel better than when they were taking medication. Although it may take time for their functioning to improve to a reasonable level, if they are patient—with careful testing, retraining, rest, relaxation, and sleep—many people can learn to function quite well without medication.

According to Dr. Cridland, there are factors that can make ADD worse. It was long thought that food additives and sugar can make children with ADD more hyperactive. A number of studies have refuted this hypothesis. However, his experience has shown that it is very valuable to put a child or adult with attention deficit disorder on a vegetarian diet derived from whole, natural foods, avoiding excess sugars and other stimulants, such as caffeine.

The most effective treatment for attention deficit disorder, says Dr. Cridland in the July/August 1997 issue of *Health Science* magazine, in addition to the appropriate training to utilize strengths to overcome weaknesses, is increased sleep. Nine or ten hours of good, deep sleep per night are usually required over a period of weeks or months, or even a year or two, to fully recover healthy neurological and emotional function. He emphasizes the necessity of slowing a child's or an adult's life down so that they don't have to push themselves quite so hard. Less sleep results in increased fatigue and a worsening of their problems. To get the sleep they need, it is essential that they slow down enough to be able to turn off the stimulation and allow themselves to experience their true energy level. For some humorous, insightful reading on the value of rest and sleep, check out book *The Art of Napping* by William A. Anthony, Ph.D. You'll never feel guilty again about napping after reading this marvelous book.

There is a place for Ritalin, says Dr. Cridland, since it enables a child to slow down and function with less disruptive behavior and more ability to complete tasks. This helps tremendously in reducing the stress on the child, their family, teachers, classmates, and others. Ritalin also can help adults to concentrate longer, enabling them to hold jobs and earn a living. But his first approach is the Natural Hygiene lifestyle and it works for many of his patients.

Q: There's a history of breast and other cancers as well as menstrual problems in my family. What can I do to have

control over my health destiny?

A: Conventional diets high in animal and dairy products provide excessive saturated fat that can increase the production of cholesterol and estrogens. Elevated estrogens can promote abnormal tissue growth. At the University of Toronto, 450 women with newly diagnosed ovarian cancer were compared with 540 demographically similar healthy women. Every ten grams of saturated fat per day increased the risk of ovarian cancer by twenty percent. Every ten grams of vegetable fiber, which can reduce the levels of cholesterol, lowered the risk by twenty percent.

In addition, a typical American diet deficient in fruits and vegetables and excessive in animal products and refined sugars can remarkably increase pathological inflammatory disturbances of normal menstrual function (painful breast tenderness and swelling, excessive bleeding, and clotting). By simply eliminating dairy and animal products and refined sugars, and eating the high-fiber, low-fat, plant-based Natural Hygiene diet, which emphasizes fruits, vegetables, whole grains, and legumes, you can significantly reduce painful menstrual responses and provide the best protection against tumor growth.

Moderate and consistent aerobic exercise also can reduce the risks associated with excess estrogens and cancer. At UCLA, 545 women under the age of forty with newly diagnosed breast cancer were compared to an equal number of disease-free women. Women who maintained three to four hours per week of aerobic exercise since menstruation had a fifty-eight percent reduction in the risk of breast cancer. Brisk walking for forty-five minutes, five times a week, can provide this level of training.

It is suggested that exercise can foster the metabolism and elimination of estrogens. Exercise also decreases the percentage of body fat and can decrease the presence of estrone, a potential tumor former and a form of estrogen produced by fat cells. It is important to realize that these effects of exercise can occur in women of all ages, even if they did not start an exercise regimen early in life. The exercise strategy mentioned above will provide major health benefits at any age, and it's never too late to start.

Q: I am very athletic, work out regularly and even compete. Is there any supplement you can recommend to enhance my performance and endurance?

A: There's an excellent supplement called Bio-Strath, which I've taken for almost twenty years. This herb supplement has been extensively tested on athletes, and it significantly enhanced their performance. The athletes were not only better able to perform, but better able to maintain a high-performance level without highs and lows. The athletes were more positive, their moods were better, and they were better able to handle strenuous exercise. Also, the results showed that the digestion and utilization of their diets were better.

One of the studies conducted with athletes was headed by S. Nuuttila (National Trainer for Finland) using seventy young athletes. The Bio-Strath-supplemented groups showed the following results:

- Better endurance during 12-minute runs.
- Improved concentration.
- A more stabilized performance record.
- Lessened negative feelings about forced tests.
- Improved sleep patterns.
- Improved bowel function.

It was concluded that chronic micronutrient deficiencies alleviated by the Bio-Strath supplementation improved athletic performance and attitudes of the athletes significantly. This is not to say, however, that only athletes should take this supplement. Anyone interested in better health would benefit.

Bio-Strath is a yeast and herb liquid with very special properties. The wild yeast strain is called Saccharomyces cerevisiae, which is a US-Pharmacological-accepted food yeast. The herbs are all wild, never cultivated, and are unsprayed. They are collected from fifteen countries to assure the finest sources available. The yeast is fermented in a slow process that takes two months. It is important to note that a yeast is as good as the media in which it is grown. The Strathmeyer yeast media (Dr. Strathmeyer started this wild yeast strain in 1948) has been developed and proven effective, and is a patented media. The assays show it to contain ten known B-vitamins, nineteen minerals, and eighteen amino acids. It's a completely natural food, free from chemicals. Additionally, this liquid, herbal yeast contains amylase, a starch-digesting enzyme; catalase, an antioxidant enzyme; pyruvate decarboxylase, an enzyme involved in glucose metabolism; and phosphatase, involved in respiration in the cells. Bio-Strath is also available in yeast-free drops. For more information, refer to Chapter Two on nutrition and the Resource Directory.

Q: Is there any way I can ensure that my brain stays healthy and alert as I age? My father has Alzheimer's disease and I want to take any steps necessary to preclude that from happening to me.

A: Fortunately, new studies are now corroborating what some scientists have long believed—that brain power in healthy people decreases very little with age. Some individuals are able to maintain alert, inquiring minds well into their nineties and beyond, says John Morris, MD, associate professor of neurology at Washington University in St. Louis.

Dr. Morris led a sixteen-year study of twenty-five people ages 71 to 95, comparing the brains of those with Alzheimer's disease to those who maintain mental clarity. His conclusion: If brain function becomes impaired, it's a result of disease, not age.

"By continuing to challenge the brain, anybody in reasonable health can improve function," says Gene Cohen, MD, director of the George Washington University Center on Aging, Health, and Humanities. "Just like your muscles, your mind needs to be exercised or atrophy will set in," adds David Morgan, MD, a specialist on neural degeneration at the University of South Florida College of Medicine.

Warner Schaie, professor of human development and psychology, and his colleagues at Penn State University have found educational levels to be less important than keeping the mind active. "Getting new experiences, reading new books, following current events," he says, "those are the best predictors about who is going to do well."

How healthy the brain stays depends to some extent (about thirty percent) on genetics. But, Cohen says, people "have enormous influence on how well they do."

Here are some tips to maintain brain power that were recommended in the 1996 April issue of the *AARP (American Association of Retired Persons) Bulletin.*

> Take care of physical health. Exercise and a low-fat, low-cholesterol diet can help keep the brain healthy. They also protect against high blood pressure, stroke, diabetes, and other illnesses that can deprive the brain of oxygen-enriched blood. Smoking and drinking immoderate amounts of alcohol, which can have a toxic effect on the brain, are to be avoided.

> Take control and reduce stress. The more you're in control of your life, the better your brain ages. Being in control helps relieve stress, which can stimulate certain disese-promoting hormones as

well as impair metabolism (the body's processing of sugar), to the detriment of brain function.

Socialize, stay involved, and keep your mind active. Activities like classes and volunteer work enhance social lives and mental dexterity. "Individuals who are at greatest risk," says Schaie, are those who retire and decide they don't have to think anymore. That's a mistake, because the way to have an active mind in the later years, he says, is "to think of education as a lifelong process."

All the people I know in their eighties or nineties who are mentally alert and exhibit impressive brain power often participate in doing crossword puzzles and/or Scrabble. That is good food for thought.

Finally, consider the following: herb and water intake. Recent scientific studies reveal that the centuries-old herb, Ginkgo Biloba, has proven effective in treating mild to severe dementia in the early stages of Alzheimer's disease. (See Ginkgo Biloba Plus in Resource Directory.)

In his thought-provoking, scientifically documented book, *Your Body's Many Cries for Water*, F. Batmanghelidj, MD writes, "In my opinion, brain cell dehydration is the primary cause of Alzheimer disease. Aluminum toxicity is a secondary complication of dehydration in areas of the world with comparatively aluminum-free water. In prolonged dehydration, the brain cells begin to shrink. Imagine a plum gradually turning into a prune. Unfortunately, in a dehydrated state, many functions of brain cells begin to get lost, such as the transport system that delivers neurotransmitters to nerve endings. One of my medical friends took this information to heart and started treating his brother who has Alzheimer's disease by forcing him to take more water every day. His brother has begun to recover his memory, so much so that he can now follow conversation and not frequently repeat himself. The improvement became noticeable in a matter of weeks." This book scientifically documents how the cause of many diseases and ailments can be traced back to chronic water dehydration. I highly recommend it.

Q: You often talk about your deep respect for the natural green world of plant-based medicine. What plants or herbs do you grow, use, or recommend?

A: In Ecclesiastics 34:4, we read, "The Lord hath created medicines out of the earth; and he that is wise will not abhor them." In a world where the damaging effects of food processing, over-medications, and agribusiness are more evident with each passing day, plants have come to stand as symbols of a more natural and healthy way of life. As described in the *Oxford English Dictionary*, all useful plants are herbs, as the term 'herb' is "applied to plants of which the leaves, or stems and leaves, are used for food or medicines, or in some way for their scent or flavor." All ancient human cultures had an understanding of 'green medicine' that was part of a life lived close to the natural world. One of the most extraordinary features of herbs is their incredible versatility. The magical biochemistry of herbs makes possible diverse properties. For example, an herb prized in cooking such as garlic, is also of value physiologically in lowering cholesterol, boosting the immune system and acting as a natural antibiotic. An herbal plant such as the elder can provide the raw material for wines, conserves, medicines, and dyes.

For more than twenty-five years, I have been studying the world of plants and herbalism and hold a deep respect for and intimacy with the natural world that characterizes plant-based medicine. Whether you live in a house or an apartment, you can grow herbs in your kitchen, patio, or garden. I grow a variety of plants (such as aloe) and herbs to use in my cooking, as medicine, or simply for their beauty. At your local health food store, you can find any number of herbal products available in a variety of different forms. Whenever possible, I choose herbal products and essential oils made by the company Frontier Natural Products Co-op. They are high-quality, organically-grown products from a company dedicated to social and environmental causes. I especially appreciate that their capsulated herbal products are from a vegetarian source. For more information about their products, please refer to the Resource Directory.

The aloe cactus, actually a desert succulent, has been touted as one of the 'miracle' green plants—and there is now good research to back many of the claims. The leaf gel and whole leaf juices are used for both internal and external healing.

The most common use of aloe vera is the application of its gel (the inside of the leaf) for burns, minor cuts, insect bites, skin irritations, and as a skin moisturizer. For more than two decades, I have been growing aloe vera plants in my yard and always have one plant available in my kitchen for quick use.

Recent research shows that the healing benefits people claim are well-founded, and can also be experienced with internal use. Aloe vera has been proven to promote rapid healing of burns, alleviate ulcers and protect the gastrointestinal lining, have strong anti-inflammatory properties, and have antiviral and mild pain-relieving properties. People also report other benefits, such as help in weight loss and chronic problems such as arthritis and irritable bowel.

The type of aloe vera used makes a big difference in whether you will receive the benefits. I enjoy Aloe Falls brand aloe juices because they are preservative-free, certified active, and even taste good (which is rare for aloe vera juices). The Aloe Falls plants are grown without herbicides or pesticides, and they produce the only aloe vera juices I have seen without preservatives (see Aloe Falls in the Resource Directory).

Q: Who are your greatest teachers or mentors?

A: Six people have made a profound, positive effect in my life. Jesus and Paramahansa Yogananda have both shown me the importance of practicing love and forgiveness, and living as a spiritual being having a human experience. My highest goal in life is to constantly live in the presence of God and to be a clear vessel to do God's will for me. I turn to their words often for inspiration. I also encourage everyone to get the Self-Realization Fellowship home study lessons of Paramahansa Yogananda for daily inspiration and motivation (see Resource Directory).

My mom, June, has also been a tremendous inspiration to me in how she lives her life with joy, enthusiasm, perseverance, and love for everything and everyone. She has a heart of gold and always instilled in me the values of high thinking, living my vision, never giving up, and following my heart. She's been a wonderful blessing in my life. My grandmother Fritzie, I would also add to this list. In many ways, she reminded me of Peace Pilgrim. She was peaceful, happy, independent and self-reliant, traveled the world, ate healthy foods, and led a simple life. By her example and loving words, she helped orchestrate my life and is still navigating with me. I feel her presence often.

Peace Pilgrim has been a great source of inspiration. Peace Pilgrim was a walking, breathing example of living peacefully. For more than twenty-eight years, she traveled the length of North America, all fifty states, the ten provinces of Canada, and parts of Mexico, sharing her thoughts about peace. Her journey was on foot, never asking for anything: food, shelter, or transportation. She walked without a penny in her pocket. All she had were the clothes she wore (pants, shirt, tennis shoes, and a short, sleeveless tunic lettered boldly on the front "Peace Pilgrim"). Her motto was as simple as her life: "This is the way of peace: overcome evil with good, and falsehood with truth, and hatred with love." There was only one thing that could inspire and support a journey of this extent and provide the strength to see it through for all those years, and that is absolute, uncompromising faith in herself and in God. It's that kind of faith I aspire to daily.

On peace, she said: "When you find peace within yourself, you become the kind of person who can live at peace with others. Inner peace is not found by staying on the surface of life, or by attempting to escape from life through any means. Inner peace is found by facing life squarely, solving its problems, and delving as far beneath its surface as possible to discover its verities and realities." (For a free book or video documentary on Peace Pilgrim, her life and philosophy, see Resource Directory.)

Finally, there's Lynn Carroll, who's the most positive and youngest eighty-something person I've ever known. She's truly an angel in human form, like my Mom, and always encourages me to look at the bigger picture and trust that Divine Love is guiding me to my highest good every step of the way, no matter what appearances are telling me. One of my most valuable life lessons I learned from Lynn has to do with the power of tithing. She helped me understand that you stay in the vibration of prosperity and abundance by giving, just as you stay in the vibration of love by loving. What you give, you received back multiplied. By the way she lives, Lynn is a shining example of the blessings of living a life rooted in the Divine.

Q: How do your feelings affect your health?

A: Letting your feelings out supports health and expresses love for yourself. Covered-up feelings cause disease. Covering up feelings is another form of lying. And like lying, we do it to protect someone we love or to protect ourselves. Warning: Covering up feelings or not being true to your feelings can be harmful to your health.

If we examine the word disease, we see that it is composed is DIS and EASE. When we are not at ease, we get disease. We are all exposed to the same viruses and germs, but the people who get sick are usually those who are under a great deal of stress.

In *Love, Medicine and Miracles,* Dr. Bernie Siegel cites the work of Dr. Caroline Bendel Thomas of Johns Hopkins University Medical School, who did a personality profile of 1,337 medical students and surveyed their health every decade throughout their adult lives. She was surprised to find that almost all of those who developed cancer "had throughout their lives been restricted in expressing emotion, especially aggressive emotions related to their own needs." According to Siegel, in order for cancer patients to get well, they need to see "how the needs of others, seen as the only ones that count, are used to cover up one's own." He goes on to say that for healing to occur, our outer choices have to match our inner desires, so that the energy that was used for these contradictions can now be used for healing.

Q: When asking questions and making important choices in daily living, how do you know if your answer is your inner guidance or merely your ego-guidance?

A: To know how to choose correctly in any given situation, we need to guide our judgments by the power of intuition. We are all endowed with this sixth sense, but most people don't use it and instead use their other five senses. These senses usually interpret things according to their own likes and dislikes rather than according to what is true and ultimately beneficial for the soul.

In learning to make right decisions, the most important thing you can do is make meditation a regular part of your daily life. In the Bible we read, "Be still and know that I am God." Few understand, says Sri Daya Mata, what that really means: the more still you become, the more you tune in with the omnipresence of God. When a question arises like, "Is this the right thing to do?" you can stand back and impartially ask yourself, "Is this something I want or is this something God wants for me?" When you have felt peace in meditation, then you will recognize that same peace which is the intuitive indicator of divine inner guidance. She recommends that you say to God, "Lord, guide me." Keep on saying it, deeply and sincerely throughout the day. Continually think of God and say: "Guide me, bless me." That keeps your mind receptive and open to inspiration, the silent guidance of God.

Yogananda said that "intuition is perceived mostly through the heart." I have found this to be true in my life. When something is not right, I get feelings and an energy change in my heart. There is an uneasiness that makes me think, "Oh, there is something wrong with that individual or with that situation." It does not make me uncomfortable, but I am conscious of a little disturbance in my heart. This is what Yogananda referred to when he said: "Whenever you are concerned about something, or trying to find the right course to pursue, calmly concentrate on the heart. Don't try to analyze the problem; just remain watching the heart...Remain calm, and then suddenly a great feeling will come over you and your intuition will point you to the right step you should take at that time. If your mind and emotions are calm and attuned to the voice of intuition within, you will be rightly guided. In your everyday life, you will meet the right people who will bring some solution to your problems, or who will help you in some way—or through their contact and counsel, you will find the right way."

Here is the great truth I encourage you to put into practice. If you persist, you will learn to recognize and be led by the 'still small voice' within. However, it doesn't happen overnight. "Through your persistent prayers for guidance and your calm receptivity," says Yogananda, "an inner sense will prompt you as to the best way to proceed. When that happens, go forward with full faith; but all the while remain flexible." Yogananda recommends to affirm: "It seems to me that this is the right way to go. But if at any time, Lord, You show me that I have made the wrong choice, I can step back; I can accept correction."

Q: Would you summarize the most important life lessons you've learned that have made the most profound difference in your life?

A: For simplicity, I'll list these in no particular order.

- Never look to another person to make you happy or believe you are responsible for the happiness of another. God is your Source and the Source of everyone you know. God knows what's best for everyone, not you. When someone really loves you, they want you to be happy. You are always in a relationship with yourself, especially in the presence of another.
- Believe in yourself, take loving care of yourself, value and respect yourself. All of your relationships are a reflection of how you're loving and honoring yourself or not loving and honoring yourself. When you come from self-love, you won't settle for less than you deserve and desire and you'll make choices that support your happiness.
- Always tell the truth—to yourself and others. That's a sign of high self-respect and self-esteem. Everyone close to you deserves to experience your honesty. Withholding your truth and feelings and lying darkens your soul and fosters deceit, leading to unhappiness for everyone involved.
- Live more from inner guidance and with faith. Stand back and let your life unfold as it was meant to be. If you stay centered, faith will find you. Sometimes you need to jump off the bridge and build your wings on the way down. Trust that unscheduled

events of your life are your own personal form of spiritual direction. In all circumstances, be grateful.

- Life is a learning experience. Pay attention. Live in the present moment. *Carpe diem*: seize the day. Spend as much time as possible in nature. That's why I hike so much. Whatever problems I think I have when I start the hike dissolve before the hike is over. You can more easily find yourself, connect with your soul, and feel the whisperings of your heart and Spirit when you spend time alone out in nature.

- Make no judgments. By letting go of the need to know why things happen as they do, you reach a state of tranquillity.

- Fear and the need to control keep you spiritually toxic. Move from fear to trust. Let go and let God guide your life instead of you believing you know what's best for you and everyone else.

- The strongest poison to the human spirit is the inability to forgive oneself or another person. Choose to practice forgiveness.

- The only path toward spiritual consciousness is through the heart. That truth is not negotiable, no matter what spiritual tradition one chooses as a means to know the Divine. If you're not happy, peaceful, fulfilled, and joyful, then you simply need to choose again because you haven't been following your heart.

- Pray every day. Meditate every day. Laugh every day. Spend an hour every day with someone you love. Fill your life with purpose and let God take charge. Make God and your spiritual life your number one priority and everything you need for your highest good will be provided.

APPENDIX

Resource Directory

Aloe Falls, Yerba Prima, Inc., 740 Jefferson Avenue, Ashland, OR 97520-3743

Aloe Falls by Yerba Prima is preservative-free, great tasting, and Certified Active, which means that Aloe Falls is laboratory verified to provide the health benefits of aloe. Found in your health food store, their Aloe Juice Formula contains fifty-percent aloe vera and a powerful herbal blend of peppermint, chamomile, and parsley to boost its soothing properties in your digestive system. They also have Hawaiian Ginger Aloe, 100 percent Whole Leaf Aloe, and light and refreshing tea and juice beverages. Write for more information.

American Natural Hygiene Society, *Health Science* magazine, James M. Lennon, PO Box 30630, Tampa, FL 33630 (813) 855-6607. Internet Web Site: http://www.anhs.org.

This wonderful organization publishes the award-winning *Health Science* magazine. Annual membership dues are $25, which includes a subscription to *Health Science*, to which I contribute articles regularly. Members also receive discounts on health books, videos, cassette programs, seminars, lectures, and more. I encourage you to write and become a member. Write or call for more information or to order.

Bionic Products, 466 Central Avenue, Suite 20, Northfield, IL 60093 (847) 441-6000, (800) 634-4667

Bionic Products markets the Elanra Therapeutic Ionizer. Elanra delivers small, ingestable negative ions essential for proper ion balance. Write or call for more information.

Bio-Strath, Nature's Answer Inc., 320 Oscar Avenue, Hauppage, NY 11788, (800) 439-2324, (516) 231-7492

Bio-Strath is an excellent liquid herbal food supplement. It's based on plasmolysed yeast and wild herbs and has been available for decades in over forty countries around the world—a result of accurate, scientifically-based work. I've included Bio-Strath in my health program for over two decades and highly recommend it. It has been found to combat fatigue, lethargy, and nervousness, and increase physical and mental efficiency, reinforce the immune defense system, and restore vitality. It's available in health food stores or call for more information.

BodySlant & Body Lift, PO Box 1667, Newport Beach, CA 92663 (800) 443-3917

The BodySlant is a superb slant board that also functions as a bed and ottoman. I recommend using it daily. The Body Lift is a simple and comfortable way to stand your body upside down so that your shoulders rest on a thick cushion, your head dangles off the floor, and your neck stretches naturally. I use the BodySlant and Body Lift daily and highly recommend them for better health, vitality, and rejuvenation. Write or call for more information or to order.

Cassettes by Dr. Susan Smith Jones

Celebrate Life! Audiocassette series by Susan Smith Jones, Ph.D. Includes seven tapes, fourteen different programs, and six guided meditations.

> 1A. The Main Ingredients: Positive Thinking and the Mind
> 1B. The Main Ingredients: Exercise, Nutrition, and Relaxation
> 2A. Get High on Life Through Exercise
> 2B. Make Your Exercise Program a Great Adventure
> 3A. Nutrition for Aliveness
> 3B. Superlative Dining
> 4A. Your Thoughts May Be Fattening
> 4B. Living Lightly, Naturally Trim
> 5A. Experience Aliveness
> 5B. Learn From Children How To Celebrate Life
> 6A. The Joy of Solitude and the Art of Serenity
> 6B. Relaxation and Meditation: Natural and Easy
> 7A. Celebrate Your Magnificence
> 7B. Affirm a Beautiful Life

Order the seven tape album for $80 or $15 per tape. Make check (US check or money order only) payable to: Health Unlimited, PO Box 49396, Los Angeles, CA 90049. For more information on the tapes, send a business size, stamped, self-addressed envelope to the above address. For credit card orders, call (800) 843-5743 (PST).

> Learn To Live A Balanced Life
> A Fresh Start: Rejuvenate Your Body
> Making Your Life a Great Adventure

The three two-tape programs above were recorded live from Susan's popular motivational workshops. Together all three make a complete program designed to show you how to live an empowered, balanced life and how to tie the physical, mental, emotional, and spiritual aspects of life together to create a holistic approach to successful living.

Order all three for $60 or $25 for each program. Make checks (US check or money order) payable to: Health Unlimited, PO Box 49396, Los Angeles, CA 90049 or call (800) 843-5743 (PST).

> How To Achieve Any Goal: The Magic of Creative Visualization—
> Living Your Vision/Commitment

A ninety-minute audiocassette by Susan Smith Jones. Includes a twenty-minute meditation you can use every day to help you realize your goals and dreams. To order, please send $15 (US check or money order only) payable to: Health Unlimited, PO Box 49396, Los Angeles, CA 90049 or call (800) 843-5743 (PST).

> Wired to Meditate: Using Meditation, Intuition, Visualization, Affirmations, and Deep Breathing to Enrich Your Life and Connect with Your Divine Source

Susan Smith Jones' *Wired to Meditate* has been recorded in a two-hour, two-tape program. This is a perfect introduction to meditation for those who are too busy to read. The program explores the fascinating relationship between the mind and the body and demystifies the process by providing practical advice on how to use meditation, deep relaxation techniques, visualization, and positive thoughts and actions to enhance your life. To order, please send $25 (US check or money order only) payable to: Health Unlimited, PO Box 49396, Los Angeles, CA 90049 or call (800) 843-5743 (PST).

Center for Conservative Therapy, Inc., 4310 Lichau Road, Penngrove, CA 94951 (707) 792-2325

This residential treatment center was co-founded by Dr. Alan Goldhamer and Dr. Jennifer Marano. The center offers an alternative approach to the restoration and maintenance of optimum health. Based

Resource Directory

on the Natural Hygiene philosophy, their focus is on helping people make diet and lifestyle changes and in certified supervising fasting. Write or call for more information.

DeSouza Chlorophyll Products, PO Box 395, Department SJ, Beaumont, CA 92220 (800) 373-5171

DeSouza's liquid chlorophyll (also in tablets and capsules) and other personal care products are very beneficial for enhancing health. I highly recommend their entire line of products. Write or call for more information or to order.

Diamond Organics, Freedom, CA (888) 674-2642

Diamond Organics offers a unique selection of all-organically grown produce including specialty greens and lettuces, Mesclun European salad greens, fresh herbs, root vegetables, seasonal fruits and flowers. No order is too small. Gift certificates in any amount are available. Their catalog even offers menu ideas and delicious recipes. Call for more information or to order. I like giving their Samplers as gifts.

EarthSave International, 600 Distillery Commons, Suite 200, Louisville, KY 40206, (502) 589-7676, (800) 362-3648

Founded by John Robbins, author of *Diet for a New America* and *May All Be Fed*, EarthSave is a nonprofit organization providing education and leadership for transition to more healthful and environmentally sound food choices, nonpolluting energy supplies and a wiser use of natural resources. Write for their catalog of books, audio and videotapes, and other products.

Ester-C Vitamin C, Inter-Cal Corporation, 533 Madison Avenue, Prescott, AZ 86301 (520) 445-8063

Inter-Cal is the manufacturer of Ester-C calcium ascorbate. Ester-C is formulated in a wide variety of nutritional supplements by many different distributors and can be found on the shelves of health food stores, drugstores, and supermarkets. Look for labels with the Ester-C logo (a small "e" enclosed in a big "C"). Write or call for more information or to order.

Excalibur Dehydrator, 6083 Power Inn Road, Sacramento, CA 95824 (800) 875-4254

The top quality Excalibur Dehydrator is an easy way to make your own dried fruits, vegetables, fruit rolls, herb seasonings, powdered vegetables, crackers, trail mix, and energy bars. The Excalibur offers the Parallexx Drying System, which means it has a heating element to warm the air, an adjustable thermostat to control the temperature, and a fan to push the air horizontally over each tray. It's also very easy to clean. I recommend this dehydrator for everyone. It's an important part of my health regimen. To receive a twenty-page color catalog full of recipes and helpful hints on dehydrating or to order, please write or call the number above.

Fortified Flax, Omega-Life, Inc. PO Box 208, Brookfield, WI 53008-0208 (414) 786-2070, (800) 328-3529

Fortified Flax is one of the best sources of Omega-3 fatty acids, along with soluble and insoluble fiber, plus a great source of lignins. This brand is fortified with the proper vitamins and minerals to help the essential fatty acids in flax metabolize properly, as well as keep the ground seed fresh. Write or call for more information or to order.

Frontier Natural Products Co-op, 3021 78th Street, PO Box 299, Norway, IA 52318, (800) 669-3275. Internet Web site: http://www.frontiercoop.com.

As I recommend at the end of Chapter Five on chlorophyll and greens, Frontier makes top-quality, certified organically-grown herbal products and essential oils that are available in natural food stores. I especially appreciate that their capsules are from a vegetarian source. Write or call for more information on their products, a catalog, or to order.

Green Foods Corporation, 320 N. Graves Avenue, Oxnard, CA 93030, (800) 777-4430, ext. 13

This excellent company offers a top quality line of barley grass juice products that are sold at health food stores and nutrition centers. Some of their products include Green Magma, Veggie Magma, Magma Plus, Barley Dog, and Barley Cat. Green barley juice is a perfect balance of vitamins, minerals, enzymes, protein and chlorophyll. This company's barley juice products are the best on the market. They are organically grown, and the company takes the utmost care in transferring live essential nutrients to an easy-to-use, convenient form that is easily and quickly assimilated by our system. I highly recommend all their products. Write or call for more information or to order.

HealthForce Regeneration Systems, 16921-C Via de Santa Fe, Box 5005, Rancho Santa Fe, CA 92067-5005, Information: (619) 756-5292. Orders only: (800) 357-2717. Internet Web Site: http://www.healthforce.net.

Owned and operated by Jamey Dina, ND and Kim Sproul, ND, HealthForce Regeneration Systems offers a wide variety of holistic products, including their wonderful all living foods, totally vegetarian recipe book titled *Uncooking with Jamey & Kim*. It contains over 100 unique recipes including dips, dressings, soups, crackers, veggie burgers, puddings, pies, nut milkshakes, and even pizza and candy bars! They also offer a large assortment of healthful food preparation equipment and other products including juicers, dehydrators, Vita-Mix Nutrition Center, air purifiers, whole food supplements (superfood alternatives to conventional isolates/synthetics), and more. HealthForce goes the extra distance to ensure that people get the best in terms of quality products and value. Their prices are excellent and they ship anywhere. Write or call for a catalog or visit their web site.

Health Mate, 7175 Orangethorpe Avenue, Buena Park, CA 90621-3309, (800) 946-6001

As I wrote in Chapter Eight on taking saunas, this practice has been an important part of my health program for more than twenty years. Health Mate Sauna makes a unique, top quality, portable sauna for home or office. It's excellent for weight control, skin cleansing, pain relief, stress reduction, stiff joints, and cardiovascular fitness. I highly recommend that you call for more information or to order. An investment in your health is the best investment you can make.

JMS Steam Cooker, JMS Estheshape, Inc., PO Box 171654, Miami, FL 33017, (305) 362-0411

The JMS Steam Cooker is a top quality stainless steel, three-piece steam cooker. Steam cooking preserves vital nutritional elements in foods, such as vitamins, trace elements, proteins, and mineral salts. This beautiful, large steam cooker can play a major role in preventing disease and promoting radiant health. It is not available in stores. Write or call for more information.

Juice Plus+, North County Healing Arts Center, 1054 2nd Street, Suite 1, Encinitas, CA 92024 (800) 530-9963

Juice Plus+ is a live food concentrate of pesticide-free fruits and vegetables that have been picked ripe and juiced—with the water and sugars extracted—and the remaining powder encapsulated. Each capsule contains many vitamins and minerals, antioxidants, fiber, enzymes, and phytonutrients—all the things nature gives us in seventeen raw fruits and vegetables! This whole food supplement has been tested in major bio-availability studies and findings are very impressive. This is not a processed, fragmented vitamin-mineral pill nor is it an extraction. Juice Plus+ combines the latest advances in nutritional science and food processing technology to give you added daily nutrition from fresh, raw fruits and vegetables in an easy-to-use capsule or chewable form for adults and children! I take and highly recommend this product. It's not available in health food stores. Write or call for free literature, cassette tape, or to purchase.

Keys Fitness Products, 11220 Petal Street, Dallas, TX 75238, (888) 340-0482

Keys Fitness offers a variety of top-quality, award-winning treadmills for your home or office. Their treadmills are made in the USA and utilize an assortment of useful functions and features including easy-to-use push button electronics, window display, a variety of user-friendly programs, and speeds ranging from 0 to 15 mph with a power incline of 0 to 12 percent, and a high efficiency five horsepower motor. Using a treadmill is one of the easiest and safest ways to get an aerobic workout and help promote radiant health. I use and recommend their treadmills. Call or write for a catalog or more information.

Kyolic Aged Garlic Extract, and **Gingko Biloba Plus**, Wakunaga of America Co., Ltd., 23501 Madero, Mission Viejo, CA 92691, (800) 825-7888

As I wrote in Chaper Two, these are excellent nutritional supplements available in your health food store. I've taken Kyolic for twenty years because of its efficiency in promoting optimum health and well-being. Write or call for more information or free samples of these products.

LivingArts, 2434 Main Street, Santa Monica, CA 90405, (800) 722-9347

LivingArts is recognized as a premier resource for audio and video media that support the lifestyle changes people seek today to experience new levels of mental, physical and spiritual fitness. They have an extensive catalog showing their award-winning audio and video titles as well as other health items such as books, fitness and yoga clothing, and other products to help you live a more healthful lifestyle. Write or call for their catalog.

Mori-Nu Silken "Lite" Tofu, Morinaga, 2050 West 190th Street, Suite 110, Torrance, CA 90504

This is a very healthy source of low-fat protein and an excellent health food. For more information and delicious recipes, send a self-addressed stamped envelope.

Mountain Valley Growers, 38325 Pepperweed Road, Squaw Valley, CA 93675, (209) 338-2775

Since its inception in 1983, Mountain Valley Growers has been testing new herb varieties so only the most flavorful and prolific plants will make it to the customer. Over 400 varieties of organically grown plants can be shipped anywhere in the US. Write or call for more information and a catalog.

North County Healing Arts Center, 1054 2nd Street, Suite #1, Encinitas, CA 92024 (760) 634-0840

Paulette Suzanne, BA, NC, is Director of the North County Healing Arts Center and Founder of Whole Person Health Services in Encinitas, California. Paulette is a Certified Nutritionist, Iridologist, Rebirther, Flower Remedy Practitioner, and Body Electronics Practitioner with twenty years experience in private practice. Write or call for more information or an appointment at the above number.

Omron Healthcare, Inc., 300 Lakeview Parkway, Vernon Hills, IL 60061, (800) 634-4350. Internet Web address: http://www.omron.com.ohi

As I mentioned in Chapter Three on creating a fit, lean body, I use and recommend the Omron Body Logic Model HBF-301. Omron's Body Logic is a hand-held bio-impedance body fat analyzer. Just set your height, weight, age, and sex, grip the silver electrode handles and press start. Within seconds, body fat percentage and the weight of your body's fat are displayed on the clear digital panel. Write or call for more information or to order.

Peace Pilgrim, Friends of Peace Pilgrim, 43480 Cedar Avenue, Hemet, CA 92544, (909) 927-7678

To receive a free thirty-two page booklet, *Steps Toward Inner Peace*, a free 216-page book, *Peace Pilgrim*, a free marvelous video documentary titled "The Spirit of Peace" or an inspiring newsletter, write to the above address. Friends of Peace Pilgrim is a nonprofit, tax-exempt, all-volunteer organization.

Physicians Committee For Responsible Medicine, 5100 Wisconsin Avenue, NW, Suite 404, Washington, DC 20016, (202) 686-2210

Become a member of PCRM and keep up with nutritional developments through their twenty-four-page quarterly magazine, *Good Medicine*. PCRM consists of approximately 3,400 physicians and 60,000 laypersons. They are a non-profit educational organization promoting nutrition, preventive medicine, ethics in human research, medical care for disenfranchised groups, and alternatives to animal experimentation. Basic membership is $20 a year. Write or call for more information or to order.

PMRI Residential Retreats, 900 Bridgeway, Suite One, Sausalito, CA 94965 (800) 775-7674, ext. 221

PMRI stands for Preventive Medicine Research Institute. This non-profit public institute offers Dr. Dean Ornish's week-long residential retreats to teach comprehensive lifestyle changes to individuals. Dr. Ornish attends each of the retreats giving lectures and answering questions about his program. Gourmet low-fat, low-cholesterol meals and cooking instruction are also provided.

PowerBar, PowerFood, Inc., 2150 Shattuck Avenue, Berkeley, CA 94704, (800) 587-6937. Internet Web Site: http://www.powerbar.com.

The PowerBar Performance is a delicious sustained-energy bar for endurance athletes and active people. It's also low in fat. PowerBar Harvest captures the goodness of whole grains, chunks of real fruit, and natural sweeteners, yet is low-fat and contain no artificial colors or flavors. My favorite flavors are Strawberry, Apple Crisp, and Cherry Crunch. PowerBars are moist and crunchy and available in health food and fitness stores and some supermarkets. Write for more information or to order, or visit their web site.

Premier One Products, Inc., 1500 Kearns Boulevard, Park City, UT 84060, (800) 373-9660

Premier One provides top-quality honeybee products in their raw, whole state. They have a variety of products—including Raw Energy and BeeVive—for energy and rejuvenation. Write or call for more information and a catalog.

Self-Realization Fellowship, 3880 San Rafael Avenue, Los Angeles, CA 90065, (213) 225-2471

Write for more information on Paramahansa Yogananda, his books, meditation, home study lessons, the locations of the Self-Realization Fellowship centers, or a catalog of their books, tapes, quarterly magazine, and other products.

Spectrum Naturals, Inc., 133 Copeland Street, Petaluma, CA 94952, (800) 995-2705

Producers of Veg Omega-3 Organic Flax Seed Oil, Spectrum Spread, Wheat Germ Oil, natural vegetable oils, pure pressed without chemicals, and a variety of natural, delicious condiments. Write for their information and consumer education series on healthy oils.

Sun Chlorella, Sun Wellness, Inc., 4025 Spencer Street, Torrance, CA 90503-2417, (800) 829-2828. Internet Web site: http://www.superhealth.com.

Sun Chlorella and Sun Siberian Ginseng are excellent products I take to promote radiant health. As I wrote in Chapter Five on chlorophyll and greens, chlorella is a nutrient-dense, natural super-food noted for its ability to detoxify pollutants. Studies reveal chlorella's efficiency in treating hypertension, diabetes, hypoglycemia, asthma, constipation, and elevated cholesterol levels. Recent research also indicates that substances in chlorella stimulate the natural immune system to protect the body against cancer. Sun Wellness produces the best chlorella on the market because it's the only one that is truly digestible, which means your body can assimilate it more easily, insuring that you get more of the essential nutrients from the chlorella. Call or write for a free sample and magazine on Sun Chlorella.

SunSmile Fruit and Vegetable Rinse, Sunrider International, 1625 Abalone Avenue, Torrance, CA 90501, (301) 781-3808

Sunrider's SunSmile Fruit and Vegetable Rinse is an all-natural rinse which cleanses fruits, vegetables, and even counter tops and cutting boards from bacteria, waxy coatings, pesticides, fungus, and parasites and their eggs. This rinse maintains the natural brilliant colors of produce, eliminates offensive odors, and prevents premature dehydration of fruits and vegetables. SunSmile Fruit and Vegetable Rinse is highly concentrated, and free of animal by-products or animal testing. This rinse is a must for any commercially-grown or imported produce.

Trace-Lyte, Nature's Path, Inc., PO Box 7862, Venice, FL 34287 (800) 326-5772, Fax (941) 426-6871

Nature's Path manufactures a top quality crystalloid electrolyte formula, Trace-Lyte, which I take and recommend. It took over thirty years to develop Trace-Lyte and takes approximately one week to make. The liquid is tasteless, colorless, and odorless. You simply put a few drops in your water or juice. This liquid promotes homeostasis in the body. Nature's Path manufactures a number of other quality products that synergistically combine with electrolytes. Write or call for more information or to order Trace-Lyte or their other excellent products.

Tree of Life Seminars and Rejuvenation Center, 171 N. 3rd Avenue, PO Box 1080, Patagonia, AZ 85634, (520) 394-2520

Tree of Life is a metaphor for a way of being in the world that supports one's own spiritual evolution in an integrated, balanced, and harmonious way. A variety of seminars and rejuvenation retreats are conducted by Nora and Gabriel Cousens, MD. Write or call for a brochure.

Unity Village and Retreat Center, 1901 NW Blue Parkway, Unity Village, MO 64065-0001, (816) 524-3550

Unity Village offers wonderful retreats ranging from one day to two weeks to rejuvenate body, mind, and spirit. *The Daily Word* is published monthly by Unity School of Christianity, Unity Village. The subscription price is only $6.95 a year and offers a daily inspiration message and affirmation you'll think was written just for you. For more than twenty years, I've started my day with *The Daily Word*. Write or call for more information. I have also often relied on their Silent Unity, where twenty-four hours a day, 365 days a year, you can call and someone will pray with you. There is no charge and all prayer requests are treated with reverence. The Silent Unity telephone number is (816) 969-2000.

Vita-Mix Total Nutrition Center and Neova, Vita-Mix Corporation, 8615 Usher Road, Cleveland, OH 44138, (800) 848-2649

For seventy years the Vita-Mix Corporation has been dedicated to improving lives with quality products. Substituting devitalized, packaged food with health-building, whole food nutrition is fast and convenient with the Vita-Mix Total Nutrition Center. Turn fruits and vegetables into whole food juices in less than four minutes. Freeze a half gallon of all-fruit ice cream in less than sixty seconds. Grind whole wheat into flour for bread or pancake batter in seconds. The machine performs thirty-five processes in all. The Vita-Mix TNC delivers to your body the balanced nutrition found only in whole foods, which ultimately can improve the way you look and feel. I've used my Vita-Mix for over twenty years and consider it an essential part of my health regimen. Neova is a top quality, stainless steel cookware that I use and highly recommend. Please mention this book when writing or calling for more information or to order.

White Wave Inc. 1990 N. 57th Court, Boulder, CO 80301, (303) 443-3470. Internet Web Site: http://www.whitewave.com.

White Wave is one of the top producers of tofu and the largest producer of tempeh in North America. An innovator in the vegetarian foods market, this high-integrity company offers a variety of healthy, delicious foods including reduced fat and baked tofu, seitan, dairyless soy yogurt, and beverages. One of my favorite products is their soy beverage called Silk™. It's a delicious lactose free, low-fat, refrigerated soy milk made from soybeans that appeals to vegetarians as well as mainstream consumers who are looking for a fresh, non-milk product for their breakfast cereal and cooking or baking. Silk is available in chocolate (soy) and rice. White Wave products are available in the refrigerator section of your natural foods store. Write or call for more information and free recipes, or refer to their web site.

Workshops, Lectures, Seminars, Retreats, Keynote Addresses by Susan Smith Jones, Ph.D., contact Universal Speaker's Bureau, (800) 644-4144, or write Health Unlimited, PO Box 49215, Los Angeles, CA 90049, Attn: Director

If you would like to schedule Dr. Susan Smith Jones to give a motivational presentation to your corporation, community, church, or school group, call the above number or write to Health Unlimited.

ABOUT THE AUTHOR

Susan Smith Jones is a leading voice for health, fitness, and peaceful living in America today. She not only teaches wellness, she lives it. In 1985, Susan was selected as one of ten "Healthy American Fitness Leaders" by The President's Council on Physical Fitness and Sports, and in 1988, the President's Council designated Susan as National Master in weight training.

Susan's credentials include a doctorate in health sciences, a master's degree in kinesiology, a bachelor's degree in psychology, and a teaching credential. She has been a fitness instructor to students, staff, and faculty at UCLA for over 25 years. She is probably best known as an advocate of healthy, peaceful living and positive thinking. She is the author of ten books, appears regularly on radio and television talk shows, and has written more than 500 magazine articles with her picture on several covers.

Susan also travels internationally as a health and fitness consultant and motivational speaker for community, corporate, and church groups. Her inspiring keynote presentations and workshops are often scheduled one to two years in advance. As a health and fitness trainer and coach, she develops personalized wellness programs for individuals, families, and specialized groups.

Susan is founder and president of Health Unlimited, a Los Angeles-based consulting firm dedicated to the advancement of human potential, health education, and peaceful living. She has acquired the nickname of "Sunny" and lives in Brentwood, Los Angeles.

If you would like to schedule Dr. Susan Smith Jones to give a motivational presentation on a variety of topics to your corporation, business, or community group, please call Universal Speaker's Bureau at (800) 644-4144.

Index

A

Abdominal exercises, 128–131
Acceptance, 162–164
Acupressure, 146–147
ADD, 278–279
Adrenaline, 121
Adversity
   reactions to, 183–184, 196
   turning to advantage, 234–235
Aerobic exercise, 52–53, 124. *See also* Exercise
Affirmations, 177–178, 184, 218–219
Aging
   Alzheimer's disease and, 39, 282–283
   brain power and, 282
   enzymes and, 31
   garlic and, 39
   undernutrition and, 56
   vitamin C requirement and, 37
Airola, Paavo, 136
Alcohol
   effect of, on brain, 282
   effect of, on metabolism, 61
Alfalfa sprouts, 59, 113
Aliveness Program, 51–67
Allen, James, 1, 9
Almond milk, 22
Aloe Falls, 285, 290
Aloe vera, 284–285
Alpha-linolenic acid. *See* LNA
Aluminum toxicity, 283
Alzheimer's disease, 39, 282–283
American Heart Association, 20, 46
American Natural Hygiene Society, 277, 290
Amylase, 30–31

Anderson, Bob, 132
Anger, 3, 8
Animals
   experiencing and embracing life, 163
   protein from, 18–22
Anorexia, 45
Anthony, William A., 279
Antioxidants, 33–35, 76, 80, 107
Aphrodisiacs, 89, 124
Apples, 107, 112, 113–114, 119
Arachidonic acid, 89
Arthritis, 118
Arugula, 103
Ascorbate supplements, 36–38
Asparagus, 114, 118
Astragalus, 39–40
Athletes
   flax seed oil consumption by, 90
   massage and, 142–145
   supplements for, 280–281
   sweating and, 138
Athlete's foot, 98
Attention deficit disorder (ADD), 278–279
Attwood, Charles, 25
Audiocassettes, 215, 291–292

B

Bach, Richard, 185
Back pain, 274
Bailey, Covert, 120
Baking, 80
Bandy, William D., 132
Barley Cat, 34, 294
Barley Dog, 34, 294
Barley grass, 34
Barnard, Neal, 25

Batmanghelidj, F., 62, 283
Beet greens, 104
Beets, 113, 114
Belgian endive, 104
Benson, Herbert, 9, 207
Berge, Geir, 37
Berries, 114
Beta-carotene, 33, 118
bGH. *See* Bovine growth hormone
Bienenfeld, Joel, 144
Bile, 82–83
Bionic Products, 290
Bio-Strath, 33–34, 272, 273, 280–281, 290–291
Blaming, 225
Blueberries, 107, 114
BMI. *See* Body Mass Index
Boca Burgers, 21
Body
   connected with the mind, 3–6
   listening to, 228
   role of, in self-mastery, 228–229
Body fat. *See* Fat (body)
Body Lift, 291
Body Mass Index (BMI), 46–48
BodySlant, 274, 291
Borysenko, Joan, 3, 5, 210, 216
Bovine growth hormone (bGH), 23
Bowel toxicity, 83, 99–100
Brain power, maintaining, 282–283
Breakfast
   healthy, 57
   skipping, 56
Breast cancer, 6, 38–39, 84
   dairy products and, 23
   exercise and, 122–123, 279–280
Breath, mediation and, 209–210
Broccoli, 28, 107, 113, 114, 118
Bromelain, 117
Brown, L. Phillips, 37
Brussels sprouts, 114, 119

Budwig, Johanna, 87, 89
Bulimia, 45
Buscaglia, Leo, 152, 156
Butter, 74–75, 76, 269
Butterhead lettuce, 104
Butterworth, Eric, 239

C

Cabbage, 29, 107, 114–115, 118, 119
Calbom, Cherie, 119
Calcium, 21–22, 119
Calories
   defined, 50
   while dieting, 55
   from fat, 19, 42
   minimum, 56
Campbell, Colin, 18, 19, 20, 21
Campbell, Joseph, 212, 229–230
Cancer
   animal protein correlated with, 19
   antioxidants and, 33, 107
   breast, 6, 23, 38–39, 84, 122–123, 280
   colon, 32, 84
   exercise and, 122–123, 279–280
   flavonoids and, 40
   fruits and vegetables and, 28–29, 107, 114, 115, 116, 118
   garlic and, 38–39
   LNAs and, 87
   macrophages and, 101
   saturated fat and, 19
   skin, 67, 77
   sweating and, 138
   unexpressed emotions and, 286–287
   visual imagery and, 4
Cantaloupe, 107, 115, 118, 119
Carbohydrates, complex, 32, 57

Carnegie, Dale, 168
Carper, Jean, 29
Carroll, Lynn, 182, 286
Carrots, 29, 113, 115, 118, 119
Carruthers, Malcolm, 120
Castelli, William P., 46, 48, 49
Cauliflower, 115
Celery, 115, 119
Cellulite, 62–63
Center for Conservative Therapy, 292–293
Change, ongoing personal, 267
Chard, 105, 115
Chen Junshi, 18
Cherries, 107, 115
Chicory, 104
Childlike
  being more, 11, 152–167
  childish vs., 153–155
Children
  books on raising healthy, 25
  experiencing and embracing life, 163
  fantasies of, 157–160
  as inspiration and teachers, 152–167
  living in the present, 11, 160–162
  meeting someone new, 156–157
  obesity in, 49–50
China Oxford Cornell Project, 18–19
Chlorophyll, 96–103
  benefits of, 101–102
  as a cleanser, 98–100
  in green juices, 110
  healing with, 97–98
  history of, 96–97
  immune system boosted by, 100–101
  liquid, 102–103, 293
  similarity to hemoglobin of, 96–97
Cholesterol
  animal protein and, 19
  HDL vs. LDL, 121
  plant protein and, 19
  trans-fats and, 72–73
Choosing, principle of, 171–172
Chopra, Deepak, 4, 224
Chymopapain, 117
Circulation, law of, 176–177
Citrus flavonoids, 40
Citrus fruit, 107, 118
Claire, Thomas, 147
Clark, Linda, 100
Co-creators, 264
Cohen, Alan, 1, 199, 212, 223
Cohen, Gene, 282
Coincidence, 262
Cole, Candia Lea Cole, 22
Collards, 104, 115, 118, 119
Colon cancer, 32, 84
Commitment
  meaning of, 268
  power of, 233–234
  to putting values first, 227
  statement, personal, 236–237
Complex carbohydrates, 32, 57
Concentration, law of, 172
Concentrative meditation, 209–210
Conscious mind, 171–172
Constipation, chronic, 99
Cookbooks, 25
Cooking, 30–31, 79–80, 108
Cornell, Joseph, 214
Correspondence, law of, 172
Cousens, Gabriel, 25, 300
Cousens, Nora, 300
Cousins, Norman, 4
Cranberry juice, 116
Crawford, Amanda, 101

Cridland, Ronald G., 279
Cross-training, 128
Crunches, 129–131
Cucumbers, 116

D

Dairy products
   alternatives to, 22, 270–271
   health risks of, 23, 41, 269–270
Dalai Lama, 195
Dandelion greens, 104, 116
Davis, Roy E., 212
Davis, T. Carroll, 97
Day, Jackie, 148, 149, 150
Daydreaming, creative, 157–160
De Angelis, Barbara, 146, 189
Death
   causes of, 17
   cellular, 69
Decision making, 287–288
Dehydrated foods, 277–278
Dehydrators, 277–278, 293–294
Demos, Steve, 276
Deodorants, 99
Depression, 8
DeSouza, Paul, 96, 102–103
DeSouza Liquid Chlorophyll, 102–103, 293
Despres, Jean Pierre, 48
De Vries, Herbert, 121
Diabetes, 88–89
Diamond, Harvey, 25, 276
Diamond, Marilyn, 25, 276
Diamond Organics, 293
Diet. *See also* Nutrition
   books on, 25
   changing, 20, 23–26
   Chinese vs. Western, 18–19
   deficiencies of modern, 15–16, 85–86
   low-fat, 69
   reasons for poor, 26
   recommended by the American Heart Association, 20
   standard American, 32, 72
   supplementing, 33–35, 36–38, 39–40
   vegetarian, 18, 20, 23–26, 41
Dieting, 45, 50, 55, 67. *See also* Weight control
Digestion
   aids for, 107, 117
   enzymes and, 29–31, 271
   fiber's role in, 32
Dina, Jamey, 295
Discipline, 266
Divine surrender, 217–218
Doctors, choosing, 229
Dossey, Larry, 202, 212, 225
Downing, George, 150
Dreams
   compromising, 223
   importance of, 182–183
   turning into reality, 157–160, 168–185, 264
Drugs, 16, 17–18
Duke, James, 29, 87
Duncan, John, 52
Dyer, Wayne, 176, 224–225

E

EarthSave International, 293
Eating disorders, 45
Eating habits, 63–66
Edema, 58, 90
Edison, Thomas Alva, 186
EFAs. *See* Essential fatty acids
Einstein, Albert, 18
Elanra Therapeutic Ionizer, 290
Elgin, Duana, 192
Ellagic acid, 29
Emerson, Ralph Waldo, 186

Emotions
  biology of, 3–6
  health and, 286–287
  negative, 4, 8
  nonexpression of, 3, 8, 286–287
  power of, 174–176
Endive, 104
Endocrine system, 5
Endorphins, 5
Energy bars, 274–275, 298
Enig, Mary, 72
Enkephalin, 120
Enzymes, 29–31, 109, 271
Erasmus, Udo, 79, 82, 86, 93
Escarole, 104
Essential fatty acids (EFAs), 68–71, 73, 76–78, 85
Ester-C, 36–38, 273, 293
Estrogen, 84, 280
Evans, William, 123
Excalibur Dehydrator, 277–278, 293–294
Exercise, 120–135
  abdominal, 128–131
  aerobic, 52–53, 124
  benefits of, 120–124, 143
  breaking up, 53
  cross-training, 128
  endurance, 54
  heart rate during, 126–127, 128
  individual programs for, 124–126
  intense, 53–54
  lack of, and obesity, 50
  massage and, 142–145
  motivating yourself, 133–135
  overtraining, 144
  resistance training, 122, 123, 125–126
  sweating and, 138
  walking, 52, 126–128

F

Failure
  begetting failure, 175
  not being afraid of, 162
Fantasy, 157–160
Fast food, 80, 86
Fasting, 112, 119
Fat (body)
  advantages of losing excess, 45
  -burning supplements, 63
  converted from dietary fat, 61
  gaining, with age, 51
  grazing and, 54–56
  location of, 48
  losing, 128–129
  measuring, 49
  optimal percentage, 49
Fat (dietary)
  calories from, 19, 42
  converted to body fat, 61
  diseases and, 68
  essential fatty acids (EFAs), 68–71, 73, 76–78, 85
  GLA (gamma-linolenic acid), 61, 77
  hydrogenated, 43, 71–75
  LA (linoleic acid), 61, 76–77, 85–86
  LNA (alpha-linolenic acid), 61, 76–77, 85–94
  monounsaturated, 70, 71
  polyunsaturated, 69–70, 71
  saturated, 69, 70, 76
  structure of, 69
  superunsaturated, 70, 71
  trans-, 43, 72–75, 76
  unsaturated, 69, 71
Fatigue, 6, 121
Fear, 9, 265
Feelings. *See* Emotions
Felix, Clara, 90

Fevers, 138
Fiatarone, Maria, 123
Fiber, 24, 31–33, 58, 82–83, 108
Field, Tiffany, 141–142
Finland
  heart disease in, 16–17
  saunas in, 136
Fisher, Hans, 96–97
Fish oils, 86
Flavonoids, 40
Flax meal, fortified, 94–95, 294
Flax seed, 61, 80–85
Flax seed oil, 61, 77, 87–94
Flexibility
  increasing, 131–133
  massage and, 143–144
Folic acid, 118
Food chain, eating low on, 40–41
Foods. *See also individual foods*
  colors of, 40
  combining, 112
  cooked, 30–31, 79–80, 108
  dehydrated, 277–278
  disease-preventing properties of, 28–29, 107
  fried, 79–80
  low vs. high glycemic index, 57–58
  nutritional labels on, 41–43, 74
  raw, 30–31, 108–109, 271–272
  saturated fats in, 76
  trans-fats in, 75, 76
Foot/hand reflexology, 147
Ford, Henry, 223
Forgiveness
  health benefits of, 202
  in relationships, 166
  unconditional love and, 166–167
Fortified Flax, 94–95, 294
Frankl, Victor E., 165
Free radicals, 33, 75–76

Fried foods, 79–80
Friendship, health benefits of, 203–204
Frisch, Rose E., 122
Fruits. *See also individual fruits*
  citrus, 107, 118
  disease-preventing properties of, 28, 107
  juices from, 110
  recommended servings of, 28, 108
  washing, 111
  when to eat, 57
Fry, William F., 10
Fuhrman, Joel, 25
Fungus infections, 98

G

Gamma-linolenic acid. *See* GLA
Gandhi, Mahatma, 81, 240
Garlic, 38–39, 107, 116, 119
Gerson, Max, 87
Gibran, Kahlil, 201
Ginger, 107, 116, 119
Ginkgo biloba, 283, 296
Giving, 176–177
GLA (gamma-linolenic acid), 61, 77
Glycemic index, 57–58
Goals
  visualizing, 9, 178–179, 265–266
  writing down, 179
God
  concept of, 263
  meditation and, 216–217
  putting first, 227
  relationship with, 13
  seeing presence of, 13, 168–169, 221–222, 230
  surrender to, 185, 217–218, 231
  thanking, 179
  trusting in, 173–174

Index

Goldhamer, Alan, 17, 18, 25, 292
Gordon, Jay, 25
Gout, 107, 115
Grapefruit, 111, 116
Grapes, 29, 107, 116
Gratitude, 11, 166–167, 185, 218
Grazing, 54–56
Green Foods Corporation, 272, 294
Green juices, 110
Greenland Eskimo study, 88
Green Magma, 34, 272–273, 294
Greens
   salads of, 103
   storing, 111
   varieties of, 103–105
   washing, 103
Guppy, Helen, 198–199, 201

H

Haas, Elson, 25, 83, 112
Happiness
   exercise and, 120–121
   through service, 193
Hauser, Gayelord, 274
HDL cholesterol, 73, 121
Headaches, 24
Healing
   body's natural drive for, 4–5, 277
   with chlorophyll, 97–98
Health
   emotions and, 286
   forgiveness and, 202
   friendship and, 203–204
   kindness and love and, 202–203
   main ingredients for, 269
   meditation and, 207–209
   Natural Hygiene, 26–27, 276–277, 279, 290
HealthForce Regeneration Systems, 295

Health Mate saunas, 139, 295
Health Unlimited, 301
Heart disease
   EFA deficiency and, 77
   exercise and, 121
   flavonoids and, 40
   garlic and, 39
   LNAs and, 87–88
   meditation and, 208
   obesity and, 46–47
   prevention of, 16–17
   trans-fats and, 72
   vegetarian diet's reversal of, 20–21
Heart rate
   maximum, 126, 128
   measuring, 127
   target, 126–127, 128
Heinerman, John, 119
Hemoglobin, 96–97
Herbicides, 40–41
Hesperidin, 40
Hill, James O., 48
Hill, Napoleon, 168
Homeostasis, 35, 300
Honesty, 12
Hotchkiss, Joseph, 29
Howell, Edward, 30, 31, 271
Humor, 10, 164–166
Hydrogenated fats, 43, 71–75
Hygienic approach, 27
Hyperactivity, 279
Hypertension, 73, 207

I

IgA. *See* Immunoglobulin A
IGF-1, 23
Immune system
   chlorophyll boosting, 100–101
   garlic's effect on, 39
   macrophage cells in, 100–101

negative emotions and, 8
small pleasures' effects on, 201–202
trans-fats' effects on, 73
vitamin C's role in, 36
Immunoglobulin A (IgA), 203
Inflammatory conditions, 89
Ingredient lists, 42
Inner child, 11, 152–167
Integrity, living with, 12
Intentional living, 226
Inter-Cal Corporation, 293
Interferon, 101
Intimacy, 146
Intuition
    developing, 10, 262
    faith in, 228
    guiding judgments by, 285–286
Ionizers, 290
Isenberg, Daniel, 227
Issels, Josef, 138

J

Jensen, Bernard, 83, 107
Jesus Christ, 285
JMS Steam Cooker, 295
Juice fasts, 112, 119
Juice Plus+, 31, 34–35, 272, 295–296
Juicers, 110–111
Juices, 107–119
    advantages of, 107–108, 109
    books about, 119
    categories of, 110
    contraindications to, 119
    fruit, 110
    green, 110
    making, 110–111, 112–113
    nutrients in, 118–119
    protein from, 111–112
    vegetable, 110

Jung, Carl Gustav, 13

K

Kabat-Zinn, Jon, 208–209, 211
Kafka, Franz, 230–231
Kale, 104, 116, 118, 119
Kazantzakis, Nikos, 183
Keane, Maureen, 119
Keller, Helen, 185
Kenton, Leslie and Susannah, 108
Keyes, Ken, Jr., 238
Kidney stones, 101
Kime, Zane, 67, 77
Kindness
    examples of, 194–195, 197, 198–201
    health benefits of, 202–203
    to oneself, 201–202
    random acts of, 195–201, 205–206
    showing, daily, 11–12, 204–206
Kitchen appliances, 43–44, 273–274
Kiwi fruits, 111
Klaper, Michael, 25, 269
Kordich, Jay, 107, 119
Kornfield, Jack, 195, 216, 265
Kriya Yoga, 210, 263
Kubler-Ross, Elisabeth, 204
Kum Nye, 147
Kyolic aged garlic extract, 38–39, 273, 296

L

LA (linoleic acid), 61, 76–77, 85–86
Labels, nutritional, 41–43, 74
Lamb, Lawrence, 121
Lard, 76
Larson, Joan Matthews, 94
Laughter, 10, 164–166
LDL cholesterol, 72, 121
LeBoyer, Frederick, 151

Leeks, 107
Lemon, 107, 116–117
Lettuce
  butterhead, 104
  romaine, 105
Lidell, Lucinda, 150
Life
  accepting, 162–164
  embracing, 204
  finding purpose in, 264–265
  interconnectedness of, 237–239, 241
  inventory of your, 224–225
  most important lessons for, 288–289
  reverence for, 12
  simplifying, 10, 191–192
  steps to a balanced, 6–14
  taking charge of, 169–170
Lifestyle
  heart disease and, 16–17
  wellness, 6–7
Lifestyle Heart Trial, 20–21
Lignans, 84
Lignins, 84
Li Junyao, 18
Lin, Robert I-San, 39
Linoleic acid. *See* LA
Lipase, 30–31
Lipids. *See* Fat (dietary)
LivingArts, 296–297
LNA (alpha-linolenic acid), 61, 76–77, 85–94
Loneliness, 175, 187
Longevity
  exercise and, 124
  undernutrition and, 56
Love
  child's, 166–167
  health benefits of, 202–203
  self-, 13, 229–230
  unconditional, 166–167
Lwoff, Andre, 138
Lycopene, 118

M

Maas, James B., 7
Macrophage cells, 100–101
Magma Plus, 34, 273, 294
Magnesium, 119
Mandino, Og, 223
Manson, JoAnn E., 46
Marano, Jennifer, 292
Margarine, 74–75, 76
Maslow, Abraham, 224
Massage, 140–151
  benefits of, 140–142
  clothes and, 149
  conditioning, 142–146
  equipment for, 147–148
  essential points, 148–150
  getting started, 150–151
  intimacy through, 146
  types of, 146–147
Mata, Sri Daya, 212, 218, 287
Maya, 221
McClelland, David, 202
McDougall, John, 25
McDowell, Margaret, 50
McGuire, Karen, 148
Meals, skipping, 55–56
Meat, 18–22
  biological concentration of poisons in, 21, 41
  lean cuts of, 20
  substitutes for, 21, 275–276
Meditation, 207–222
  balancing, 231
  books on, 212
  breath and, 209–210
  concentrative, 209–210
  daily, 9, 230–231, 287

ending, with prayers, 219–221
exercise and, 124
health benefits of, 207–209
how to begin, 212–214
location for, 211–212
making a priority, 221, 230–231
mindfulness, 210–211
in nature, 214
spiritual blessings from, 215–217
stillness, 214
time for, 212
white light, 214–215
Melons, 117
Menstrual problems, 101, 279–280
Mental health
exercise and, 120–121
meditation and, 208
Metabolism
alcohol's effect on, 61
defined, 50
increasing, 50–58, 67, 90
sunlight and, 67
MetLife height and weight tables, 46
Milk
alternatives to, 270–271
health risks of, 23, 269–270
"low-fat," 42
Milner, John, 39
Mind
-body connection, 3–6
components of, 171
controlling, 169, 171–172
Mindfulness meditation, 210–211
Mistakes, not being afraid of, 162
Mitochondrial bioenergetics, 58
Monounsaturated fats, 70, 71
Montagu, Ashley, 150
Moran, Victoria, 25, 44, 45
Morgan, David, 282

Mori-Nu Silken "Lite" Tofu, 297
Morris, John, 282
Motion sickness, 107
Motivation
exercise and, 133–135
weight control and, 66–67
Mountain Valley Growers, 297
Mucilage, 83
Multiple sclerosis (MS), 90
Murray, Michael, 119
Muscles
importance of, 51–52
losing, with age, 51
massage and, 142–145
resistance training and, 51–52, 123
soreness of, after exercise, 143
Mustard greens, 104
Myss, Carolyn, 223, 225

N

Nader, Ralph, 86, 196
Naps, 7, 279
National Cancer Institute, 28
Natural Hygiene, 26–27, 276–277, 279, 290
Nature
meditation in, 214
walking in, 188
Neova cookware, 273, 300–301
Neuropeptides, 5
Newman, N. Lee, 37
Nixon, Peter, 5
Norepinephrine, 120–121
North County Healing Arts Center, 297
Nowakowski, John, 25
Null, Gary and Shelly, 119
Nurses' Health Study, 46–47
Nut milks, 22
Nutrition. *See also* Diet; Fat

(dietary)
  animal protein, 18–22
  antioxidants, 33–35, 76, 80
  beta-carotene, 33, 118
  books on, 25
  calcium, 21–22, 119
  enzymes, 29–31
  fiber, 31–33
  flavonoids, 40
  folic acid, 118
  magnesium, 119
  potassium, 119
  reading labels, 41–43, 74
  selenium, 33, 119
  under-, 56
  vitamin B_6, 118
  vitamin C, 33, 35–38, 118
  vitamin E, 33, 84, 118
  vitamin K, 101, 118
  zinc, 119
Nuuttila, S., 281

O
Obesity. *See also* Weight control
  central, 48
  heart disease and, 46–47
  in infancy and childhood, 49–50
  lack of exercise and, 50
  overweight and, 49
Oils
  cooking with, 79–80
  essential fatty acids in, 77
  flax seed, 61, 77, 87–94
  olive, 78
  organic, 78
  refined, 78
  saturated fats in, 76
  trans-fats in, 76
Olive, Diane, 25, 108
Olive oil, 78
Omega-3 fatty acid. *See* LNA

(alpha-linolenic acid)
Omega-6 fatty acid. *See* LA (linoleic acid)
Onions, 107, 113
Oranges, 111, 117, 118
Organic farming, 102–103
Ornish, Dean, 20, 25, 67, 208, 211–212, 225
Osteoporosis, 21–22, 122, 270
Outwater, Jessica, 23
Overtraining, 144

P
Paffenbarger, Ralph, 124
Pain relief
  through massage, 141
  through meditation, 208–209
Pancreatitis, 99
Papain, 117
Papayas, 111, 117, 118
Parsley, 104–105, 113, 117
Parsnips, 117
Patience, 173–174, 183–184
Pauling, Linus, 35
Peace meditation prayer, 220–221
Peace of mind, 14
Peace Pilgrim, 194, 285–286, 297
Peas, 119
People, meeting new, 156–157
Peppers, 117, 118, 119
Pesticides, 40–41
Peto, Richard, 18
Physicians Committee for Responsible Medicine, 23, 298
Phytochemicals, 28–29
Pierson, Herbert, 38, 94
Pineapple, 107, 117
Pinto, John, 38
Placebo effect, 5
PMRI residential retreats, 298
PMS, 77

Polarity therapy, 147
Polyphenols, 107, 114
Polyunsaturated fats, 69–70, 71
Positive meditation prayer, 219–220
Positive thinking, 168, 172
Potassium, 119
Potter, John, 29
PowerBars, 274–275, 298
Prayer. *See also* Meditation
   books on, 212
   daily, 221–222, 230–231
   examples of, 219–221, 222
   making a priority, 221, 230–231
   meditations ended with, 219–221
   of surrender, 217–218
Premier One Products, 298
Present, living in, 11, 160–162
Proskauer massage, 147
Prosperity, 178–179
Prostaglandins, 87
Protease, 30, 99
Protein
   animal, 18–22
   danger of excess, 21
   from flax seed, 82
   from juices, 111–112
   plant, 275
"Psychology of being," 224
Pycnogenol, 40

Q
Quercetin, 40

R
Radicchio, 104
"Random acts of kindness," 195–201, 205–206
Rapp, Doris, 94
Raspberries, 29

Raw foods, 30–31, 108–109, 271–272
Reeve, Vivienne, 39
Reflexology, foot/hand, 147
Reichian massage, 147
Relationships
   forgiveness in, 166
   with God, 13
   massage and, 146
   with yourself, 156
Relaxation techniques, 7–8. *See also* Meditation
Resistance training
   benefits of, 125
   for the elderly, 123
   increasing muscle mass through, 51–52
   osteoporosis and, 122
   program for, 125–126
Responsibility, taking, 224–225, 234–235
Rhubarb, 113
Ridpath, Robert, 97
Ritalin, 278–279
Robbins, Anthony, 172
Robbins, John, 25, 261, 293
Rolfing, 147
Romaine lettuce, 105
Roquette. *See* Arugula
Rosch, Paul, 4
Rose, Seth, 36
Rudin, Donald O., 85, 90
Rutabaga, 113
Rutin, 40, 114

S
Sacred space, personal, 212
SAD. *See* Standard American Diet
Santillo, Humbart, 25, 31, 272
Satori, 231
Saturated fats, 69, 70, 76

Saunas, 136–139, 295
Schaie, Warner, 282–283
Seasons, celebrating, 165–166
Selenium, 33, 119
Self-esteem, 13, 229–230
Self-love, 13, 229–230
Self-mastery, 223–239
    begins with life inventory, 224
    importance of God for, 227
    keys to, 267–268
    mind-set for, 225–226
    role of body in, 228–229
Self-Realization Fellowship, 210, 218, 263, 285, 299
Selye, Hans, 208
Separateness, illusion of, 237–239
Serenity, 186
Serure, Pamela, 25, 112
Service, happiness through, 193
Serving sizes, 43
Sexual disorders, 89
Shiatsu, 146–147
Siegel, Bernie, 225, 286
Siguel, Edward N., 68, 77
Silence, 9, 186–190
Silent Unity telephone number, 300
Silliness, importance of, 164–166
Silverstein, Steven, 37
Simonton, O. Carl, 3
Simplifying, 10, 191–192
Sit-ups, 128
Skin cancer, 67, 77
Skin conditions, 89
Slant boards, 274, 292
Sleep
    for ADD, 279
    apnea, 45
    getting enough, 7
Smiling, power of, 164, 198
Smith, June B., 201, 285

Smith, Lendon H., 16, 25, 26
Sodium, 42
Solitude, 9, 186–190
Sorbitol, 107, 114
Sorrel, 105
Soy products, 275–276, 301
Spectrum Naturals, 77–78, 93, 299
Spectrum Spread, 74, 76, 297
Sperling, Caroline, 3, 4
Spinach, 105, 113, 117, 118
Spiritual health
    exercise and, 124
    food and, 67
    mediation and, 230–231
Sports. *See* Athletes; Exercise
Spot reducing, 128
Sproul, Kim, 295
Sprouts, 59–60, 113
Standard American Diet (SAD), 32, 72
Steam rooms, 136–137
Stillness meditation, 214
Stir-frying, 80
Stoddard, Alexandra, 140
Stone, Arthur, 202
Strawberries, 29, 111
Strength training. *See* Resistance training
Stress
    back pain from, 274
    exercise and, 121
    LNAs and, 89
    meditation and, 207–209
    negative vs. positive, 208
Stress points, 143
Stress Reduction Clinic, 208
Stretching, 131–133
Strickland, John, 181
Stroke, 39
Subconscious, 171–172
Success, 169, 175, 227–228

Sugars, 42, 43, 279
Sulforaphane, 28
Sunlight, 67
Superunsaturated fats, 70, 71
Supplements
   Bio-Strath, 33–34, 272, 273, 280–281, 290–291
   Ester-C, 36–38, 273
   fat-burning, 63
   Green Magma, 34, 272–273, 294
   Juice Plus+, 34–35, 272, 295–296
   Kyolic aged garlic extract, 38–39, 273, 296
   LNA, 90–92
Surrender, Divine, 217–218
Suzanne, Paulette, 271, 272, 297
Sweating, 136–139
Swiss chard, 105

T
Talalay, Paul, 28
Teresa, Mother, 9, 12, 197, 202
Thinness, excessive, 48
Thomas, Caroline Bendel, 286
Thoughts
   becoming reality, 172–173
   choosing, 8, 169, 171–172, 177–180
Throats, sore, 107
Tithing, 176, 286
Tofu, 275–276, 297, 301
Tomatoes, 29, 118, 119
Touch, importance of, 142, 150
Touch Research Institute (TRI), 141
Toxicity
   in the body, 58
   bowel, 83, 99–100
   decreasing, 58, 109
Trace-Lyte, 300
Tracy, Brian, 168, 178

Trager massage, 147
Trans-fats, 43, 72–75, 76
Tree of Life, 300
Tremblay, Angelo, 54
TRI. *See* Touch Research Institute
Trigger points, 143
Triglycerides, 121
Turnip greens, 104, 118, 119
Turnips, 29, 113, 118, 119

U
Ulcers, 73, 107
Unity Village and Retreat Center, 300
Unsaturated fats, 69, 71
Urinary tract infections, 114, 116

V
Vegetables. *See also individual vegetables*
   dark orange, 107
   disease-preventing properties of, 28, 107
   green, 103–105, 107
   juices from, 110
   recommended servings of, 28, 108
   washing, 103, 111
Vegetarian diet
   advantages of, 18, 25–26, 41
   changing to, 20, 23–25
Veggie Magma, 34, 273, 294
Veg Omega-3 Organic Flax Oil, 93
Verlangieri, Anthony, 36
Visualization, creative, 3, 9, 177–179, 183, 184, 265–266
Vitamin B_6, 118
Vitamin C, 33, 35–38, 118
Vitamin E, 33, 84, 118
Vitamin K, 101, 118

Vita-Mix Total Nutrition Center, 273, 300–301

W
Waist/Hip Ratio (WHR), 48–49
Walford, Roy L., 25, 56
Walker, N. W., 119
Walking
  for exercise, 52, 126–128
  in nature, 188
Wallace, R. Keith, 207
Walpole, Hugh, 203
Warren, Dianne, 25
Water
  health benefits of, 62
  retention, 58, 90
Watercress, 105, 118
Weight, healthy, 45–50
  Body Mass Index (BMI), 46–48
  MetLife height and weight tables, 46
  Waist/Hip Ratio (WHR), 48–49
Weight control. *See also* Dieting
  exercise and, 123–124
  motivation and, 66–67
  principle of choosing and, 171–172
  saunas and, 137
  steps for, 51–67
Weight lifting. *See* Resistance training
Weil, Andrew, 225
Weindruch, Richard, 56
Wheat grass, 60, 118
White blood cells, 4
White light meditation, 214–215
White Wave Silk, 22, 23, 270–271, 276, 301
White Wave Vegetarian Cuisine Company, 276, 301
WHR. *See* Waist/Hip Ratio

Wilkie, Diana J., 141
Willett, Walter, 74
Williamson, Marianne, 224, 268
Willstatter, Richard, 96
Wilson, Roberta, 62
Winfrey, Oprah, 225
Women
  breast cancer, 6, 23, 38–39, 84, 122–123, 279–280
  cellulite, 62–63
  exercise and, 122–123
  heart disease, 46–47
  menstrual problems, 101, 279–280
  osteoporosis, 21–22, 122, 270
  PMS, 77
Words
  choosing, 177–182
  following through on your, 181–182
Workshops, 301
World
  accepting as is, 162–164
  intense pace of, 264
  view of, 268–269

Y
Yeast, 281
Yerba Prima, 290
Yoga, 131
Yogananda, Paramahansa, 27, 186, 191, 193, 207, 210, 212, 218, 225, 263, 285, 287, 299

Z
Zable, Werner, 148
Zinc, 119
Zone therapy, 147